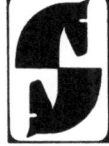

Recent Results in Cancer Research

Fortschritte der Krebsforschung

Progrès dans les recherches sur le cancer

23

Edited by

V. G. Allfrey, New York · M. Allgöwer, Basel · K. H. Bauer, Heidelberg
I. Berenblum, Rehovoth · F. Bergel, Jersey · J. Bernard, Paris · W. Bernhard, Villejuif · N. N. Blokhin, Moskva · H. E. Bock, Tübingen · P. Bucalossi, Milano · A. V. Chaklin, Moskva · M. Chorazy, Gliwice · G. J. Cunningham, Richmond · W. Dameshek, Boston · M. Dargent, Lyon · G. Della Porta, Milano · P. Denoix, Villejuif · R. Dulbecco, La Jolla · H. Eagle, New York
R. Eker, Oslo · P. Grabar, Paris · H. Hamperl, Bonn · R. J. C. Harris, London
E. Hecker, Heidelberg · R. Herbeuval, Nancy · J. Higginson, Lyon
W. C. Hueper, Fort Myers · H. Isliker, Lausanne · D. A. Karnofsky †, New York · J. Kieler, København · G. Klein, Stockholm · H. Koprowski, Philadelphia · L. G. Koss, New York · G. Martz, Zürich · G. Mathé, Villejuif
O. Mühlbock, Amsterdam · W. Nakahara, Tokyo · V. R. Potter, Madison
A. B. Sabin, Cincinnati · L. Sachs, Rehovoth · E. A. Saxén, Helsinki
W. Szybalski, Madison · H. Tagnon, Bruxelles · R. M. Taylor, Toronto
A. Tissières, Genève · E. Uehlinger, Zürich · R. W. Wissler, Chicago
T. Yoshida, Tokyo

Editor in chief

P. Rentchnick, Genève

Springer-Verlag New York · Heidelberg · Berlin 1969

W. A. Fuchs · J. W. Davidson · H. W. Fischer

Lymphography in Cancer

With Contribution by

G. Jantet · H. Rösler

With 189 Figures

Springer-Verlag New York · Heidelberg · Berlin 1969

Sponsored by the Swiss League against Cancer

ISBN 978-3-642-87386-7   ISBN 978-3-642-87384-3 (eBook)
DOI 10.1007/978-3-642-87384-3

Preface

Lymphography is an established procedure in the diagnosis of malignant disease. Major scientific meetings, numerous publications and several postgraduate courses on this subject have been presented during the past ten years. However, perusal of the literature will convince any critical reader of the need for a comprehensive presentation of lymphography in cancer. Fundamental knowledge of the anatomy and physiology of the lymphatic system, pharmacology of the contrast media, possible complications and in particular understanding of the clinical behaviour of malignant tumors place high demands on the physician. For this reason the personal experience of five authors and the most important data published in the literature have been compiled in this volume. It should give the reader up to date information on the indications for clinical lymphography and its interpretation, thereby demonstrating the limits of its diagnostic accuracy and stressing the great importance of the method for the evaluation of cancer patients.

It has been a fortunate circumstance to draw on the experience of four distinguished contributors whose cooperation has enabled this attempt at a thorough coverage of clinical lymphography in cancer.

W. A. FUCHS

Acknowledgements

It is a pleasure to thank CHARLES HYAMS, cand. med. for his invaluable help in editing the english manuscripts of chapters 1, 2, 5, 6, 7, 9 and 10. Without his stimulating cooperation this work would have been impossible. The contribution of Miss CHARLOTTE KÜPFER, who has done a vast amount of secretarial work is gratefully appreciated. I also wish to thank Mr. P. SCHNEIDER for the drawings, and Mrs. M. RENTSCH and Mr. E. GROB for the photographic work.

W. A. Fuchs

The tables in the section "Lymphography in Malignant Lymphomas" were assiduously prepared by Dr. E. AILEEN CLARKE, Research Assistant in Diagnostic Radiology, The Ontario Cancer Institute. It is a pleasure to thank Dr. T. C. BROWN and his staff of the Department Pathology for their invaluable assistance, and Dr. W. D. RIDER for help with the manuscript. The contributions of Miss RUTH MACLEAN, who typed this manuscript, and Mrs. M. GAETTENS and her staff of the Department of Photography, The Ontario Cancer Institute, are gratefully acknowledged. This work was in part supported by Grant 41—15 of the Ontario Cancer Treatment and Research Foundation.

Permission and courtesy of Dr. ROBERT J. LUKES and MESSRS. LEA and FEBIGER, Philadelphia, is gratefully acknowledged for the use of Figure 2.

J. W. Davidson

The authors express their gratitude to the publishers, *Springer-Verlag*, for their spirit of cooperation and great attention to fine details.

Contents

Contents

List of Authors

JAMES W. DAVIDSON, M.D., Department of Diagnostic Radiology, The Ontario Cancer Institute, 500 Sherbourne Street, Toronto 5/Canada.

HARRY W. FISCHER, M.D., Director, Department of Radiology, Wayne County, General Hospital, Eloise, Michigan, and Professor of Radiology, Department of Radiology, University of Michigan School of Medicine, Ann Arbor, Mich./USA.

WALTHER A. FUCHS, M.D., Professor of Radiology, University of Bern, Department of Radiology, University Hospital, Inselspital, Bern/Switzerland.

GEORGES JANTET, M.B., F.R.C.S., Consultant Surgeon, Department of Surgery, King Edward Memorial Hospital, London W. 13/Great Britain

HELMUT RÖSLER, M.D., Department of Radiology, University Hospital, Inselspital, Bern/Switzerland.

Chapter 1

Historical Survey

W. A. Fuchs

The Ancient Greeks knew of the existence of the lymphatic system: HIPPOCRATES spoke of "white blood" and ARISTOTLE of "tubules with colorless fluid"; in the 4th century, the Alexandrian school described the lymphatic system in animal and human anatomy. However, during the following 1300 years, this knowledge was lost.

The forgotten lymphatic vessels were found again by GASPARO ASELLI, an Italian anatomist, who in 1622 vivisected an apparently well-nourished dog and found white channels in the mesentery from which a milky fluid could be obtained. In 1647 PECQUET of Montpellier described the cisterna chyli and thoracic duct in a dog, and five years later both structures were identified in the human body by VAN HOORN of Leyden.

It was at about this time that two researchers, working independently, described the lymphatic system in detail. Thus, THOMAS BARTOLINUS of Copenhagen gave the system its present name "vasa lymphatica", and OLOF RUDBECK at the Swedish University of Uppsala is credited with the first description of the valves of lymph vessels, the relationship between the vessels and the thoracic duct, and the juncture of the thoracic duct with the great veins. It was Rudbeck's opinion that edema and ascites could be produced by an occlusion of the lymphatic vessels, and it was his thesis that the lymphatics constitute a circulatory system separate from the blood circulation—a thesis not accepted by The Royal Society of London until 1751. ANTON NUGG introduced the method of injecting the lymphatics with mercury in 1692 and throughout the next century his method and similar techniques were used to trace the entire anatomy of the lymphatic system. MASCAGNI and CRUISHANK developed a method of filling the lymph vessels that is still unsurpassed for quality and accuracy. However, mercury injection was difficult and time consuming, and many workers searched for simpler techniques. In 1896, GEROTA described a combined cinnabar and mercury procedure which, after several modifications, found universal acceptance. This new technique enabled BARTHELS (1909) and JOSSIFOW (1930) to undertake their comprehensive classical studies of the human lymphatic system.

After the discovery of x-rays, attempts were made to visualize the lymphatic system radiographically. Experiments were made first on cadavers to obtain a better understanding of the topography of the lymphatics and lymph nodes. Later, experiments on animals were performed to study the physiology of the lymphatic system. Contrast agents were injected subcutaneously, intraarticularly, intraperitoneally, intrapleurally and intrapericardially. A variety of contrast media were tried, such as heavy metal salts, iodides, water-soluble agents, iodized oil and colloidal solutions. At first the subcutaneous injection of Thorotrast seemed most promising. This agent is absorbed almost selectively by the subcutaneous lymphatics. During the 4th International Congress of Radiology in Zurich in 1934 CARVALHO reported the results of lymphography with Thorotrast and discussed the potential value of the method for the diagnosis of malignant lymphatic invasion. However, Thorotrast-lymphography as a clinical practice was short-lived. Owing to its radioactivity, its slow excretion and consequent carcinogenic effect, Thorotrast was abandoned quickly. Interest in the radiologic examination of the lymphatic system diminished. On March 25th, 1954 J. B. KINMONTH, the British vascular surgeon, described his now classical method of lymphography in a Hunterian Lecture to the Royal College of Surgeons. His technique is based on McMASTER's (1932) observation that certain dyes are taken up almost selectively by the lymphatics after their subcutaneous injection. KINMONTH reasoned that the stained lymphatics could be dissected. Injection of contrast agents directly into the dissected lymphatics enabled radiological demonstration of the lymph vessels and lymph nodes. The work of KINMONTH paved the way for the development of today's techniques which are being used widely in clinical work and in experimental research.

Lymphography was at first applied to study the etiology of lymphedema. Publications on pathological changes in lymph nodes by COLLETTE (1957, 1958), KAINDL and THURNHEER (1958), FUCHS, DEL BUONO and RÜTTIMANN (1959), LEENHARD and COLIN (1959), MALAMOS et al. (1959) soon followed. TJERNBERG (1956, 1959, 1962), and FISCHER and ZIMMERMANN (1959) and MALEK and BELAN (1959) conducted classical animal experiments investigating the possibilities of tumor diagnosis by lymphography using various contrast substances. Originally water-soluble contrast agents were used for radiological demonstration of lymph vessels and lymph nodes. The introduction of oily contrast substances enabled further progress. First reports of its use came from BRUUN and ENGESET (1956), PROKOPEK and KOLIHOVA (1958) and ZHEUTLIN and SHANBRON (1958), who injected the contrast agent directly into pathologically enlarged lymph nodes infiltrated by neoplastic disease. Later PROKOPEK and KOLIHOVA (1959), SHEEHAN et al. (1961) and WALLACE et al. (1961) introduced oily contrast media directly into the lymphatic vessels. Since then a great number of publications on the applications of lymphographic techniques for tumor diagnosis have appeared and extensive references are made throughout the text to facilitate the reader's comparisons and critical analysis.

Chapter 2

Investigation Techniques

W. A. Fuchs

With 3 Figures

Radiological demonstration of lymph vessels and lymph nodes in man may be achieved only by *Direct Lymphography,* which is performed by injecting contrast material directly into lymph vessels, lymph nodes, or occasionally into lymph cysts. *Indirect Lymphography* is used only in animal experimentation, and the contrast agents in this technique are introduced outside the lymphatic system either orally or by injection subcutaneously, intramuscularly, into joints, serous cavities or into solid organs. No contrast agent for indirect lymphography of the human body exists, and therefore clinical lymphography demonstrates only those lymph vessels and nodes connected with the subcutaneous lymphatics of the extremities and the retro-auricular region. Radiological investigation of the lymphatic system of the internal organs remains completely outside the range of diagnostic possibilities for the present.

Clinical lymphography is performed essentially according to the direct technique of KINMONTH (1954, 1955) in which injection of *contrast material* is preceeded by the subcutaneous injection of a *vital dye* which serves to facilitate visualization of the lymph vessels during the surgical cutdown procedure required for their direct puncture. Percutaneous puncture of normal sized lymph vessels is not possible because their diameter does not exceed 1 mm. Retrograde contrast-filling of the lymphatic system is also impossible because numerous valves prevent retrograde flow.

Instruments and Material

Sterile and non-sterile instruments and material are carefully prepared prior to lymphography.

The *non-sterile material* consists of: Ether to clean the skin, skin disinfectant, Patent Blue Violet 2% (ampules of 2 ml), Procaine 2% witout adrenalin, syringe and needles for drawing up Procaine, contrast medium (Lipiodol UF, ampules of 5 ml), silk 000 and 00, Polybactrin-Spray (containing Neomycine, Polymycine, Bactracine), elastoplast gauze, bandages, scissors, razor, magnifying eye glasses.

The *sterile trolley* includes the following material and instruments: bowl with skin disinfectant, bowl with normal saline, bowl with Procaine 2% without adrenalin for local anaesthesia, 5 ml syringe with needles for drawing up and injecting local anaesthesia, scalpel, 2 curved arterial clamps, 1 pair of fine scissors, 1 fine and 1 large dissecting forceps, 1 large surgical forceps, 2 towel clips, 3 types of special lymphography needles 35/100 mm, 40/100 mm, 55/100 mm, silk: 000 for guide loop around the lymph vessel and for fixation of the needle, 2 10 cc syringes with Luer lock, 1 18-gauge drawing up needle for contrast medium, 2 polythene tubes (PE 205) 30 cm long with Luer locks, 1 needle-holder and needles for closing incision, sterile towels, gauze, pads, swabs, 2 pairs of sterile rubber gloves.

After the investigation all instruments which have been in contact with the oily contrast medium are thoroughly cleaned and then soaked in ether for 24 hours. All instruments are sterilised in accordance with current practice.

Needles and Catheters

Several types of needles and catheters are used for puncture of the lymphatic vessel.

The needle designed by RÜTTIMANN and DEL BUONO (1962) consists of two parts and is similar to a trocar. The needle is about 2.5 cm long and has a blunt conical tip. The stylet is 2 mm longer and has a close connection with the conical needle tip. However, there is always a small ridge left between stylet and needle tip which has to be introduced into the vessel lumen using gentle rotating movements. The tip of the needle is roughened for a length of 2 mm to prevent its slipping out of the vessel lumen. The diameters of the needles are 55/100 mm and 40/100 mm for normal sized lymphatics and 35/100 mm for fine lymph vessels. The puncture needle described by DE ROO (1966) is based upon the same principle but has a small spring attached at the place where the stylet locks into the needle. The spring releases the stylet when the needle is placed within the lymph vessel. Ordinary sharp 27-gauge or 30-gauge needles have the disadvantage that the posterior wall of the lymph vessel can be easily perforated.

Other investigators prefer to use a polythene catheter: TJERNBERG, 1959, 1962; FISCH and DEL BUONO, 1963; FISCH, 1966; TRAPP, 1966; KROPHOLLER et al., 1968. The catheter is prepared as follows: a 50 cm long polythene tube (PE 10) is heated over a flame or electrocautery. As soon as the polythene starts to melt, the tube is taken away and reduced by gentle tension to a diameter of 0.1 mm. Two catheters of about 20 cm length are cut. Stretching of a polythene tube without heating does not produce good results.

Automatic Injectors

Special automatic injectors have been constructed for perfusion and therefore slow and continuous injection of the viscous oily contrast material (CLEMENTZ and OLIN, 1961; RÜTTIMANN and DEL BOUNO, 1962; DE ROO, 1966). They consist of three main parts: a motor complete with gear box, a carrier with thrust rods and a syringe holder. The drive is an electric motor with a friction coupling which comes into action above an injection pressure of 2 kg/cm². The power from the electric motor is transmitted to a screw by a low speed gear. The variable voltage transformer regulating the motor permits fine adjustments of the gear speed, and with this arrangement the rate of the thrust into the syringe can be varied continuously between 0.015 ml/min and 5 ml/min. The injection pressure is approximately 0.2 to 0.6 kg/cm². The syringe holder accommodates up to three 10—20 ml syringes of all standards types. This type of apparatus has the advantage that the quantity injected is automatically adjusted to the prevailing pressure within the lymph vessels, and accidental bursting of a lymph vessel consequent to excessive pressure is avoided. Injection by hand or by simple injector, which utilizes weights, cannot precisely control the injection pressure and is therefore not advisable. Provision is made to keep the contrast agent at body temperature.

Special Instruments

A low power binocular magnifying eye glass is of great help for preparation and puncture of the lymphatic vessels.

Preparation of the Patient

Normally, special premedication of the patient is not required. Sedation with barbiturates may be necessary occasionally for children or apprehensive patients, but informing the patient beforehand that the procedure is nearly painless is usually comfort enough. For infants, however, deep sedation or general anaesthesia is used. Every patient should have a light meal prior to the investigation, as lymphography lasts 2—3 hours. Furthermore, the patient may suffer from loss of appetite and nausea on the day following the procedure and may not be able to eat. Also the patient may be allowed to read to help pass the long time of injection more quickly.

Not only the patient, but all those concerned, should be informed of the discolorations consequent to the use of the dye. The skin, especially the facial area, and the urine will be somewhat blue for 1—2 days, and the site of the injection will remain a patchy-blue for 1—2 weeks.

Preparation and injection of the lymph vessel follow careful positioning of the patient on a well upholstered table, an x-ray table not being needed until later provided that water-soluble contrast medium is not being used. Moreover, preliminary control films may be taken conveniently with mobile x-ray equipment, leaving the x-ray room free.

Vital Staining of Lymph Vessels

Lymph vessels are stained to enable their visualization and dissection, and the staining results from the subcutaneous injection of a vital dye. Only the lymphatics absorb the dye, and a few minutes after injection they are visible through the skin as fine greenish-blue streaks. A 1⁰/o dye solution is prepared by diluting one part 2⁰/o Patent Blue-Violet with an equal part of 2⁰/o Procaine without adrenalin. The recommended volumes to be injected and the dye concentration of 1⁰/o must be closely adhered to, otherwise local necrosis and excessively severe, generalized discoloration of the skin will follow. The sites of injection are precisely described under the appropriate heading for each regional investigation, but generally speaking, correspond to those areas, like the interdigital webs, where a great number of lymphatics find their source (Fig. 1). Active or passive movements of the extremity or region injected increase lymph flow and speeds up dye absorption.

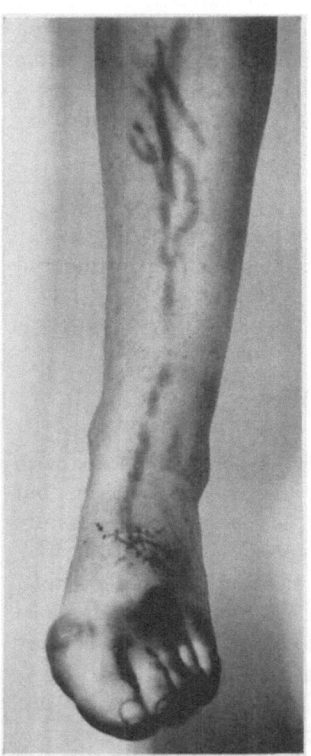

Fig. 1. *Subcutaneous lymphatics of the antero-medial group* visible as greenish-blue streaks due to vital staining of 2% Patent Blue-Violet after interdigital injection

Surgical Procedure and Injection of Contrast Medium

The vital dye injection sites are swabbed with skin disinfectant, and the subcutaneous injections are made. The skin of the region to be studied is then shaved and cleaned with ether and alcohol, then draped with sterile towels. Although it is possible to begin the cutdown of the lymph vessel immediately, as it takes only a few seconds to fill the lymphatics, it is preferable to wait 5—10 minutes to allow for better definition, which simplifies the surgery involved. When the subcutaneous lymph vessels are sufficiently stained so as to be recognized as fine blue-green streaks through the skin, the procedure may be started. A low power binocular dissection microscope will prove to be helpful in preparing and puncturing the lymphatic vessel. The area of incision is chosen at a place where the stained lymphatics are clearly seen and where it affords the largest lymphatics in the region as well as a stable seating for the needle. A local anaesthetic is injected subcutaneously, and a superficial, transverse incision, 2—4 cm long, is made (Fig. 2 a). The transverse incision exposes more lymphatics than a longitudinal incision. The skin is raised with surgical forceps, and the subcutaneous tissue is carefully dissected. The subcutaneous lymphatics become visible as fine blue-green vessels within the subcutaneous tissue. They are lifted up with curved forceps and the adherent fat and fibrous tissue are stripped away with fine pincers (Fig. 2 b). The lymph vessels must be cleaned thoroughly over a distance of 1—2 cm. Complete stripping is essential for a successful puncture: it insures that the needle-tip lies in the lumen of the vessel and not in surrounding tissue. A loop of silk thread is then placed around the vessel near the proximal border of the incision, and the lymphatic is pulled upwards slightly by the silk, thereby producing a fold which obstructs the vessel (Fig. 2 c). By massaging the region just distal to the incision, lymph fluid may be milked up against the silk loop thereby dilating the vessel. With curved forceps—held in the left hand—the dilated lymph vessels is raised and stretched slightly (Fig. 2 d). While—with the right hand—the tip of the puncture needle is placed exactly over the upper edge of the curved forceps and introduced into the lumen of the vessel with a gentle rotating movement (Fig. 2 e). When both the stylet and the blunt needle tip have been placed within the lumen of the vessel, the curved forceps are discarded. Holding the needle with the left hand, the stylet is withdrawn with the right, witout moving the blunt needle tip situated within the vessel lumen (Fig. 2 f). Stretching the vessel again with the curved forceps, the blunt tip of the needle is advanced carefully up the vessel. The needle is carefully set down, the curved forceps are removed, and the silk knot is

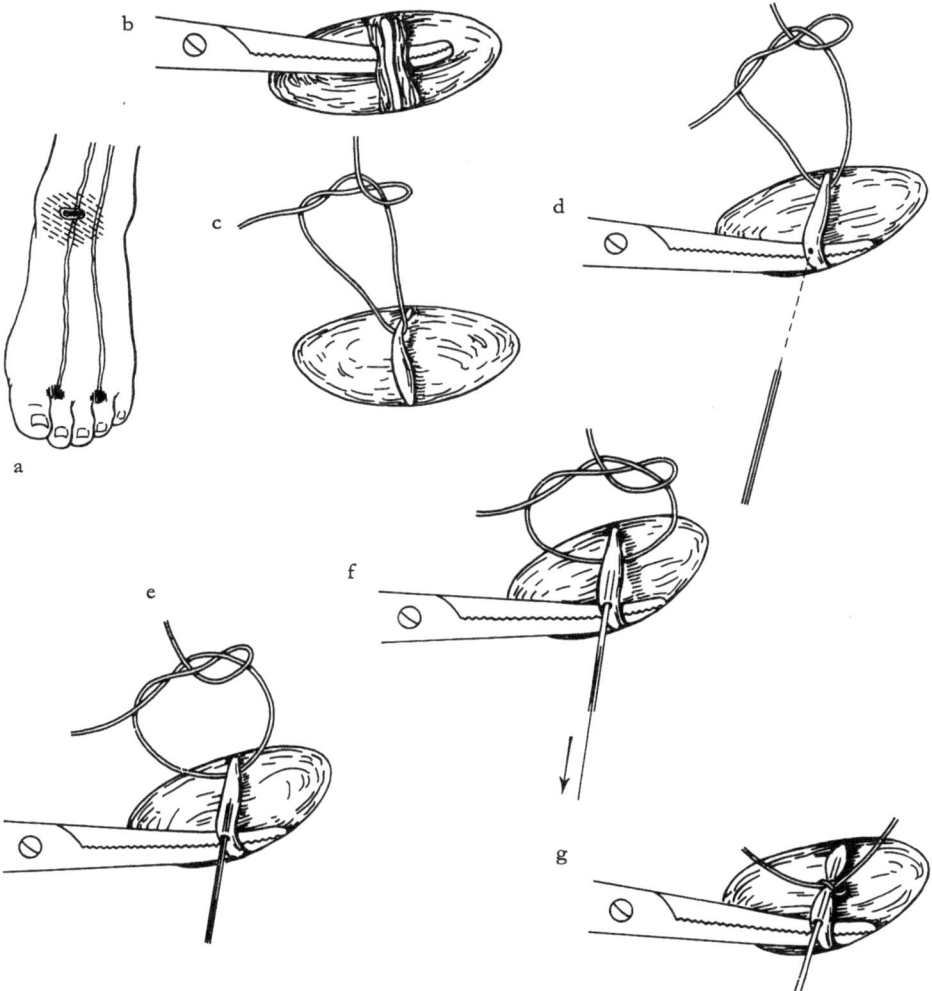

Fig. 2. *Schematic presentation of the lymphographic investigation technique.* a Interdigital injection of a vital dye. Local anaesthesia. Transverse incision of the skin. b A lymph vessel is lifted up with a curved forceps and the adherent fat and the fibrous tissue are stripped away. c A silk loop is placed around the lymphatic and is pulled upwards to obstruct and dilate the vessel. d Stretching of the lymphatic by a curved forceps. e Puncture of the lymphatic on the edge of the forceps. f Withdrawl of the stylet. g The blunt needle tips is advanced within the vessel and a silk knot is tightened over the rough part of the needle

tightened over the rough part of the needle, 2—5 mm from the tip (Fig. 2 g). In this way, the needle is placed securely within the lumen of the vessel. Care must be taken to prevent the needle from sliding sideways.

A soft 30 cm long polythene tube (PE 205), which has been pre-filled with contrast medium, is then connected with the needle by means of a Luer lock and to the syringe, which has been placed in position on the automatic injector. The polythene tube is fastened to the sterile towels with a clip at toe level (Fig. 3). The use of stiff tubing

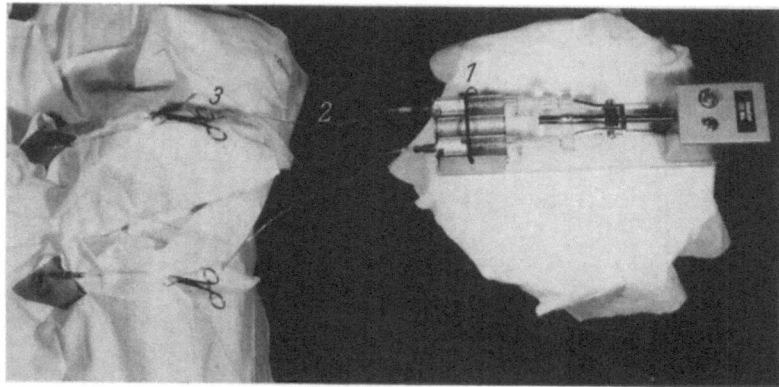

Fig. 3. *Lay-out for clinical lymphography*. 1 Automatic injector; 2 Polythene tubes (PE 205); 3 Clips to fasten the polythene tubes connected with the puncture needles inserted into the lymph vessels

is not recommended as it is prone to dislocate the needle, thereby perforating the vessel wall. Use of the above technique minimizes the probability of needle slippage.

Other investigators use special clamps with rubber covered tips instead of a silk loop to hold and to distend the lymph vessel and to prevent back-sliding of the needle (DE ROO, 1966). Also, clips consisting of two metal arms have been contructed for fixation of the lymphatic (YOUKER, 1966).

The syringe on the automatic injector has been filled with the oily contrast medium (Lipiodol UF, Ethiodol), the injection rate and pressure are set and the injection commenced. Higher rates of injection than those recommended below may cause painful rupture of the lymphatics and extravasation. Also, use of greater volumes of contrast medium significantly increases the amount which enters the blood circulation. During the time of the injection, usually about 1¹/₂ hours, the incision is covered with sterile towels and the patient is left alone, but is checked frequently. Flow of the contrast material is indicated when the lymph vessel dilates and when a yellow-transparent tinge appears above the tip of the needle. There should be no leakage at the site of puncture if the needle has been inserted correctly. If the intralymphatic pressure should increase because of an obstructed vessel, the contrast material will be observed oozing through the vessel wall. In this case the material is recognizable because of its oily consistency and tendency to form droplets.

When a second puncture is necessitated, the use of a different vessel is preferable. Otherwise, the second puncture must be made proximal to the first to avoid leakage during the injection with the disadvantage that the original puncture prevents dilatation, because lymph will leak out through the hole during massage for insertion of the needle. When the injection is completed, the needle is withdrawn carefully, taking particular care not to tear the vessels. The silk loop is removed and the vessel left without ligature. The incision is then swabbed with disinfectant, injected with a local anaesthetic, sprayed with an antibiotic and closed with several closely-spaced sutures. The patient is then taken to the x-ray room on a stretcher. After the films have been taken, the patient may go home, but should be escorted. Instructions are given that he should go to bed immediately. A slight fever is commonly experienced after the procedure, and the patient should be advised of this.

Use of water-soluble contrast media requires alteration of some procedures: the volumes of contrast material injected are much greater, and the material is injected at a faster rate. By way of example, unilateral injection of the leg requires 20—30 ml injected at a rate of 3—4 ml/min. Also, because the water-soluble media diffuse through the vessel walls within 5—10 min of injection, serial radiographs at one-minute intervals are made. The patient suffers from slight discomfort caused by the sudden dilatation of the lymph vessels and by the diffusion of the material into surrounding tissues. The discomfort may be sensed along the entire length of the injected group of lymph vessels.

Radiographic Techniques

The standard 90 KV exposure is considered to be correct when the structure of the lymph nodes is shown in good detail. In the majority of cases the routine exposures are made twice, once immediately after the contrast injection (filling phase) and a second time 24 hours later (storage phase). In addition, a standard chest film is taken with the second series to demonstrate if lung changes have been caused by the contrast material.

The following special techniques deserve comment:

Preliminary screening with image intensifier and TV is necessary in special cases to observe the extent of filling obtained.

Roentgen cinematography may be applied for a dynamic study of lymph flow.

Tomography is valuable as a supplementary method to distinguish between fused and superprojected lymph nodes. In obese patients and in the event of the super-projection of bony structures, the lymphographic pattern of lymph nodes is demonstrated in detail. Tomography localizes marginal filling defects and in special cases is necessary to establish the exact topographic position of lymph nodes. The tomograms are made with a rectilinear tube and film motion, a focus film distance of 1.50 m and an angle of 40 degrees. The distance between each section is 0.25—0.5 cm (DE ROO, 1965, 1966; BELTZ and THURN, 1966). Hypocycloidal tomography has the advantage of not producing linear unsharpness (DONINI et al., 1965). Cut sections of 0.1 cm give more detailed information about structural changes of lymph nodes.

Direct roentgenographic magnification with an x-ray tube combining a high x-ray output with a fine focal spot produces very sharp images at two to three times linear magnification. This technique yields exquisite definition of nodal architecture and therefore increases the accuracy of diagnostic lymphography (LOVE and TAKARO, 1966; DITCHEK and SCANLON, 1967).

Logetronic detail enhancement by photographic or television technique yields additional definition of the structural pattern of lymph nodes, because small details are accentuated.

The subtraction technique cannot be applied for lymphography since it is practically impossible to obtain roentgenograms of identical position both prior to the investigation and after the lymph nodes are contrast filled.

Stereoscopy is not used because no additional diagnostic information is obtained after standard oblique projections.

Foot Lymphography

Vital Staining

1—2 ml of 1% dye solution are injected subcutaneously into each of the first and forth interdigital webs. Demonstration of both the antero-medial and antero-lateral subcutaneous lymphatics is achieved (Fig. 1). When a second or third study is performed on the same limb at a later date, it is necessary to inject all the webs.

Surgical Dissection

The region of the first metatarsal bone is usually the most appropriate site for incision because the antero-medial lymphatics are easily dissected, and the needle rarely slides away from the flat mid-foot surface. In addition, the lymphatics here are of larger diameter than those of the antero-lateral group.

Contrast Injection: Dosage and Settings

For adults, a 6 ml injection is used on each side in bilateral visualization. The unilateral injection dose is 8 ml with provision thus being made for some contralateral filling of the aortic lymph nodes. For children, 1—4 ml are sufficient to fill the entire retroperitoneal lymph system unilaterally. The injection rate is set at 0.1—0.15 ml/min at a pressure of 0.4 atm.

Roentgenographic Technique

Films of the lower extremities are required only in case of edema following malignant invasion.

The following routine exposures are made twice, immediately after injection and 24 hours later:

Inguinal and pelvic region: (a-p, 30×40 cm)
Thoracic duct, thoracic region: (a-p, 30×40 cm)
Optional: upper abdominal region (lateral projections)
24 hours only: standard chest roentgenogram

Arm Lymphography

Vital Staining

0.5 ml of the 1% dye solution is injected into each of the interdigital webs of the hand.

Surgical Dissection

The group of lymphatics demonstrated, i. e. either the radial or the ulnar group, corresponds to the side of the carpus chosen as the site for incision and injection. Because lymphatics of the arm are of small diameter (0.1—0.5 mm), generally smaller than those of the leg, it is possible that no lymphatics suitable for puncture will be found in the carpal region. In such cases, dissection of lymph vessels in the cubital fossa may be attempted.

Contrast Injection: Dosage and Settings

For demonstration of the lymph vessels and nodes of the upper extremity and axilla, 4—5 ml of oily contrast material are required. The speed of injection should not exceed 0.1 ml/min to prevent rupture of the delicate lymph vessels.

Roentgenographic Technique

The following routine exposures are made twice, immediately after injection and 24 hours later:

Forearm: (a-p, lateral)
Upperarm: (a-p, lateral)
Axillary and supraclavicular regions: (a-p, right and left oblique with an angle of 25°)
24 hours only: Standard chest roentgenogram

Cervical Lymphography

The technique of cervical lymphography has been established by FISCH and DEL BUONO (1963). The investigation is performed with the patient lying in an ordinary hospital bed to insure a comfortable position.

Vital Staining

Three subcutaneous injections of 0.5 ml each of 1% dye solution are made behind the ear.

Surgical Dissection

The incision of the skin in the mastoid region is "C-shaped" and is situated at the lower margin of the retroauricular muscles and above the insertion of the sterno-cleidomastoid muscle. The retroauricular lymphatics located here have a diameter of 0.1—0.5 mm. A lymph vessel suitable for injection is carefully dissected, and a silk loop is placed 2—3 mm distal to the site of puncture. The anterior wall of the lymphatic is incised and elevated with the hooked tip of an ordinary puncture needle. The tip of a specially prepared polythene catheter with a diameter of 0.1 mm is now introduced within the lumen of the lymph vessel. The catheter is fastened with a silk knot and connected to the syringe on the automatic injector.

Contrast Injection: Dosage and Settings

4—6 ml of oily contrast material are injected at the slow rate of 0.067 ml/min.

Roentgenographic Technique

Roentgenograms in a-p and lateral projection of the neck are made twice, immediately after injection and 24 hours later. Also a standard chest roentgenogram is made at 24 hours after injection.

References

BELTZ, L., u. P. THURN: Die Tomographie des Lymphadenogramms. Röntgen-Bl. 19, 181 (1966).

BÉLANGER, R., C. HARD, D. ONIMET-OLIVA et L. KATZ: Téchnique de la lymphographie par cathéter. J. Canad. Ass. Radiol. 16, 237 (1965).

CLEMENTZ, B., and T. OLIN: Apparatus for controlled infusion of saline in angiography and contrast medium in lymphography. Acta radiol. (Stockh.) 55, 109 (1961).

DE ROO, T.: An improved, simple technique of lymphangiography. Amer. J. Roentgenol. 98, 948 (1966).

—, P. THOMAS, and R. W. KROPHOLLER: The importance of tomography for the interpretation of the lymphographic picture of lymph node mestastases. Amer. J. Roentgenol. 94, 924 (1965).

—, and A. E. VAN VOORTHUISEN: The indications for selective supplementary angiographic examination in lymphography. Amer. J. Roentgenol. 97, 957 (1966).

DITCHEK, T., and G. T. SCANLON: Direct magnification lymphography. J. Amer. med. Ass. 199, 654 (1967).

DONINI, J.: Radiographic and tomographic structural analysis in neoplastic lymphopathies explored by means of lymphography. Radiol. med. (Torino) 51, 1265 (1965).

FISCH, U.: Lymphographische Untersuchungen über das zervikale Lymphsystem. Basel-New York: Karger 1966.

—, u. M. S. DEL BUONO: Zur Technik der cervicalen Lymphographie. Schweiz. med. Wschr. 93, 994 (1963).

JING, B. S.: Improved technique of lymphangiography. Amer. J. Roentgenol. 4, 952 (1966).

KINMONTH, J. B., R. A. HARPER, and G. W. TAYLOR: Lymphangiography by radiological methods. J. Fac. Radiol. (Lond.) 6, 217 (1955).

—, and R. KEMP HARPER: Lymphangiography. A technique for the clinical use in the lower limb. Brit. med. J. 1955, 940.

KINSK, H., and W. P. PANNING: A simple, practical technic of lymphography. Radiology 88, 576 (1967).

KROPHOLLER, R. W., J. M. H. BLOM, and I. IRTÓ: Lymfografie met behulp van een polytheen-catheter. Ned. T. Geneesk. 112, 696 (1968).

LOVE, R. W., and T. TAKARO: Lymphangiography with direct roentgenographic magnification. Radiology 87, 123 (1966).

MADDISON, F. E.: Lymphatic cannulation without dye. Technical notes. Radiology 88, 362 (1967).

RÜTTIMANN, A., u. M. S. DEL BUONO: Die Lymphographie mit öligem Kontrastmittel. Fortschr. Röntgenstr. 97, 552 (1962).

TJERNBERG, B.: Lymphography as an aid to examination of lymph nodes. Acta Soc. Med. upsalien. 61, 207 (1956).

— Lymphography. An animal study on the diagnosis of Vx2 carcinoma and inflammation. Acta radiol. (Stockh.) Suppl. 214 (1962).

TRAPP, P.: Technik der Kunststoffschlaucheinführung in Lymphgefäße. Röntgen-Bl. 19, 1 (1966).

TURNER, A. F.: Lymphographic needle clamp. Amer. J. Roentgenol. 96, 1053 (1966).

VIAMONTE, M., and R. C. STEVANS: A new trocar for lymphatic cannulation. Radiology 86, 934 (1966).

YOUKER, J. E.: A clamp to facilitate lymphangiography. Brit. J. Radiol. 39, 556 (1966).

Chapter 3

Contrast Media

Harry W. Fischer

With 3 Figures

Historical

The first radiographic visualizations of the lymphatic structures in the late 1920's and early 1930's were performed largely with contrast media which were injurious to tissue. Such materials given a trial were red lead, bismuth subcarbonate, collargol, and cinnebar. Another early contrast material, colloidal thorium dioxide (Thorotrast) was not damaging to tissue initially, but later when it was found to be long retained in the body and to induce neoplasia and scarring and fibrosis, it also fell into disrepute. Early lymphography was mainly by indirect technique, that is, interstitial injection or by injection of contrast media into body cavities and joints in which colloidal or particulate materials served best. A defect of the indirect technique of lymphography was that a major portion of the contrast material remained at the injection site, even though some did pass up the lymph trunks to the nodes. The combination of unsatisfactory contrast media and deficient technique resulted in no essential progress in lymphography until KINMONTH [26] and co-workers in 1952 injected directly surgically exposed lymph trunks made visible by the interstitial injection of blue dye. Thus the modern era of lymphography was begun. Water soluble organic iodide compounds were successfully used by them for the demonstration of the lymphatics of the extremities in patients with lymphedema but the desire to visualize the nodes as well as trunks led to the adoption of the iodinated oily contrast agents. In several aspects, the widely used radiopaque oil is an eminently satisfactory contrast material.

Contrast Medium

The standard, widely used contrast medium for lymphography is an iodized oil, known commercially as Ethiodol in the United States, and as Lipiodol Ultra-Fluid in European countries. It was originally introduced as a contrast medium for hysterosalpingography, sialography, and injection of sinus tracts [6, 7]. Iodized oils, Iodipin, Lipiodol and Ethiodol were first used for lymphography by direct percutaneous injection into enlarged lymphomatous nodes [4, 35, 52].

Ethiodol was evaluated as a direct lymphographic contrast medium in animals in comparison to water soluble agents and other materials by FISCHER [13, 19], and then used successfully in direct lymphography in man despite its undesirable characteristics of formation of oil emboli in the lungs and high viscosity, recognized in the experimental work [40, 50]. Ethiodol was demonstrated to be much superior to the

Ethyl diiodostearate

$$CH_3-(CH_2)_4-\underset{\underset{I}{|}}{CH}-(CH_2)_3-\underset{\underset{I}{|}}{CH}-(CH_2)_7-COOC_2H_5$$

Ethyl monoiodostearate

$$CH_3-(CH_2)_7-\underset{\underset{I}{|}}{CH}-(CH_2)_8-COOC_2H_5$$

Fig. 1. The chemical structure of the major components of Ethiodol or Lipiodol Ultra-Fluid, the ethyl esters of monoiodo and diiodo stearic acid are shown here. Together these two compounds comprise about 88% of the oily lymphographic contrast medium, with the uniodinated saturated and unsaturated components about 12%. The iodine content of the medium is 37%

water soluble media in visualizing the lymph nodes, and in visualizing well lymph nodes and trunks at a distance from the site of injection. In addition the oil did not diffuse from the lymph trunks. Opacification of the nodes was not fleeting, the oily contrast medium remaining in the nodes for months [19, 40, 50].

Table 1. *Viscosities of some contrast media used for lymphography, at room temperature (approximately 25° C). The figure on the experimental Ethiodol emulsion is included as an example of viscosity reduction*

	Flow time (OSTWALD) seconds	Viscosity (BROOKFIELD)
Distilled Water	90	
Cholegrafin 52%	506	
Ethiodol	2454	48.5 cent.
Ethiodol Emulsion 23-10		10.9 cent.

Ethiodol is synthesized from the natural oil of poppyseeds, the oil consisting of the glyceryl esters of several fatty acids, namely oleic, linoleic, linolenic, palmitic and stearic. Iodination of the poppyseed oil is obtained by treatments with hydrioic acid, the iodine entering at the double bonds of the unsaturated fatty acids converting linoleic acid to diiodostearic acid component and oleic acid to monoiodostearic acid component (Fig. 1). After iodination, the ethyl group is substituted for glycerol moiety, the resultant iodinated ethyl esters of the fatty acids having a greatly lowered viscosity compared to the glycerol ester preparation (which is known commercially as Lipiodol). The diiodo portion is about 80%, the monoiodo portion about 12% of the whole, with the uniodinated saturated and unsaturated components about 8% [6, 7].

Ethiodol is yellow or amber colored, having a specific gravity of 1.280 at 15° C. Viscosity is about 55 centipoises at 20° C, about 30 centipoises at 37° C (Table 1). The iodine content is 37%.

Stored in the closed ampules and protected from light Ethiodol is stable. It decomposes with liberation of iodine when heated strongly; contract with air also leads to liberation of iodine. The assuming of a darker color indicates its decomposition and the material should not be used under these conditions [1] [6, 7].

Ethiodol injected directly into a peripheral lymphatic fills initially the lymph vessels and nodes. At 3 days post-lymphography in the dog, 23% of radioactively tagged I-131 Ethiodol was found in the nodes, when a dose of 0.6—0.8 ml/kg of

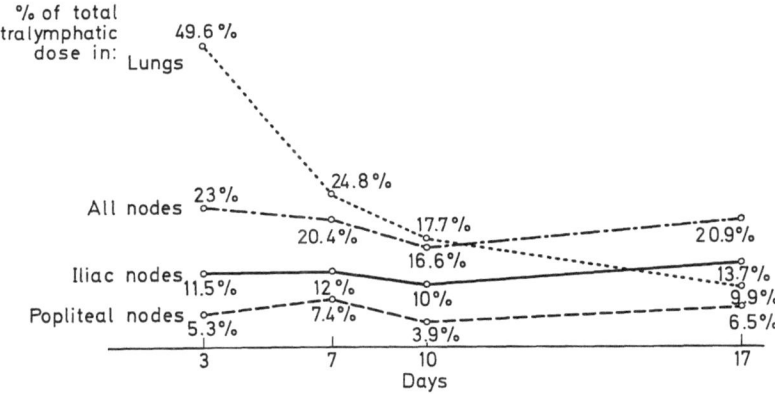

Fig. 2. The body distribution of Ethiodol after intralymphatic injection of 0.06 to 0.08 ml/kg body weight in the dog, based on the data of KOEHLER, 1964. This is a dose larger than the customary human dose of 0.35 ml/kg. In man there are proportionately more nodes than in the dog, and the portion of Ethiodol in the nodes probably is higher, and the portion in the lung lower

body weight was injected, a dose larger than the customary human dose of 0.35 ml/kg. With the use of a smaller dose in humans, and proportionately more lymph nodes, the per cent retained in the nodes is probably much higher, and the portion in the lungs lower. The amounts in the nodes remain essentially the same at 7, 10 and 17 days [27] (Fig. 2). In man the opaque material remains in the nodes for long periods of time. Much of the radiopacity is retained for several months and it is not unusual to find opaque material still present a year or more later. Using radioactive tagged I-131 Ethiodol, the half life in the node was found to be about six days for

---

[1] (Ethiodol is marketed by E. Fougera & Co., Hicksville, N. Y., Lipiodol Ultra-Fluid by Laboratories Andre Guerbet, Paris, France).

the dog's popliteal or pelvic nodes [15], but it is suspected the labelled I-131 moves out of the node faster, that is becomes free of the oil faster than the non-radioactive iodine.

Contrast medium in excess of that retained in the nodes enters the systemic veins via the thoracic duct or by way of lymphatico-venous communications. From the great veins, it passes through the right heart chambers into the pulmonary artery and its branches to be distributed in the lung capillaries. At 3 days post-lymphography with the 0.6—0.8 ml/kg dose, almost 50% of the injected Ethiodol was in the lungs. Thereafter the lung content dropped rapidly until it was less than 10% at 17 days [27]. Some of the contrast material is removed via the circulation and some enters the macrophages in the alveolar spaces. It is the later which is removed in part via the sputum [1]. At postmortem examinations of man there was no measurable radio-activity in the lungs several weeks post-lymphography with radioactive tagged con-trast medium [32, 39]. The biological half life of I-131 Ethiodol in the lungs is com-paratively short, 2.2 days [39].

Following injection of doses in the 0.6—0.8 ml range in the dog, the lung acts as a fairly efficient filter, allowing little spillover so that no other organ or system receives more than a few percent of the injected dose [27]. With increase in size of administered dose the lung becomes a less efficient filter for the oil particles and the amount initially reaching other organs is higher [42]. In the kidneys, Ethiodol has been visualized in the glomerular and peritubular capillaries. The spleen too has contained the fat vacuoles [38].

After an injection of radioactive I-131 Ethiodol, the radioactivity is initially in lipid form but later it has been determined as in the plasma fraction but not ether extractable [39], as absorbed on red cells, and in plasma in both aqueous and lipid phases [46], and inorganic form [27]. The evidence is fragmentary but it appears that the lipid form rapidly is converted to the inorganic one, presumably by esterases in tissues and in the blood and body fluids and then excreted renally. Virtually all the renally excreted iodine is in the iodide form [27]. Ethiodol in the circulating blood is never at a high level. At most in the dog about 0.9% and in man 0.5% [39], of the injected dose can be found in the blood at any one time. Urinary excretion has not exceeded 3% of the injected dose per day for the dog [27], and 2.5% for man [39], and generally is considerably less. At 17 days, about 35% of the injected dose of the tagged iodine has been excreted [27].

Low concentrations of iodine reported in the thyroid as revealed by I-131 studies may be in error, for thyroid saturation may take place with non-radioactive iodine I-127 which is liberated from Ethiodol [27].

Postmortem examinations in man after several weeks post-lymphography have shown no measurable radioactivity from tagged Ethiodol in liver, kidney, spleen, thyroid, and lung. Serial complete blood counts and platelet counts bi-weekly for several weeks after radioactive Ethiodol have shown no change [39].

Scanning of the body in vivo following radioactive lymphography shows distri-butions which do not differ greatly from studies on nodes removed surgically [12].

Toxicity: The fatal dose of Ethiodol injected intralymphatically in dogs averaged 3.62 ml/kg of body weight with a range of 2.92 to 4.40 ml/kg. The fatal dose for intravenous administrations is understandably less, averaging 1.58 ml/kg, with a range of 1.21 to 1.90 ml/kg. The contrast medium was administered at a rate of 0.2 ml/min through a No. 27 needle while the animals were under light pentobarbital anesthesia [45]. The fatal dose for rabbits averaged 0.97 ml/kg [21], or 1.0 ml/kg [42]. The LD_{50} for the mouse is 1.8 ml/kg. It is fruitless to apply these figures to limitations for man, for it has now become clear a dose of 0.35 ml/kg body weight, 12 ml for each lower extremity for a 70 kg individual, seldom if ever needs to be exceeded to insure a good clinical examination. It should be remembered the animal data refers to acute, rapid injection studies until the animal becomes immediately, severely incapacitated or succumbs. No figures are available for subacute toxicity, for example, for a 30 day survival period.

The pattern of toxicity in the dog is rapid, shallow respirations beginning at approximately 60% of the fatal dose level proceeding to short, labored breathing, and death. The cause of the respiratory disability and death is diffuse massive embolization of the lung capillaries by the oily medium [20, 21, 45]. Airless, dark ecchymotic zones in the lung are seen at autopsy, which have the characteristics of pulmonary infarcts microscopically [20]. Although some fat globules may lodge in other organs [45] their number is few and an unlikely contribution to acute toxicity or death. Ethiodol when injected in 1½ cc amount in the hind leg muscle of mice produced sarcoma in an occasional animal from 6 to 18 months after injection [51].

Acute toxicity as described above is interwoven with the signs and symptoms of acute, subacute and chronic toxidity in man, and will be further discussed under the heading of "Complications".

Dosage: To perform lymphography of the leg and trunk so that inguinal, iliac, and aortic-abdominal nodes are visualized, seven to eight ml of Ethiodol are injected into each side in an adult male. For the adult female who is of generally smaller size, four to seven ml is sufficient per lower extremity. Depending upon the size of the child, two to five ml should be used. There is a better correlation between suitable dose and body length than body weight. Doses expressed as ml per kg of body weight are therefore not too meaningful; the dose of 16 ml for a 70 kg patient calculates to 0.23 ml/kg. To perform lymphography of the arm and visualize the axillary nodes, 2 to 4 ml are required.

Rate of administration recommended is forty to eighty minutes for an 8 ml dose, or 0.1 to 0.2 ml per minute. A pressure of 0.4 atmosphere is advised [36]. High injection speeds and pressures predispose to rupture of the lymph trunk and extravasation.

Testing for Sensitivity to Ethiodol: In the United States, there is no standard, well-used pre-lymphography test for sensitivity to iodine or Ethiodol. Patients are asked about previous reactions to iodine, and questioned about allergies in general. If a positive history of iodine sensitivity is obtained, lymphography is contraindicated. A strong history of allergy should alert the lymphographer to proceed with caution, for it is generally recognized that patients with an allergic history have a high incidence of untoward reactions to other intravascular contrast media and presumably will react more frequently to Ethiodol.

A test for sensitivity to iodine used to some extent on the continent is to give the patient 5 ml of potassium iodide or 1 ml of lipiodol ultrafluid orally one day prior to planned lymphography. If signs of hypersensitivity occur (nausea, fever, skin reactions, impaired general condition) lymphography is not performed.

Ethiodol with Chlorophyll: Ethiodol in which chlorophyll had been dissolved was for a time utilized in lymphography. The rationale for its use was to aid the surgeon in visual recognition of nodes at the time of operative dissection. The agent has not gained a sound place in the armamentarium, for often the nodes at operation are still obscured by the surrounding fatty tissues. Its value is further diminished by the chlorophyllated medium being associated with a more intense, earlier developing tissue reaction and slower removal from the lymph vessels [23, 31]. An increased incidence of groin tenderness and palpable inguinal adenopathy has been observed. The prolonged stasis of the chlorophyll-Ethiodol in the trunks makes radiographic interpretation more difficult because nodal outlines were obscured by the overlying material [31].

Water Soluble Media: The angiographic-urographic water soluble organic iodide contrast agents may be used for lymphography. Diatrizoate compounds, both the sodium and methylglucamine salts being in wide usage, have been most commonly pressed into service as lymphographic agents. Water soluble materials have two serious disadvantages, they diffuse rapidly from lymph channel and node, obscuring details of structure, and they do not demonstrate lymph nodes at a distance from the site of injection adequately. Water soluble agents can be injected with much greater speed than the oily materials, but films must be made without delay before diffusion of the medium takes place. A warm or burning sensation accompanying the flow of the fluid up the leg is usual with water soluble agents which are hypertonic.

Comparison studies in animals have shown the cholangiographic agent iodipamide (Cholegrafin, Biligrafin) to be a superior contrast medium of the water soluble type [3, 19, 24, 48]. The lesser tendency to pass through the lymphatic wall and diffuse has been attributed to a higher molecular weight than other compounds [24].

Water soluble agents are now seldom used. Occasionally they find usage when it is desired to only visualize lymphatics of the leg as in patients with congenital lymphedema, but the approach is not completely rational since the status of the inguinal and more proximal nodes may bear on the problem of the swollen leg and any contrast media which does not demonstrate all the nodes well is inadequate.

Experimental Lymphographic Agents: The dissatisfaction with the high viscosity of Ethiodol and the oil embolization of the lungs has led to several attempts to find a better contrast medium.

Emulsions of Ethiodol have been reported upon [3, 11, 17, 37, 43, 44] with varying degrees of enthusiasm as solving the problems of viscosity and embolism, yet avoiding diffusion from the lymphatic system. At the present time, there is no emulsion of Ethiodol being made available on other than an experimental trial basis. With the improvement in some characteristics, other defects of new contrast media have been encountered. Emulsification has led to a heightened tissue response to the iodinated oil [3, 25, 44], to a less prolonged opacification of the nodes, and to a hypotensive response [17]. Whether pulmonary dysfunction is entirely eliminated by use of an emulsion has been called into question [18]. The characteristics of response of the experimental animal to Ethiodol and its emulsions may be misleading for differences have been noted between dog and man [25]. Other approaches have been unsuccessful, either because of physical characteristics [8, 49], or unsatisfactory interaction with lymph and lymphatic tissue [16, 19].

Earlier, TJERNBERG [48], using rabbits and dogs had tested materials of several types as lymphographic agents: suspensions of acetrizoic acid, lead-EDTA solutions, proprietary preparations of water soluble organic iodides such as Diodrast, Per-Abrodil M, Urokon, Hypaque, Urografin, Miokon, Biligrafin, Endografin, Thorotrast, emulsion of Pantopaque, Immetal. Of these, Thorotrast produced the best quality lymphograms, but was considered unsatisfactory because of its radioactivity. Highly viscous materials such as the highly concentrated water soluble agents required too high injection pressure. The water soluble media have the tendency to extravasate, but of these tested Urografin had the least marked tendency to do so in the rabbit, while in dogs Urografin, Biligrafin, and Miokon were equally satisfactory. Diodrast and Urokon showed the most extravasation. Oily media were initially condemned on the basis of the risk of fat emboli, local toxic action, and high viscosity.

Indirect Lymphography: At present a satisfactory contrast medium for indirect lymphography does not exist. Thorotrast injected into tissue visualizes regional lymphatics and lymph node to a certain extent, but the visualization is quite deficient compared to direct lymphography. The nodes and lymph vessels are less well opacified, and there is less regularity and completeness of node filling [14]. Water soluble agents such as the current angiographic media have been used for indirect lymphography [9, 33], but with these materials even with hyaluronidase or with increase of the tissue pressure, node and lymph vessels visualization is much inferior to direct lymphograph [14]. Moreover, some of these agents can cause damage when injected interstitially [14, 18].

Ethiodol emulsion has been used for indirect lymphography in animals with inconsistent results [37]. Ethiodol has been used for an attempt at indirect lymphography in humans, that of injection into the base of the broad ligament with the intention of visualizing hypogastric and obturator nodes. Sufficient evidence was not provided of the indirect techniques visualizing all nodes of the region and in one of five patients a moderately severe granulomatous reaction with parametritis occurred [34].

In another indirect method, emulsions of iodinated oils (Ethiodol) [37] and (Angiopac) [2] have been tested for visualization of substernal nodes by injection of the contrast material in the peritoneal cavity. A fair degree of success was realized but thus far the investigation is limited to experiments in small animals and the dog.

A modified indirect technique consisting of retrograde injections of water soluble medium retrograde into a peripheral vein, while the vein is kept proximally occluded and tissue pressure is raised by inflation of a pneumonic cuff around the extremity has been reported to produce good lymphograms in the experimental animal [30]. No clinical application has resulted, however.

Visualization of lymphatic structures by oral administration of contrast media has been obtained, but the technique has not reached a stage of clinical efficiency or acceptance. An emulsification of iodinated propylester of poppyseed oil (Lipiodol) was utilized [41].

Vital dyes

To make visible the lymphatic trunks for the technique of cannulation and direct lymphography, a blue dye is injected intradermally or subcutaneously. For a lower extremity and trunk lymphogram the dye is injected between the toes and for an arm and axillary lymphogram between the fingers. The blue dye enters the lymphatics, coloring the lymph a greenish-blue, allowing the clear identification of the lymphatic.

Patent Blue V

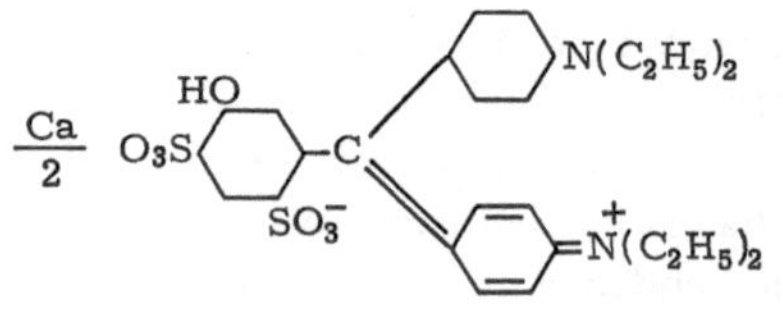

Fig. 3. The chemical structure of Patent Blue V, a diamino derivative of a triphenylmethane dye, officially termed Blue 3 by the Colour Index. (See reference to Colour Index in text.) Alphazurine 2 G is a closely similar compound, frequently listed as identical to Patent Blue V

KINMONTH [26] originally used a blue dye, Patent Blue V, also known as Patent Blue Violet, because of early work which had shown certain dyes when injected into the tissue entered the lymphatics, clearly delineating them [22].

Patent Blue V is a triphenylmethane dye, officially termed Acid Blue 3, and having the number 42051 in the Colour Index [2]. Its molecular weight is 1159.4 and the chemical formula $Ca(C_{27}H_{31}N_2O_7S_2)_2$. Its molecular structure is given in Fig. 3.

Alphazurine 2 G is a blue dye which has been frequently used in the United States. It has at times been listed as identical to Patent Blue V. However the manufacturer of Alphazurine 2 G gives its structure as being similar to C. I. Acid Blue 1, Colour Index No. 42045 [3].

A 11% water solution of Patent Blue V or Alphazurine 2 G is isotonic with body fluids. The prepared dye solution should be made sterile by autoclaving in sealed ampules.

Other dyes which have been used are Evans Blue, Brilliant Blue F.C.F. (F.D. and C. Blue No. 1), direct sky blue and prontosil rubrum.

Dose: 0.1 ml of 11% solution is injected intradermally between the toes and fingers; or 0.2 to 0.5 ml of 11% solution is diluted in 1.5 to 3 ml of 1% procaine or other local anesthetic and injected subcutaneously in the web space between toes or fingers.

Metabolism: Patent Blue V after interstitial injection is absorbed and transported from the tissue not only by lymphatics but by blood vessels as well. In normal subjects, 10% of the 0.1 ml of 11% solution, the usual injected dose, is excreted in the urine, half of which was excreted in the first $2^{1}/_{2}$ hours [47]. The blue coloration progressively clears from the injected area and is essentially gone at two weeks.

Toxicity. Toxicity has been manifested by skin reactions. See "Complications".

---

[2] Colour Index, 2nd Ed., 1956. Published by the Society of Dyers and Colourists, and Amer. Assoc. of Textile Chemists and Colourists, Bradford, Yorkshire, England, and Lowell, Mass., USA, Vol. III.

[3] Alphazurine 2G is manufactured in the U.S. by Allied Chemical Corporation, Morristown, N. J.

Testing for Sensitivity to Blue Dye: Testing for sensitivity to blue dye prior to lymphography is seldom performed in the United States. Should the lymphographer desire to test, it is recommended 0.02 ml of a 0.1% solution of Alphazurine 2 G (Patent Blue V) be injected intradermally on the arm. A wheal and flare reaction within 20 minutes contraindicates the use of the blue dye [29].

References

[1] BELIN, R. P., M. A. SHEA, N. H. STONE, and W. O. GRIFFEN: Iodoliposputosis following lymphangiography. Report of a case. Dis. Chest 48, 543—544 (1965).

[2] BENNETT, H. S., and A. A. SHIVAS: The visualization of lymph nodes and vessels by ethyl iodostearate (Angiopac) and its effect on lymphoid tissue. J. Fac. Radiol. 5, 261—266 (1954).

[3] BISMUTH, V., M. GUERBET, J. P. DESTREZ-CURELY, A. GLUCKMAN, and R. BOURDON: Lymphangiography with new oily contrast media. Presented at the Second International Congress of Lymphology, March 1968, Miami, Fla. To be published.

[4] BRUUN, S., and A. ENGESET: Lymphadenography. Acta radiol. 45, 389—395 (1956).

[5] Communication from Allied Chemical Co., Specialty Chemicals Div., Morristown, N. J., 1968.

[6] Communication from E. Fougera and Co., Inc., Hicksville, N. Y., 1968.

[7] Communication from Laboratories Andre Guerbet, Paris, France, 1968.

[8] DANESE, C. A.: Experiments with new lymphographic agents. In: International Symposium on Lymphology, Proceedings, Zurich, Switzerland, July 19—23, 1966, p. 342.

[9] DANESE, C. A., J. M. HOWARD, and R. BOWER: Lymphangiography by subcutaneous injection of water soluble radiopaque medium. The role of interstitial pressure. Ann. Surg. 155, 614—619 (1962).

[10] DUMONT, A.: Roentgenography of the diaphragmatic and retrosternal lymphatics by intraperitoneal injection of contrast media. In: International Symposium on Lymphology, Proceedings, Zurich, Switzerland, July 19—23, 1966, p. 394.

[11] ELKE, M., G. WOLF, and G. HARTMANN: Experiments with an emulsion of Lipiodol-UF (Guerbet) to avoid pulmonary embolism. In: International Symposium on Lymphology, Proceedings, Zurich, Switzerland, July 19—23, 1966, p. 336—337.

[12] FAVA, G., and L. RONCORONI: Autopsy investigations of the distribution in various organs of radioactive lipiodol introduced through the lymphatic system. Radiol. med. 50, 653—659 (1964).

[13] FISCHER, H. W.: Lymphangiography and lymphadenography with various contrast agents. Ann. N. Y. Acad. Sci. 78, 799—808 (1959).

[14] — A critique of experimental lymphography. Acta radiol. 52, 448—454 (1959).

[15] — Intralymphatic therapy for lymph node metastases of carcinoma of the cervix. An analysis of the proposition and presentation of pertinent experimental data. Cancer 18, 1059—1065 (1965).

[16] — Microcrystals of ethylipodate as a lymphographic agent. In: International Symposium on Lymphology, Proceedings, Zurich, Switzerland, July 19—23, 1966, p. 343.

[17] — Experiences in seeking an Ethiodol emulsion for lymphography. Invest. Radiol. 1, 29—36 (1966).

[18] —, K. A. FEISAL, and W. C. STEVENS: Lung function studies after the intralymphatic injection of emulsions of Ethiodol in dogs. Lymphology, in press (1968).

[19] —, and G. R. ZIMMERMAN: Roentgenographic visualization of lymph nodes and lymphatic channels. Amer. J. Roentgenol. 81, 517—534 (1959).

[20] GOLDBERG, M. E., and S. B. FEINBERG: Pulmonary infarction following lymphangiography in dogs. Its implications in human studies. Radiology 81, 479—483 (1963).

[21] GUINEY, E. J., M. H. GOUGH, and J. B. KINMONTH: Lymphography with fat-soluble contrast media. J. cardiovasc. Surg. 5, 346—354 (1964).

[22] HUDACK, S., P. D. McMASTER: Permeability of the wall of the lymphatic capillary. J. exp. Med. 56, 223—238 (1932).

[23] JACKSON, R. J. A.: Chlorophyllated Lipiodol ultrafluid as a contrast medium; An explanation for the disadvantages attending its use. Presented at the Second International Congress of Lymphology, March 1968, Miami, Fla. To be published.

[24] JACOBSSON, S., and S. JOHANSSON: Method of lymphography. Kungl. fysiografiska sällskapets i Lund Förhandl. 29, 57—63 (1959).

[25] JOHANSSON, S., N. H. STERBY, G. THEANDER, and L. WEHLIN: Iodinated oil emulsion for lymphography. Acta radiol. 4, 690—704 (1966).

[26] KINMONTH, J. B.: Lymphangiography in man. Method of outlining lymphatic trunks at operation. Clin. Sci. 11, 13—20 (1952 a).
—, R. A. K. HARPER, and G. W. TAYLOR: Lymphangiography by radiological methods. J. Fac. Radiologists 6, 217—223 (1955 b).

[27] KOEHLER, P. R., W. A. MEYERS, J. F. SKELLEY, and B. SCHAFFER: Body distribution of Ethiodol following lymphangiography. Radiology 82, 866—871 (1964).

[28] — Radiographic visualization of the substernal lymph nodes. Radiology 85, 565—567 (1965 a).
— Radiographic visualization of retrosternal lymph nodes. In: International Symposium on Lymphology, Proceedings, Zurich, Switzerland, July 19—23, 1966 b, pp. 389—392.

[29] KOPP, W. L.: Anaphylaxis from Alphazurine 2G during lymphography. J. Amer. med. Ass. 198, 200—201 (1966).

[30] LAINE, J. B., R. S. TODD, and J. M. HOWARD: An experimental method of intravenous lymphangiography. Brit. J. Surg. 50, 866—869 (1963).

[31] LEMMON, W. T., JR., A. S. KETCHAM, J. D. MACHOWRY, and J. HERDT: Surgical applications of Ethiodol with chlorophyll in lymphangiography: Histopathologic, radiographic, and clinical disadvantages in 36 cases. Ann. Surg. 164, 114—122 (1966).

[32] LIEBNER, E. J.: An appraisal of radioactive therapeutic lymphography. Amer. J. Roentgenol. 93, 110—121 (1965).

[33] MALEK, P., u. J. KOLC: Die indirekte Lymphographie mit zeitweiligem Verschluß der Blutkapillaren. Acta radiol. 49, 361—368 (1958).

[34] PATTILLO, R. A., D. V. FOLEY, and R. F. MATTINGLY: Internal pelvic lymphography. Amer. J. Obstet. Gynec. 88, 110—122 (1964).

[35] PROKOPEC, J., and E. KOLEHOVA: Lymphadenography in clinical practice. Fortschr. Röntgenstr. 89, 417—424 (1958).

[36] RUTTIMANN, A.: Errors in lymphography. Radiol. austriaca 16, 77—86 (1966).

[37] SANEN, F. J., and L. K. THOMPSON, III.: A physiological and simple approach to lymphography. An experimental study. Radiology 87, 450—456 (1966).

[38] SCHAFFER, B., P. R. KOEHLER, C. R. DANIEL, G. T. WOHLE, E. RIVERA, W. A. MEYERS, and J. F. SKELLEY: A critical evaluation of lymphangiography. Radiology 80, 917—930 (1963).

[39] SEITZMAN, D. M., R. WRIGHT, F. A. HALABY, and J. H. FREEMAN: Radioactive lymphangiography as a therapeutic adjunct. Amer. J. Roentgenol. 89, 140—149 (1963).

[40] SHEEHAN, R., M. HRESHCHYSHYN, R. K. LIN, F. P. LESSMAN: The use of lymphography as a diagnostic method. Radiology. 76, 47—53 (1961).

[41] SOHN, N., and A. E. DUMONT: Roentgenography of the thoracic duct in man by oral administration of contrast media. Proc. Soc. exp. Biol. Med. 112, 901—903 (1963).

[42] SZABO, G.: Oil embolism studies. In: International Symposium on Lymphology, Proceedings, Zürich, Switzerland, July 19—23, 1966, pp. 320—321.

[43] TAKASHIMA, T.: Experimental lymphangiography, with special reference to search for adequate medium. Thesis. University of Kanazawa, Japan.

[44] TEPLICK, J. G., M. E. HASKIN, J. SKELLEY, G. T. WOHL, and F. SANEN: Experimental studies with a new radiopaque emulsion. Radiology 82, 478—485 (1964).

[45] THOMPSON, L. K. III, and W. G. ANLYAN: Toxicologic study of an iodinated oil following intralymphatic and intraveneous administration in dogs. Surg. Gynec. Obstet. 121, 107—111 (1965).

[46] THREEFOOT, S. A., and R. CUSH: Fate of oil in the lungs after lymphography. In: International Symposium on Lymphology, Proceedings, Zurich, Switzerland, July 19—23, 1966, pp. 321—322.

[47] — Urinary excretion of Patent Blue V after intradermal injection in man. Proc. Soc. exp. Biol. Med. 103, 815—819 (1960).

[48] TJERNBERG, B.: Lymphography. An animal study on the diagnosis of Vx2 carcinoma and inflammation. Acta radiol. suppl. 214, 1962.

[49] VIAMONTE, M.: Compounds unsuitable for lymphography. In: International Symposium on Lymphology, Proceedings, Zurich, Switzerland, July 19—23, 1966, pp. 343—344.

[50] WALLACE, S., L. JACKSON, B. SCHAFFER, J. GOULD, R. R. GREENING, A. WEISS, and S. KRAMER: Lymphangiograms: Their diagnostic and therapeutic potential. Radiology 76, 179—199 (1961).

[51] WEXLER, H., J. P. MINTON, and A. S. KETCHAM: A comparison of survival time and extent of tumor metastases on mice with transplanted, induced and spontaneous tumors. Cancer 18, 985—994 (1965).

[52] ZHEUTLIN, N., and E. SHANBROM: Contrast visualization of lymph nodes. Radiology 71, 702—708 (1958).

Chapter 4

Complications of Lymphography

Harry W. Fischer

With 2 Figures

Wound Complications

The incidence of infection of the wound following lymphography is low, approximately 1%. It is no greater than the infection rate for other small superficial wounds, such as the incisions for placing a catheter or needle directly into a peripheral vein for infusions. Wound infections can be kept to a minimum level by adequate cleansing of the skin, and by performing lymphography with strict adherence to aseptic technique. Separate instruments, needles, and tubing should be used for each extremity to avoid cross-contamination. The needles and syringes used for injecting the blue dye should not be used for any other portion of the technique since the area between the toes is most difficult to render aseptic. It is preferable to dispose of the tubing after only one use to avoid the problems of sterilizing plastic tubing. It is also preferable to have the doses of blue dye in separate ampules so that there is no possibility of accidental contamination from one lymphogram to the next by this route.

Necrosis of the skin about the lymphography wound is rare. The phenomenon is not encountered with lymphography any more often than with other small wounds of the extremities.

Lymphangitis of an infectious nature is also uncommon. It occurs more frequently in the extremities which are already lymphedematous. Swelling of the extremity after lymphography occurs on occasion, more often in patients who are found to have diseased lymph nodes, such as then enlarged nodes of lymphoma. Usually the swelling is temporary and not of consequence.

Delayed wound healing of a foot wound is seen in a small percent of the cases, probably as a result of excessive activity of the patient during the healing phase. Precise apposition of the skin edges by the suturing, and allowing the sutures to remain in place longer than seven days helps insure a well healed wound. Seldom is it necessary to place subcutaneous sutures in addition to skin sutures to obtain secure wound closure. Persistent leakage of lymph from the wound is not often encountered even in view of the fact the lymphatic is usually not ligated before skin closure.

Pain in the extremity is occasionally experienced by the patient during the course of the injection. It is brief and not severe, resulting presumably from distention of the lymph vessels. With water soluble materials the hypertonicity of the contrast agent may be a factor. Pain and tenderness in the inguinal nodes has been rarely seen. Deep pain in the trunk region is thought to be related to distention of lymphomatous nodes by contrast medium.

Extravasation of the contrast media from the lymphatic or the node is not uncommon. With water soluble agents it is generalized after the first few minutes and is one of the undesirable features of the use of this type of contrast medium, leading to poor definition of lymph structures. Extravasation of oily contrast medium is thought to be related to injection at excessive pressure or to excessive pressure developing in the lymphatic system when obstruction is present. In the arm, where the lymphatics are considered more delicate, extravasation is more frequent [4]. It must be admitted, however, that the phenomenon is not completely understood. It may be due to defects in the lymphatic wall secondary to trauma or disease. Extravasation is of importance for contrast material lost into the tissue is not available for visualizing lymphatic structures. An inadequate lymphogram may result if the loss is great. Extravasated oil is also a potential hazard for it is absorbed slowly from the tissues, although no ill effects have thus far been documented. Extravasated water soluble contrast material is rapidly absorbed and except for some brief, irritation action on adjacent tissue, the modern contrast media produce no harm.

Histological Complications in Lymph Nodes

Within a few hours after lymphography, the lymph nodes show dilatation of the marginal and intermediary sinuses and giant cell reaction [39]. The foreign body reaction consists of diffuse reticulocytosis and sinus-histiocytosis. Diffuse plasmocytosis, an increase in number of eosinophils, and hypervascularization is also seen [30]. About the 10th to the 14th day the giant cells which had been increasing in number until that time become smaller in size and fewer in number. The overall response is then at its height. The amount of contrast media in the marginal sinuses decreases at the same time until at 3—6 months dilated sinuses are few in number. The increase in size of nodes observed radiographically in the first days post-lymphography can therefore be accounted for by these two processes, dilated sinuses filled with contrast media and the cellular inflammatory response [27].

The oily contrast material is seen as droplets or vacuoles in the sinuses and the pulp region. Surrounding the droplets is a margin of reticulum cells. In time, both phagocytosis and possibly other metabolic processes reduce the size and number of the droplets. KRAUS [30] reports significant decrease in phagocytic reaction after several weeks. Although substantial amounts of oil are found in the nodes for many months post-lymphography, the lipid material is eventually absorbed. Foreign body giant cells have almost completely disappeared by six months [18], and the reaction changes have mainly disappeared by 12—15 months [30, 34]. The only irreversible changes reported are small circumscribed fibrous scars in the marginal sinuses and area of capsular fibrosis, or fibrous encapsulation of some of the droplets occasionally is seen [30, 34]. At 14 months post lymphography, FRISCHBIER [18] could not recognize any differences is node structure compared to hypogastric nodes which had not contained contrast medium.

The histologic changes described in the nodes for an Ethiodol emulsion were quantitatively similar to those for Ethiodol in both patients and in the experimental animal, the dog, but a more intense histologic response was noted with emulsion. In one patient a groin node removed seven days post-lymphography with emulsion showed some areas of necrosis and areas of necrosis were seen in dog nodes at 8 days with emulsion [24]. Clinically the reaction of the nodes to emulsion in some patients was more than that usually resulting from Ethiodol, but was not a cause for alarm. Regional nodes became swollen and tender, and in four of fifty patients a lymph-angitis was encountered, a higher incidence than with Ethiodol [24].

More histological response was associated with lymphography in the dog than in man with various contrast media [24].

When examined by a second lymphography several months later undiseased nodes are of the same size and opacity pattern as at original lymphogram.

With any procedure utilized for the diagnosis of neoplasm, the question must be asked, "Does the procedure cause spread or extension of the neoplasm?" Clinical evidence has been difficult to obtain, only three pieces of evidence being available on this point: 1. tumor cells were found in the circulating blood following lymphography in one patient [38]; 2. Reed-Sternberg cells in increased number have been found in the thoracic duct in a patient with Hodgkin's disease after lympho-graphy [14]; 3. following lymphography in a patient with melanoma of the foot, metastases developed along the medial aspect of the thigh [11]. None of these three is very strong evidence. On many other attempts, no tumor cells could be demonstrated after lymphography [38] and the importance of circulating Reed-Sternberg cells to the spread of Hodgkin's disease is questionable. As for the spread of melanoma, it is well known that metastases on the same extremity are not unusual in cases in which no lymphography has been performed.

Evidence from the laboratory consequently has been sought to reassure lympho-graphers of the safety of the procedure. Utilizing experiments with the transplantable Vx2 tumor in rabbits, lymphography with oily contrast medium did not increase the number of metastases [13, 38] and the lymphography rabbits lived longer than the controls [13]. Oily contrast medium did not influence the filter function of the lymph nodes, as tested with macroaggregates of human serum labeled with I-131. Although filled with contrast medium, nodes were still able to filter 100×10^6 particles of protein of cell size from the lymph stream in 20 minutes, nor did injected contrast medium cause the macroaggregates to leave the node [7].

ENGZELL [15] and co-workers found also that lymphography did not promote migration of prior injected rabbit Vx2 tumor cells, but cells injected after lympho-graphy passed through the nodes into the efferent lymph in some animals. An explana-tion for the above described behavior is afforded from experiment in which red cells were used to study efficiency of node filtration. The dog's popliteal node was found to be an efficient (nearly 100%) filter for small quantities of intralymphatically injected red cells but not for larger quantities. Phagocytosis is the prime method of filtration when small quantities are handled. With large quantities, mechanical trapping and sedimentation in the sinuses predominate [42]. The node opacified with Ethiodol is known to be enlarged initially, in part due to dilated contrast medium filled sinuses. It is these dilated sinuses which may allow tumor cells to pass through the node.

The correlation of tumor cells passing through a node to actual increased incidence of metastases is not yet proven, but it is reasonable to think there is such a relationship For the present, we must await further evidence of this aspect of lymphography.

To date, there are no clinical or laboratory experimental reports of an increased incidence of infection or evidence of interference with host resistance to infection following lymphography.

Reactions to Contrast Media and to Iodine

Like any other material introduced into the body, the lymphographic contrast media have the potential for inducing an untoward reaction due to the chemical nature of the material itself. Reactions to the oily contrast media were recorded in 40 of 32,000 lymphograms, an incidence of 1 per 1000, approximately [28].

A dermatitis, erythema, swelling and tenderness was observed in three patients by REDMAN [35]. The dermatitis was considered a local drug reaction of the vascular type, related to the Ethiodol which had extravasated into the leg along the lymphatic channels. This is not to say the extravasation was the cause of the reaction for extravasation is fairly frequent, but dermatitis is rare. In one of the patients a later lymphogram led to a similar more rapid response. The dermatitis was thought to be the type which occurs following the administration of drug to which the patient becomes sensitive. The presumed causative factor is iodine, although it could be the fatty acids or their esters.

A rash was encountered in five patients in a series of 522 lymphographies, the exanthem involving the limbs consisting of papular or wheal and erythema response with pruritis [12], while in two patients in another large series of cases an erythematous pruritic skin reaction was seen [31].

Corticosteroids and antihistaminics have been utilized with effectiveness for the dermatitic reactions.

Another type of reaction in lymphography is iodine sialadenitis seen in two patients of 522 lymphographies [12]. This reaction too is assumed to be a hypersensitivity of the salivary gland to iodine, for iodine is excreted by the glands usually without event.

Reactions to the Blue Dye

Adverse reactions to the blue dye are infrequent. In 32,000 lymphograms, 57 reactions to blue dye were reported [28], an incidence of one for seven hundred examinations. The occurrence of a non-fatal, anaphylactic reaction to alphazurine 2G (Patent Blue V or Patent Blue Violet) in two patients has been reported in detail [29]. One patient noted immediate itching of the legs, nasal congestion, and choking immediately after the injection of 0.25 ml of a 11% solution of the blue dye in both feet. Generalized urticaria and syncope developed. The other patient immediately experienced generalized urticaria, edema of the eyelids and lower lip, and choking immediately after injection of 2 ml of a 11% solution of blue dye in both feet.

The symptoms responded gradually to epinephrine, diphenhydramine and hydrocortisone. Alphazurine 2G at a concentration of 100 mcg/100 ml caused a wheal and flare reaction to the skin prink test in each patient. A negative test for liodcaine was obtained. Both patients also responded positively to skin testing with two other triphenylmethane dyes, as well as to a second lot of alphazurine.

The evidence is therefore very strong for anaphylactic hypersensitivity to Alphazurine 2G, but it is not known how sensitization is acquired. The suspicion nevertheless remains of the hypersensitivity reaction being related to the use of local anesthetics with the blue dye, although the urticarial reaction has been observed without local anesthetic. In KINMONTH's [25] series no toxic effects have been encountered in 14 years of use, but a general anesthesia is used. An interesting feature of the reaction is bluish coloration of the skin wheals.

A complication of blue dye usage is the long term bluish discoloration of the injected part. In extreme cases, this caused considerable dissatisfaction to the patient. With Patent Blue Violet 10% of the dye is excreted in the first 24 hours [44]. Long term discoloration does not occur with Patent Blue Violet, although the time for return of the skin to normal coloration varies from a few days to a few weeks. With one other dye, Direct Sky Blue, long term skin discoloration is seen, decreasing the usefulness of this compound.

A transient complication is a generalized blue discoloration of the skin seen within the first few hours after the injection of blue dye. It is thought due to rapid absorption of excessive amounts of dye which is distributed systematically before being excreted. Children and young adults seem to be more predisposed to the phenomenon. We have not seen this persist longer than one day. The bluish-green discoloration of the urine is observed for several hours to a few days post-lymphography, and represents only the usual process of excretion of the dye by the kidney.

Lung Complications

The lung complications of lymphography with oily contrast agents are in incidence most common, and in significance most important of all complications of lymphography. They account for the majority of deaths which have been suffered. The lung complications of lymphography are caused by embolization of the iodized oil into the pulmonary capillaries and the subsequent disturbances.

With each performance of a lymphogram with Ethiodol, some oily globules invariably enter the venous circulation and travel to the lung, although the degree with which this is radiographically visible varies. Typically the droplets of Ethiodol cause a diffusely stippled pattern of fine opacities in the lung. Originally some workers had thought because no symptoms had occurred and the chest roentgenogram showed no fine emboli, no oil embolism had occurred, but lung scans after use of radioactive tagged contrast media have shown quite well embolism occurs in every case [37]. Even without the isotopic or histologic evidence, it is apparent lung embolization occurs in every case for any amount in excess of what the nodes will retain must enter the venous system and go to the lungs. Lung embolism of oily contrast media is tolerated by the vast majority of patients without symptoms of any kind.

Despite the absence of symptoms or any outward indication of disturbed physiology, pulmonary function studies have revealed definite abnormalities. Decrease in pulmonary diffusing capacity and pulmonary capillary blood volume was noted in seven patients examined by a battery of pulmonary function tests following lymphography. The mean time between start of injection and the first observed decrease in diffusing capacity was 13 hours, with a range of 3 to 27 hours. Maximum decrease was noted between 3 and 72 hours, (Mean 37 hours), and recovery varied from 21 to 256 hours, (mean 80 hours) [21]. The maximum change from control value for pulmonary diffusion capacity varied from a decrease of 12% to a decrease of 60%. No significant changes from control values were seen in lung volume, airway resistance, alveolar gas uniformity, venous hemoglobin concentration, end-expired carbon dioxide tensions, and arterial blood and gas studies. In each of three patients the slope of the pressure-volume curve during inspiration decreased, while the slope during expiration remained unchanged. An analysis of the several tests showed the decreased diffusing capacity was due to decreased capillary blood volume, the measured pulmonary capillary blood volume decreases being from 28 to 60%, and this suggests the number of patent pulmonary capillaries decreased [21]. The function tests correlate well with the histologic evidence of oil in pulmonary capillaries of both man and dog. The cause of the decreased pulmonary compliance during inspiration was not clear. It may be due to contraction of smooth muscle of the peripheral airways as seen after changes in the surface tension of the liquid film lining the alveoli [21] as have been noted in fat embolism [23].

Other studies have also shown a fall in diffusing capacity of the lung but no change in ventilating ability following lymphography even though the patient had no respiratory symptoms or outward disability [3, 17]. Lung biopsies revealed the oil initially in lung capillaries but some of the lipid staining material was seen a short time later in the interstitial tissues. Further evidence of passage of oil from the capillary was obtained by recovering radioactive sputum following performance of lymphography with radioactive I-131 tagged contrast medium [5, 17].

A significant fall in arterial oxygen tension, an increase in arterial pH, and a slight hyperventilation at four hours post-lymphography was reported in yet another study [16]. At 48 hours, values had returned to normal. In one patient a second lymphogram at this time resulted in a deeper and more persistent decrease in arterial pO_2. The greater disturbances in gas exchange were observed in those patients who showed parenchymatous infiltrations or interstitial edema in addition to typical micro-emboli [16].

Although in all the groups studied by pulmonary function tests, no symptoms have been present and no disability induced, and although the great majority of patients undergoing lymphography are likewise not placed in any pulmonary stress of which they are aware, pulmonary embolism of oil has been incriminated in cases of severe morbidity and death.

Patients who develop respiratory symptoms soon after lymphography are probably suffering primarily from blockage of pulmonary capillaries by oil. This may occur in a patient with previously normal lung function, but it is the patient with significant underlying pulmonary disease, with low functional reserve who is more likely to develop symptoms. If there is significant loss of pulmonary diffusing capacity prior to lymphography, followed by occlusion of more capillaries by oil, the patient is more likely to be placed in jeopardy. Previous radiation to the chest causing lung fibrosis, and involvement of lung by neoplasm are entities which make the patient particularly susceptible [26, 31]. The mechanical block of lung capillaries by oil droplets which occurs in all patients post lymphography and causes acute symptoms rarely, also leads in some patients to what has become known as the chemical phase or a chemical pneumonitis. After the initial vascular occlusive phenomena, a lung response may develop consisting of edematous and inflammatory changes as a reaction to the oil and its components in the vessels and in the lung tissue surrounding the vessels.

With endogenous fat embolism, the secondary or chemical phase when neutral fats are hydrolyzed to the more irritating fatty acids is blamed for morbidity and mortality, and probably the same factors are involved with Ethiodol embolism. The fatty acids damage the vessel endothelium and alveolar membranes, causing hemorrhage and exudate. Interference with the production of lung surfactant may also occur [23]. A marked intravascular cellular reaction in the form of histiocytes, foreign body type giant cells, and endothelial cells associated with oil emboli has been described in human lungs one to 33 days post-lymphography. When guinea pigs lungs were studied after Ethiodol embolization, a very early bronchopneumonia was found which on the second day had become an inflammatory reaction with a predominance of histiocytes. By the eighth day a granulomatous pneumonia is seen which had essentially cleared by the 32nd day [22]. Ethiodol leaves the lung in part through the vascular system and in part crosses the vessel wall probably as fatty acid and enters the alveoli. Iodine and lipid have been found in the sputum for as long as six weeks after lung reaction of lymphography [5, 17]. The chemical phase, or at least some of the clinical manifestations of it, may not become apparent until the 11th day or may occur shortly after lymphography [19].

Clinically the chemical phase is marked by fever, cough with sputum which is frequently bloody, and varying degrees of respiratory distress from minor to severe. The patient may also have tachycardia and hypotension. Laboratory studies show oxygen desaturation and if blood loss is sufficient, a low hemoglobin. With endogenous fat embolism, an elevation of serum lipase is expected, and likely this occurs in Ethiodols's chemical pneumonitis phase but is as yet undocumented [1, 2].

The radiographic appearance of the lung changes from the finely stippled pattern of opacities of uncomplicated embolism to diffusely scattered or localized patchy infiltrates. In one or more areas the infiltrates may become confluent, and often this feature has been termed an infarction. The speed of resolution is variable, eventually the radiographic appearance in the surviving patients returning to normal without residuals. In a recent survey of 32,000 lymphograms, 114 serious pulmonary complications were reported. Ten of these were listed only as hemoptysis, while the others also were instances of the chemical phase of oil embolism, but described as infarct, edema, and pneumonia [28] evidently on the basis of the radiographic appearance.

As it has become more widely known that lung complications of lymphography are related to oily contrast media embolism, efforts at minimizing the amount of oil reaching the lungs have grown, and an effort to select patients has taken place. Pulmonary function studies have been advocated on every patient before lymphography [21], but a more reasonable approach is to test pulmonary function when there is the slightest possibility of diminished reserve, allowing these patients without physical sign or symptom, or without history of lung disease to have lymphography without further delay. A history of prior radiation therapy directed to the chest, or involvement of the lung by metastatic neoplasm or lymphoma or by fibrotic disease should cause the lymphographer to be very cautious.

To minimize the amount of Ethiodol reaching the lungs, doses have been progressively lowered. Whereas formerly it was usual to inject 10 to 15 ml and even more into each leg of the adult patient, 7 or 8 ml is now thought to be sufficient for large, tall men and one-half that amount for small women.

A second approach to dose limitation is to stop the injection when the iodized oil has reached the level of the upper lumbar vertebrae, which generally allows adequate filling of all sub-diaphragmatic lymph structures. The image intensified fluoroscope is useful for this purpose. Similarly, monitoring with the image intensifier has been advocated for the purpose of detecting shunting of contrast medium from lymph system to vein. Such shunts are difficult to visualize directly, and are usually only suspected or surmised.

Fibrotic nodes which have resulted from heavy irradiation or other cause are likely to retain less contrast media than more normal modes, thus allowing more contrast media to enter the lungs. Similarly nodes largely replaced by tumor will not retain much contrast material. Low doses are appropriate if this condition can be foreseen.

Cannulation of the thoracic duct in the neck prevents the contrast medium from embolizing in the lungs [45]. The technique appears to be inappropriate because of amount of time and effort needed to be expended, except in highly selected cases. Moreover, when more than one thoracic duct enters the venous system or where lymphatico-venous anastomoses exist, the collection of contrast medium would be subtotal.

One of the most reasonable approaches for the poor risk patient, or the patient in which the lymphographer feels he must proceed with caution, is to perform a lymphogram on one lower extremity initially, then wait four days, and perform a lymphogram on the other extremity. In this way, the number of oil emboli which may reach the lungs are drastically reduced on the first injection, and the patient's pulmonary functions have the chance to return to control levels before the second shower of oil globules reach the lungs.

Procedures, such as operation and anesthesia, should not be performed in the immediate post-lymphography period when lung diffusion is diminished for the combination of two insults may be poorly tolerated, whereas either one alone does not produce symptoms, or disability of consequence.

Treatment of Lung Complications of Lymphography

Treatment of the lung complications of lymphography depends firstly on the state of lungs considered to be present and the factors assumed to be physiologically accounting for the symptoms and signs. In the first hours following injection of contrast media, the occurrence of dyspnea, tachypnea, tachycardia and cyanosis would indicate the patient is suffering from acute mechanical block of the pulmonary capillaries by the oil globules (Fig. 1), and a rise in pulmonary artery pressure as a result. If the acute vascular obstruction is extensive and compensatory adjustments are not made, the right heart may fail. Clinical shock may supervene. The treatment of these acute disturbances in pulmonary and cardiac function is to give whatever support possible to improve the exygenation of the blood and to maintain the circulation. Oxygen should be administered quickly. The patient, of course, is kept at bed rest. He must be kept under close observation and if signs of heart failure present, digitalis should be given parenterally [40]. Hypotension and shock must be treated. Tracheostomy may be necessary to maintain a clear airway. Nine of 13 cardio-pulmonary fatalities reported following lymphography were of this tpe with acute early onset [40]. This type of lung complication is dependent on the amount of Ethiodol

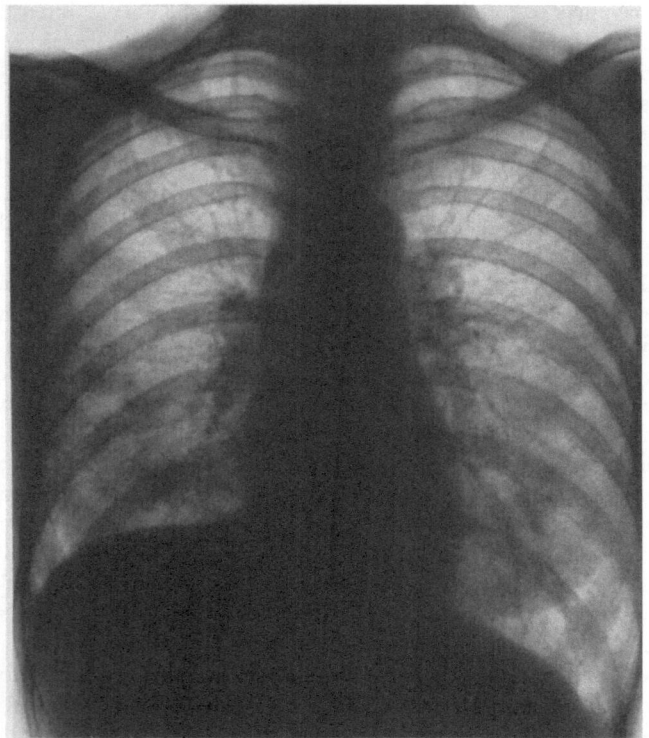

Fig. 1 a. Radiographic appearance of the chest of a patient immediately post-lymphography. The fine opacities scattered diffusely throughout both lung fields are to be noted. This is the appearance produced by many small emboli of Ethiodol. In the left lung there is no complicating pneumonia, but already in the right lung there are two areas of infiltration which probably represent pneumonia, assumed to be an early chemical stage of pulmonary oil embolism

reaching the lungs, the prior status of the lungs, the cardiac reserve, and quite likely to other factors not appreciated or understood at the present time.

Basically, relief comes from the unblocking of the capillaries, from oil globules moving on through the capillaries, by their moving through shunts to the venous system, by their passing from the capillaries into the alveoli, or by the globules being broken down by enzymatic activity.

The other type of serious, and occasionally fatal, lung complication, has a delayed onset and is characterized by fever, tachycardia, hypoxia, respiratory distress, blood in the sputum, and hypotension. The onset may be as late as the tenth day post-lymphography, but it is usually at 2 to 6 days, based theoretically on the time necessary for hydrolysis by serum lipase of neutral fat emboli to fatty acids and glycerol. Radiologically, patches of infiltrate and areas of consolidation are seen (Figs. 1, 2). Treatment is based upon evidence obtained with patients who have had endogenous fat embolism post trauma. For hypoxia and respiratory distress administration of oxygen is essential, and intermittent positive pressure respiration is advo-

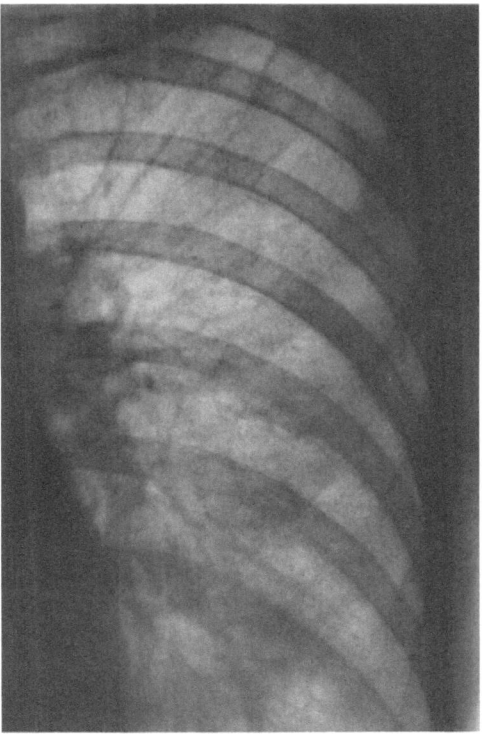

Fig. 1 b. Enlargement view of an area of lung showing the very small pulmonary emboli of opaque oily contrast media

cated [9, 33]. The blood loss from hemorrhages into the lung manifested by a low hemoglobin value must be replaced if excessive [33].

To decrease the rate of hydrolysis of the neutral fat emboli and therefore to slow the conversion to fatty acids and the progress of the chemical phase attempts to block the activity of lipase are advocated. Ethyl alcohol has been found to be a satisfactory lipase inhibitor [1] in endogenous fat embolism and presumably would be of value also in Ethiodol embolism. Intravenous administration of 2000 cc of 5% ethyl alcohol in 5% glucose intravenously is advised [1, 33], if the patient cannot be given 30 cc of 50% alcohol every three to four hours by mouth. The evidence for use of heparin in conflicting, since it has been found to increase mortality in experimental fat embolism, yet seems to have been effective at times clinically. Some value was suggested from a trial of sublingual heparin, whereby heparin retains its lipolytic property but not its anticoagulant properties [2]. To combat intravascular aggregation and clumping of the formed elements of the blood, the sludging phenomenon of the blood which occurs, low molecular weight dextran is recommended [6, 40]. For the lowering of serum calcium which may occur due to binding of and removal of calcium ions by the fatty acids, calcium is advised [40].

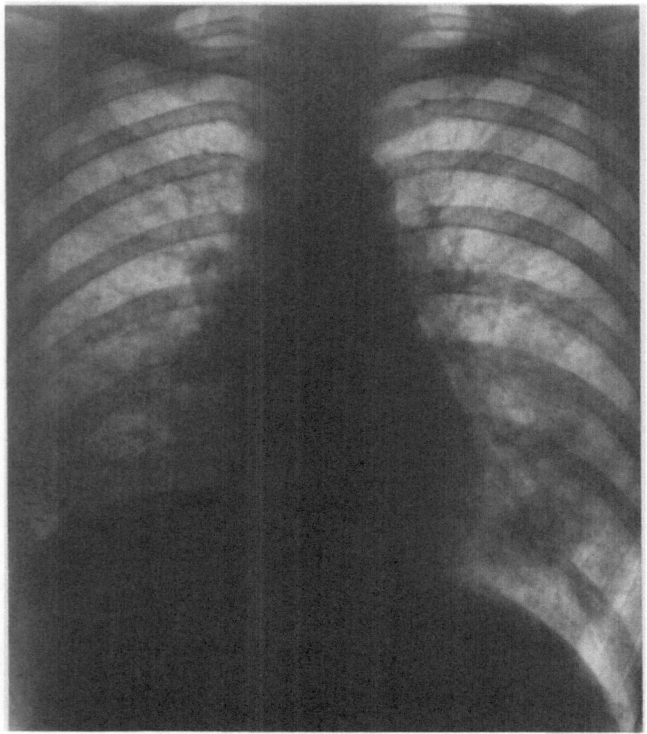

Fig. 1 c. Seven days post-lymphography, there is an extensive lower lung pneumonia on the right with pleural effusion and a moderate area of involvement by pneumonia in the left lower lung

Four of 13 cardiopulmonary deaths following lymphography were of the late onset, pneumonia-infarction type [40], while there have been a larger number who have survived this type of lung complication after a morbid period which has varied greatly in length and severity.

Sodium dehydrocholate (Decholin), hypothermia, and ether anesthesia have been suggested, but evidence is not thought sufficient to support their use.

Cerebral Embolism

Relatively few incidents have been reported which can be attributed to embolism of the droplets of oily contrast medium in the brain. Large series of cases have been performed without serious complication but five cases are known in which three fatalities occurred [32, 36].

The lung acting as a primary filter ordinarily traps the droplets entering the venous system from the thoracic duct or lymphatico-venous communications. With the increase of the dose of contrast medium injected, the lung becomes a less efficient

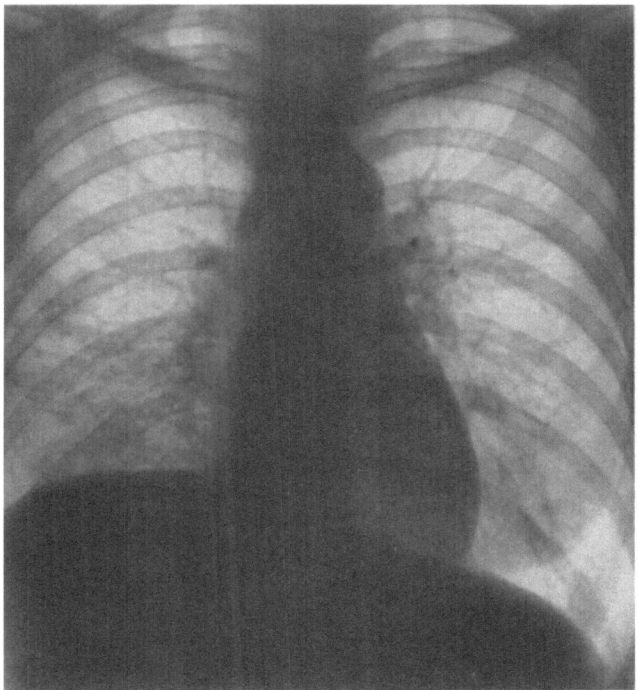

Fig. 1 d. Twenty-four days post-lymphography the pneumonia in the left lung is almost completely cleared and there has been considerable improvement in the pneumonia in the right lower lung. It is interesting to note that although the pulmonary oil embolization was diffuse and apparently equal in the various regions of the lung that only the lower lobes developed the pneumonia

filter [41]. When the number of droplets is very large as when excessive doses of Ethiodol are injected intralymphatically, when there is extensive shunting of oil from lymphatic to venous systems, or when the nodes do not retain the Ethiodol well as they do not at times in a post-irradiated or fibrotic state, or when they are extensively replaced by neoplasm the filtration capacity of the lungs is presumably exceeded and cerebral embolism is more likely to occur. Probably all three of these factors were at work in one very well documented case of cerebral oil embolism [32]. Other predisposing factors whould be the presence of right to left cardiac shunts such as septal defects or malpositioned vessels or arterio-venous shunts in the lung vasculature.

Treatment of cerebral oil embolism is similar to and interrelated to the treatment of pulmonary oil embolism (see section on treatment of lung complications of lymphography). Special care is to be given the maintaining of adequate oxygen saturation of the blood for the patient with cerebral fat embolism.

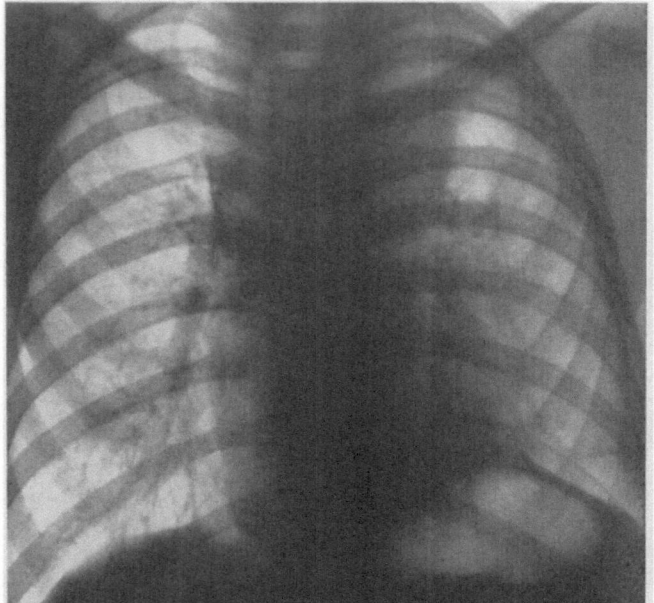

Fig. 2 a. The appearance of the lungs and mediastinum prior to lymphography are shown. The patient had had previous extensive radiation to the mediastinum and the left lung. A diagnosis of Hodgkin's disease had been made 13 years prior to this time

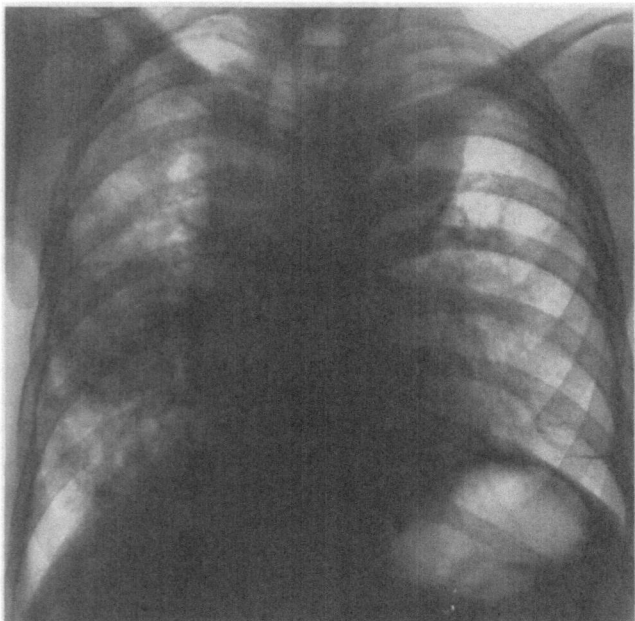

Fig. 2 b. The appearance of the lungs 3 days post-lymphography showing the confluent densities, mainly in the right lung and to a lesser extent in the left lung. Immediately post-lymphography there was evidence of emboli but not of pneumonia. There is massive pneumonic involvement of lung parenchyma on the right, considered to be the chemical phase of pulmonary fat embolism

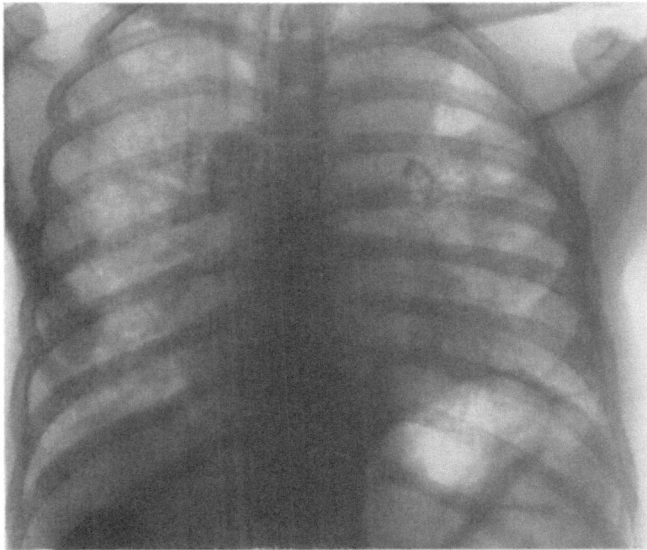

Fig. 2 c. Four days later (7 days post-lymphography) there is a moderate amount of resolution of the previously described pneumonia, but still there is considerable involvement of the lungs

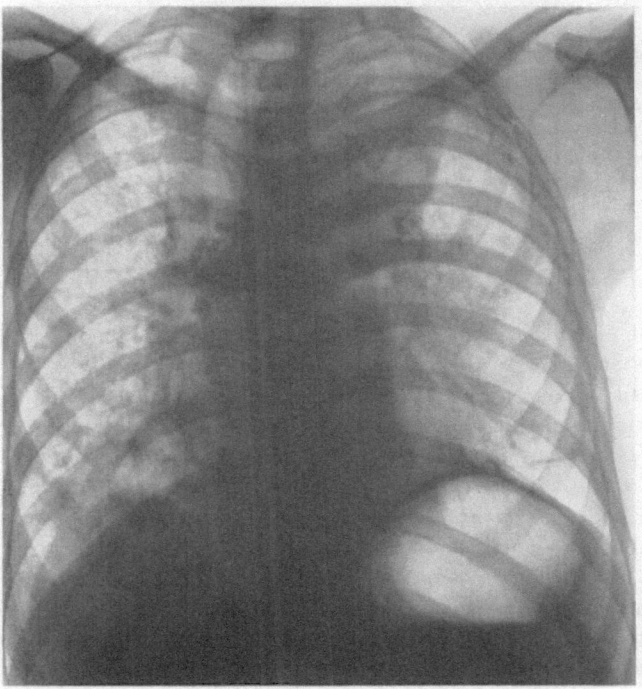

Fig. 2 d. Radiographic appearance of the lungs 20 days post-lymphography. The persistent areas of pneumonia are to be noted

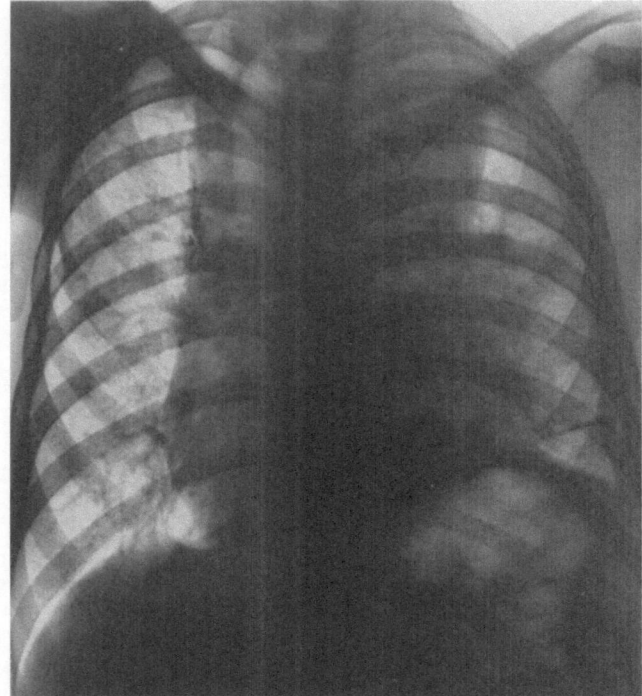

Fig. 2 e. Radiographic appearance 51 days post-lymphography. The radiographic appearance of the chest has returned almost to normal with only a few residual areas of pneumonia on the right. In the left base there are some linear markings which are considered to be linear atelectasis. The patient was in severe distress during the times that films b and c were made with clinical improvement by film d and further clinical improvement by film e

Hepatic Oil Embolism

Hepatic oil embolism seen radiographically is an uncommon complication of lymphography, one that occurs only in lower extremity injections. The existence of two interrelated conditions is necessary to the occurrence of this phenomenon: 1. severe lymphatic obstruction in the upper common iliac-lower aortic-abdominal regions, and 2. complete destruction of both proximal common iliac veins and the distal inferior vena cava [43]. In practically every case, the obstructing lesion has been extensive node metastases. The injected Ethiodol being unable to flow proximally in the iliac and aortic-abdominal lymphatics is shunted into the iliac veins, through lymphatico-venous anastomoses. Since the Ethiodol cannot course proximally in the iliac veins and inferior vena cava due to the obstruction, it flows via collateral circulation into the hemorrhoidal venous plexus and on into the portal system.

Fortunately, the complication does not produce symptoms, the only evidence of its occurrence being the fine stippled hepatic opacification. A survey of 18, 371 lymphograms has revealed 36 cases, an incidence of 0.19% [8]. Hepatic oil embolism has been produced also in the experimental animal by division and extensive stripping of the second and third lumbar lymphatics and acute ligation of the inferior vena cava, producing the same mechanism in the described clinical situation [8].

Hepatic oil deposition occurs in all lymphography according to distribution studies of radioactive tagged Ethiodol in the experimental animal [26]. No impairment of hepatocytic function as measured by maximal sodium sulfobromophthalein transfer rate and relative storage capacity could be found in eight patients following lymphography and in two patients, BSP clearance showed no change during the fifteen days postlymphography [20].

There has been no recognizable clinical liver function impairment thus far.

Miscellaneous Complications: A hypertensive episode with confusion and with clonic convulsions was observed in one patient, a hypotensive reaction in another [12], while two patients were observed to have episodes of collapse, one with loss of consciousness and profuse sweating [19].

Of the 18 deaths reported to KOEHLER [28] in his 1968 survey, two are listed as due to cardiac failure. In six additional fatalities, the cause of death is not given. In addition, the survey lists one case of acute cardiac failure, and six hypotensive crises, none of which were fatal.

Thyroiditis and enlargement of pre-existing goiters following lymphography has been reported. Hemolytic crises and signs of thrombo-cytopenic purpura may be attributed to oily medium used in lymphography [10].

Fever post-lympography is common, but is seldom of importance. To say that it is a body response to the contrast medium is not very informative. The reported incidence of fever ranges from about ten percent up to almost 100%, although some workers do not even mention it as a complication. The incidence of oil embolization in the lungs and elevation of temperature has been thought related. However frequent fever may be, it is not often more than low grade or longer lasting than 24 or 48 hours. The physician may prescribe antipyretics if he so desires.

Headache, nausea, and vomiting may sometimes be noted but these symptoms are also transient and not of consequence.

References

[1] ADLER, F., S. P. LAI, and L. F. PELTIER: Fat embolism: Prophylactic treatment with lipase inhibitors. Surg. Forum 12, 453—455 (1961).

[2] —, and L. F. PELTIER: The effect of sublingual potassium heparin (Clarin) on the serum lipase activity of patients following fractures. J. Trauma 4, 390—393 (1964).

[3] BAERT, A. L., L. BELLIET, and J. GRUWEZ: Changes in pulmonary function following lymphography. In: International Symposium on Lymphology, Proceedings, Zurich, Switzerland, July 19—23, 1966, p. 315.

[4] BAGLIANI, G., S. CHIAPPA, and G. GALLI: Some comments on the danger of direct lymphography. Radiol. med. (Torino) 50, 843—872 (1964).

[5] BELIN, R. P., M. A. SHEA, N. H. STONE, and W. O. GRIFFEN: Iodolipsputosis following lymphangiography. Report of a case. Dis. Chest 48, 543—544 (1965).

[6] BERGENTZ, S. E.: Indications for the use of low viscous dextran in surgery. Acta chir. scand. 122, 343—357 (1961).

[7] BLOM, J. M. H., and J. OORT: Lipiodol and filter function of lymph nodes. Presented at the Second International Congress of Lymphology, March 1968, Miami, Fla. To be published.

[8] CHAVEZ, C. M., J. PICARD, and D. DAVIS: Liver opacification following lymphangio-
     graphy, pathogenesis and clinical significance. Surgery 63, 564—570 (1968).
[9] DENMAN, E. E., C. S. CAIRNS, and C. K. McHOLMES: Case of severe fat embolism treated
     by intermittent positive-pressure respiration. Brit. med. J. 2, 101—102 (1964).
[10] DESPREZ-CURELY, J. P., V. BISMUTH, A. LANGIER et J. DESCAMPS: Accidents et incidents
     de la lymphographie. Ann. Radiol. 5, 577—588 (1962).
[11] DESMONS, M., and H. RAMIOUL: Perilymphatic spread of a melanoma of the foot after
     lymphography. J. Radiol. Électrol. 45, 703—706 (1964).
[12] DOLAN, P. A.: Lymphography: Complications encountered in 522 examinations. Radio-
     logy 86, 876—880 (1966).
[13] EDWARDS, J. M.: Dissemination for tumor cells by lymphangiography. In: International
     Symposium on Lymphology, Proceedings, Zurich, Switzerland, July 19—23, 1966,
     p. 309.
[14] ENGESET, A.: Dissemination of tumor cells by lymphangiography. In: International
     symposium on Lymphology, Proceedings, Zurich, Switzerland, July 19—23, 1966,
     p. 308—310.
[15] ENGZELL, U., C. Rubio, and J. ZAJICEK: The lymph node barrier against Vx2 cancer
     cells before, during and after lymphography. Presented at the Second International
     Congress of Lymphology, March 1968, Miami, Florida (to be published).
[16] FABEL, H., G. KUNITSCH, and H. ST. STENDER: Changes in pulmonary function follow-
     ing lymphoangiography. In: International Symposium on Lymphology, Proceedings,
     Zurich, Switzerland, July 19—23, 1966, p. 314—315.
[17] FRAIMOW, W., S. WALLACE, P. LEWIS, R. R. GREENING, and R. T. CATHCART: Changes
     in pulmonary function due to lymphangiography. Radiol. 85, 231—241 (1965).
[18] FRISCHBIER, H. J.: Studies on the effect on the tissues of oily contrast media. In: Inter-
     national Symposium on Lymphology, Proceedings, Zurich, Switzerland, July 19—23,
     1966, p. 331.
[19] FUCHS, W. A.: Complications in lymphography with oily contrast media. Acta radiol.
     57, 427—432 (1962).
[20] —, R. PREISIG, and H. BUCHER: Liver function after lymphography. Presented at the
     Second International Congress of Lymphology, March 1968, Miami, Fla. (to be
     published).
[21] GOLD, W. M., J. YOUKER, S. ANDERSON, and J. A. NADEL: Pulmonary function ab-
     normalities after lymphangiography. N. Engl. J. Med. 273, 519—524 (1965).
[22] HALLGRIMSON, J., and M. E. CLOUSE: Pulmonary oil emboli after lymphography. Arch.
     Path. 80, 426—430 (1965).
[23] HAMILTON, R. W., JR., and R. F. HUSTEAD, and L. F. PELTIER: Fat embolism: The effect
     of particulate embolism on lung surfactant. Surgery 56, 53—56 (1964).
[24] JOHANSSON, S., N. H. STERNBY, G. THEANDER, and L. WEHLIN: Iodinated oil emulsion
     for lymphography. Acta radiol. 4, 690—704 (1966).
[25] KINMONTH, J. B., R. A. K. HARPER, and G. W. TAYLOR: Lymphangiography by radio-
     logical methods. J. Fac. Radiol. (Lond.) 6, 217—223 (1955).
[26] KOEHLER, P. R., W. A. MEYERS, J. F. SKELLEY, and B. SCHAFFER: Body distribution of
     Ethiodol following lymphangiography. Radiology 82, 866—871 (1964).
[27] —, E. J. POTCHEN, W. R. COLE, and R. STUDER: Experimental studies of intralymphatic
     administration for radiotherapy. Radiology 90, 495—501 (1968).
[28] KOEHLER, P.: Complications of lymphography. Presented at the Second International
     Congress of Lymphology. March 1968. Miami, Florida. To be published.
[29] KOPP, W. L.: Anaphylaxis from Alphazurine 2G during lymphography. J. Amer. med.
     Ass. 198, 200—201 (1966).
[30] KRAUS, R., and J. KLEMENIC: The histologic picture of the lymph node up to 15 months
     after lymphography with Lipiodol UF.: In: International Symposium on Lympho-
     logy, Proceedings, Zurich, Switzerland, July 19—23, 1966, pp. 329—330.
[31] LEE, B. J., J. H. NELSON, and G. SCHWARZ: Evaluation of lymphangiography, inferior
     venacavography, and intravenous pyelography in the clinical staging and manage-
     ment of Hodgkin's Disease and lymphosarcoma. N. Engl. J. Med. 271, 327—337
     (1964).

[32] NELSON, B., E. A. RUSH, M. TAKASUGI, and J. WITTENBERG: Lipid embolism to the brain after lymphography. N. Engl. J. Med. **273**, 1132—1134 (1965).

[33] PIPKIN, G.: The early diagnosis and treatment of fat embolism. Clin. Orthopaedics **12**, 171—182 (1958).

[34] RAVEL, R.: Histopathology of lymph nodes after lymphangiography. Amer. J. clin. Path. **46**, 335—340 (1966).

[35] REDMAN, H. C.: Dermatitis as a complication of lymphangiography. Radiology **86**, 323—326 (1966).

[36] Reports by J. GRUWEZ, J. M. COLLETTE, and R. CARDIS: In: International Symposium on Lymphology, Proceedings, Zurich, Switzerland, July 19—23, 1966.

[37] RICHARDSON, P., E. H. CROSBY, H. A. BEAN, and D. DEXTER: Pulmonary oil deposition in patients subjected to lymphography. Detection by thoracic photoscan and sputum examination. Canad. med. Ass. J. **94**, 1086—1091 (1966).

[38] SCHAFFER, B., P. R. KOEHLER, C. R. DANIEL, G. T. WOHL, E. RIVERA, W. A. MEYERS, and J. F. SKELLEY: A critical evaluation of lymphangiography. Radiology **80**, 917—930 (1963).

[39] SIEBER, F.: Reactive changes of lymph nodes due to oily contrast media. In: International Symposium on Lymphology, Proceedings, Zurich, Switzerland, July 19—23, 1966, pp. 327—328.

[40] SIEGENTHALER, W.: Treatment of pulmonary fat embolism. In: International symposium on Lymphology, Proceedings, Zurich, Switzerland, July 19—23, 1966, pp. 318—319.

[41] SZABO, G.: Oil embolism studies. In: International Symposium on Lymphology, Proceedings, Zurich, Switzerland, July 19—23, 1966, pp. 320—321.

[42] TADA, S., D. L. BENNINGHOFF, and P. G. HERMAN: Erythrocyte filtration by the popliteal lymph node in the dog. Cancer Res. **27**, 1961—1966 (1967).

[43] THORNBURY, J. R.: Lymphatico-venous anastomoses involving the portal system. Lymphographic changes in man. Presented at the Second International Congress of Lymphology. March 1968. Miami, Florida. To be published.

[44] THREEFOOT, S. A.: Urinary excretion of Patent Blue V after intradermal injection in man. Proc. Soc. exp. Biol. Med. **103**, 815—819 (1960).

[45] TJERNBERG, B.: Cannulation of the thoracic duct in lymphography with oily contrast media. In: International Symposium on Lymphology, Proceedings, Zurich, Switzerland, July 19—23, 1966, p. 342.

Chapter 5

Normal Anatomy

W. A. Fuchs

With 43 Figures

Topographic Roentgen Anatomy

The roentgen anatomy of lymph vessels and lymph nodes is based mainly upon the classic anatomic studies of POIRIER (1898), BARTHELS (1909), CUNÉO and MAR-CILLE (1901), MOST (1917), JOSSIFOW (1930), ROUVIÈRE (1932) and REIFFENSTUHL (1957).

The roentgen anatomic descriptions by COLETTE (1958), KAINDL et al. (1958), JACOBSSON and JOHANSSON (1959), MALEK et al. (1959), FISCHER et al. (1962), DITCHEK et al. (1963), HERMAN et al. (1963), ARVAY and PICARD (1963), DARGENT et al. (1963) as well as RÜTTIMANN and DEL BUONO (1964), NELSON et al. (1964) and ABBES et al. (1964) are mainly based upon these anatomic investigations. Extensive roentgen anatomic studies on a large number of cases have been performed by GERTEIS (1966) and WIRTH (1966). In the authors studies the relationship between the different groups of lymphatics and lymph nodes and the pelvic veins, inferior vena cava, the pelvic arteries and abdominal aorta was elucidated by carrying out simultaneous lymphography, arteriography and phlebography. The various groups of lymph nodes were also localized by extraperitoneal lymph node excision and post mortem studies (FUCHS and BÖÖK-HEDERSTRÖM, 1961). The roentgen anatomy of the inguinal, pelvic and aortic lymph nodes was carefully evaluated later in 100 normal lymphograms (FUCHS and PFAMMATTER, 1969). The nomenclature of lymph vessels and lymph nodes corresponds basically to the proposals made at the First International Symposium on Lymphology in Zurich in 1966.

Lower Extremity

The lymphatics of the lower extremities consist of a subcutaneous prefascial and a deep subfascial lymph system. The lymph from the capillary network of the skin and the subcutis drains through delicate lymphatics into groups of larger, longitudinal lymph vessels situated above the fascia. They are closely connected with the largest subcutaneous veins. The deep subfascial lymph vessels collect the lymph from the muscles, fascia and joints. At present, lymphography as a routine procedure can outline only the prefascial lymphatics. The valves in lymphatics direct the flow,

contrary to veins, from the deep to the superficial lymphatic system. Roentgéno-
graphic demonstration of deep subfascial lymphatics by blocking the subcutaneous
lymph vessels as routinely performed in venography is consequently not possible.

According to their relationship to the veins, the lymph vessels of the leg are
divided into an anterior vena saphena magna group and a posterior vena saphena
parva group. The anterior group is composed of a medial and a lateral bundle of
lymphatics, which constitute most of the subcutaneous lymph vessels of the leg. The

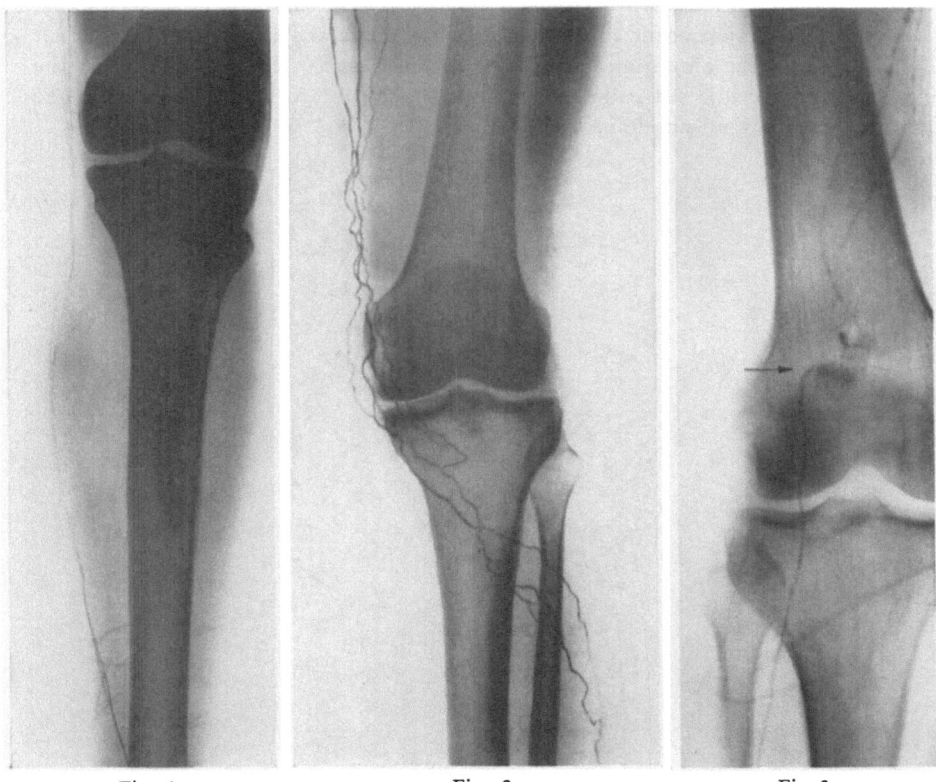

Fig. 1   Fig. 2   Fig. 3

Fig. 1. Antero-medial group of subcutaneous lymphatics

Fig. 2. Antero-lateral group of subcutaneous lymphatics

Fig. 3. Posterior prefascial group of lymphatics connected with 2 popliteal lymph nodes (→)

anterior medial group follows a straight and almost parallel course on the medial
side of the leg and comprises in the lower leg 5—6 vessels and in the thigh 10—20
vessels (Fig. 1). The vessels of the antero-lateral group of lymphatics, 5—6 in number,
lie distally on the peroneal side of the leg, cross in a wide curve toward the medial
side at the level of the knee and are then of large diameter and tortuous (Fig. 2).
Above the knee these lymphatic trunks are always situated medially in close connection with the great saphenous vein until they join the superficial inguinal lymph

nodes. The posterior prefascial lymphatic groups, accompanying the lesser saphenous vein, consist of only 1—3 prefascial collecting trunks which reach 1—3 subfascial lymph nodes in the popliteal region (Fig. 3). The latter nodes are connected to the deep inguinal or iliac node by subfascial lymphatics which follow the deep blood vessels on the medial aspect of the thigh.

The collecting subcutaneous prefascial lymph vessels branch dichotomously as they course proximally. Despite this division they retain an equal diameter of about 0.75—1 mm. Normally there are no anastomoses between the different superficial groups of vessels. Therefore, in lymphography each group must be filled separately.

In some cases injection of contrast media into a lateral lymph vessel of the foot will however fill the antero-medial as well as the antero-lateral lymphatics. If the contrast media are injected still further laterally, the antero-lateral groups and the posterior group may fill simultaneously.

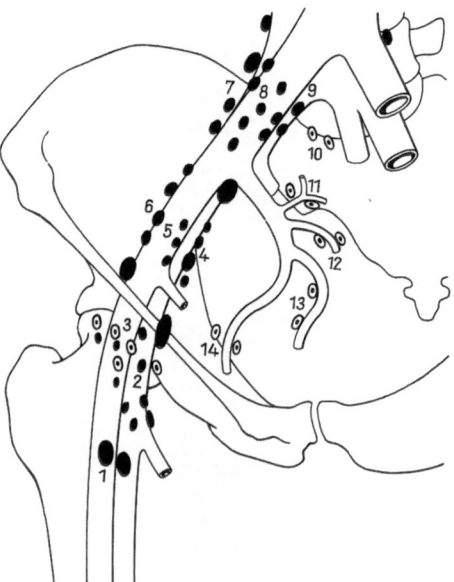

Fig. 4. Topographic roentgen anatomy of the inguinal, iliac and aortic lymph nodes (oblique projection)

Inguinal lymph nodes:

1 Inferior superficial inguinal (subinguinal) lymph nodes
2 Superior superficial and deep inguinal lymph node group
3 Superior superficial inguinal lymph nodes (perineal and genital group)

Pelvic lymph nodes:

4 Medial external iliac lymph nodes
5 Intermediate external iliac lymph nodes

6 Lateral external iliac lymph nodes
7 Lateral common iliac lymph nodes
8 Intermediate common iliac lymph nodes
9 Medial common iliac lymph nodes
10 Promontorial (subaortic) lymph nodes
11 Lateral sacral lymph nodes
12 Superior gluteal lymph nodes
13 Inferior gluteal lymph nodes
14 Obturator lymph nodes

● Routinely demonstrated by lymphography; ⊖ Inconstantly demonstrated by lymphography

The injection of contrast media into the antero-medial or the antero-lateral group of lymphatics regularly produces a characteristic pattern of lymph vessels and lymph nodes in the inguinal, pelvic and retroperitoneal regions (Figs. 4, 5). Both groups of lymphatics drain predominantly into the corresponding groups of superficial inguinal lymph nodes. The numerous afferent vessels of the inferior superficial inguinal lymph nodes are normally fine and divide into several branches before entering the sinus of the lymph nodes (Fig. 6).

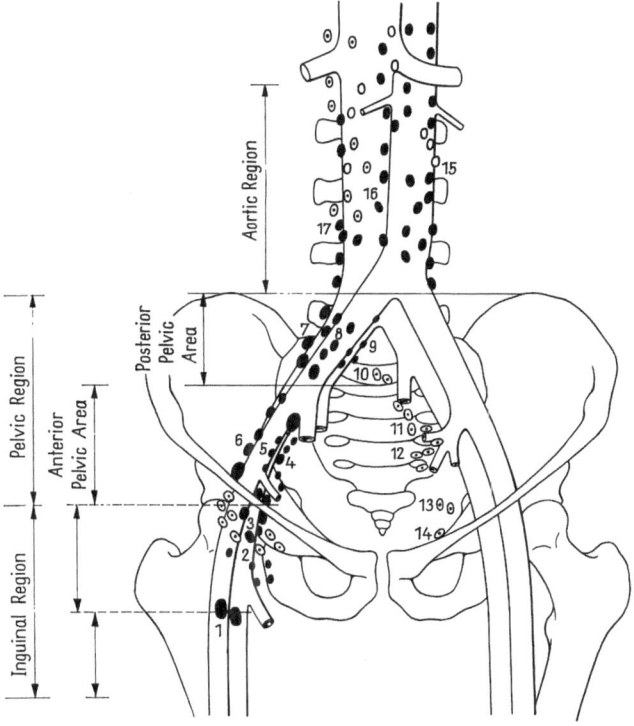

Fig. 5. Topographic roentgen anatomy of the inguinal, iliac and aortic lymph nodes
(a-p projection)

Inguinal lymph nodes:
1 Inferior superficial inguinal (subinguinal) lymph nodes
2 Superior superficial and deep inguinal lymph node group
3 Superior superficial inguinal lymph nodes

Pelvic lymph nodes:
4 Medial external iliac lymph nodes
5 Intermediate external iliac lymph nodes
6 Lateral external iliac lymph nodes
7 Lateral common iliac lymph nodes

8 Intermediate common iliac lymph nodes
9 Medial common iliac lymph nodes
10 Promontorial (subaortic) lymph nodes
11 Lateral sacral lymph nodes
12 Superior gluteal lymph nodes
13 Inferior gluteal lymph nodes
14 Obturator lymph nodes

Aortic lymph nodes:
15 Left aortic lymph nodes
16 Pre-retroaortic lymph nodes
17 Right aortic lymph nodes

● Routinely demonstrated by lymphography; ⊖ Inconstantly demonstrated by lymphography

Selective contrast filling of the posterior prefascial groups is of little value for the diagnosis of tumor metastases in the inguinal and pelvic regions as only some of the deep inguinal and external iliac nodes are contrast filled (Fig. 7). These very nodes

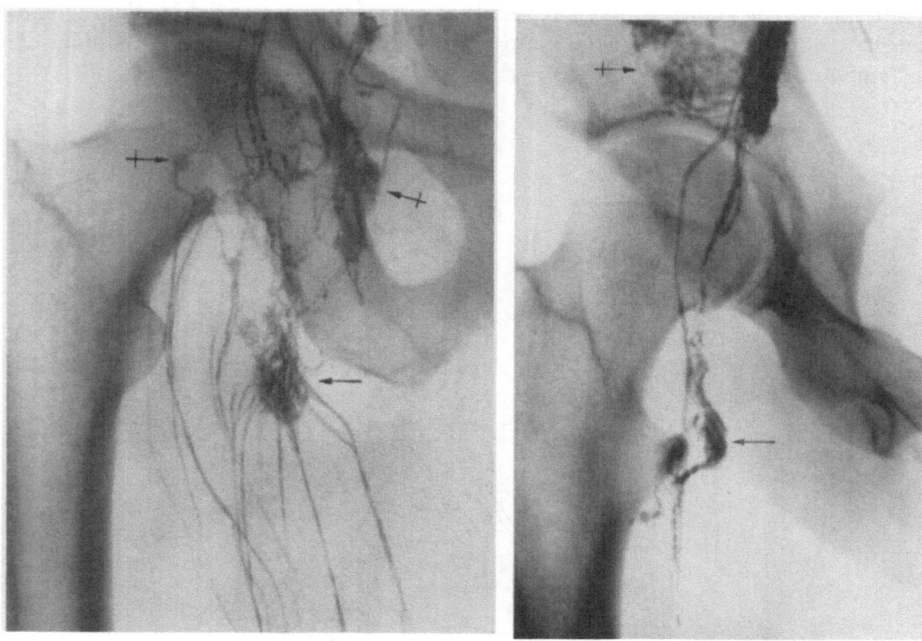

Fig. 6   Fig. 7

Fig. 6. Subcutaneous lymphatics of the antero-medial group enter inferior superficial inguinal (subinguinal) lymph nodes (→) and deep inguinal lymph nodes (+→)

Fig. 7. Lymphatics of the posterior prefascial group connected with deep inguinal lymph nodes (→), intermediate and medial external iliac lymph nodes (+→)

are not visualized when injecting contrast material into lymphatics of the anterior group (FISCHER et al., 1962; FUCHS, 1965). Consequently conventional foot lymphography does not demonstrate all the lymph nodes localized within the inguinal region. Rounded dilatations of the lymphatics are present at various intervals which represent bulbs at the distal levels of the valves. The number of valves increases proximally.

Inguinal Region

The inguinal region is demarcated from the iliac region by a line parallel to the inguinal ligament running from the anterior superior iliac spine to the pubic tubercle (Fig. 4). In the a-p projection this boundary line touches the most central part of the acetabulum; in the oblique projection it runs through the epiphysis of the neck of the femur. The lymph nodes of the inguinal region are subdivided into a superficial and a deep group (Fig. 8).

Superficial Inguinal Lymph Nodes

This node group is localized in the subinguinal region below the subcutaneous fascia and upon the fascia lata in close connection with the inguinal ligament and the terminal parts of the greater saphenous vein, the circumflex iliac vein, the external pudendal veins and the superficial epigastric vein (BARTHELS, JOSSIFOW). POIRIER divides this agglomeration of lymph nodes into a perineal group, receiving afferent lymphatics from the buttocks and skin of the lower half of the abdominal wall, a genital group in connection with lymphatics from the anal and genital region and a crural group with afferent lymph vessels from the skin of the thigh.

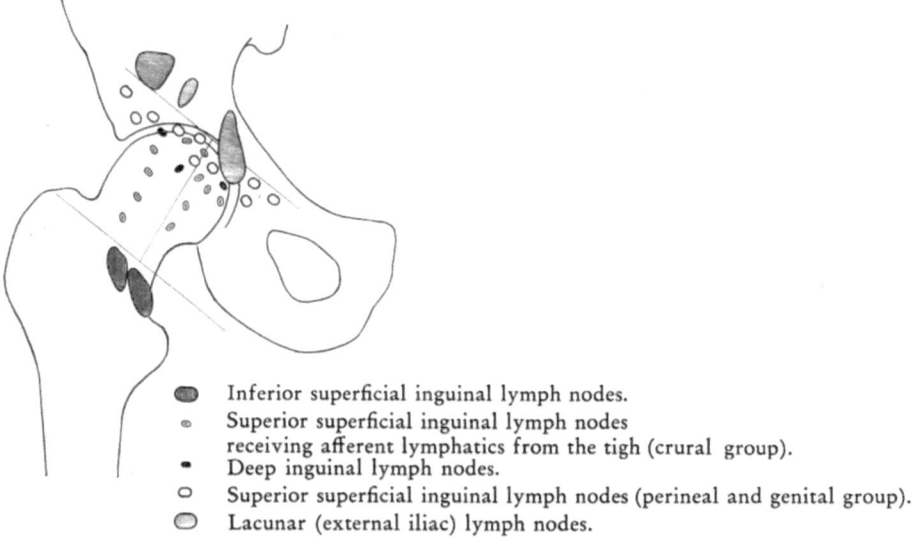

Inferior superficial inguinal lymph nodes.
Superior superficial inguinal lymph nodes
receiving afferent lymphatics from the tigh (crural group).
Deep inguinal lymph nodes.
Superior superficial inguinal lymph nodes (perineal and genital group).
Lacunar (external iliac) lymph nodes.

Fig. 8. Topographic anatomy of the inguinal lymph nodes

The superficial inguinal lymph nodes are separated into a superior and inferior group. A similar subdivision of the inguinal lymph nodes is also proposed by GINS-BERG (1957). The superior superficial inguinal lymph nodes are positioned above and below the inguinal ligament, the inferior superficial inguinal lymph nodes around the greater saphenous vein and its branches within the fossa ovalis (BARTHELS).

The number of superficial inguinal lymph nodes varies from 4 to 20 nodes according to different anatomists.

In the *lymphogram* the *superior superficial inguinal lymph nodes* are demarcated against the inferior group by an oblique boundary line running through the neck of the femur. The superior superficial inguinal lymph nodes, situated parallel to the inguinal ligament, are demonstrated in 1.75% of the author's case studies (Fig. 9). GERTEIS has observed this group in 14% of his studies. The small percentage of contrast filling of the superior superficial inguinal lymph node group is explained by the fact that these nodes are very seldom connected with afferent lymphatics from the lower extremity. As a rare variation, small lymph nodes in the symphyseal area may be filled with contrast material.

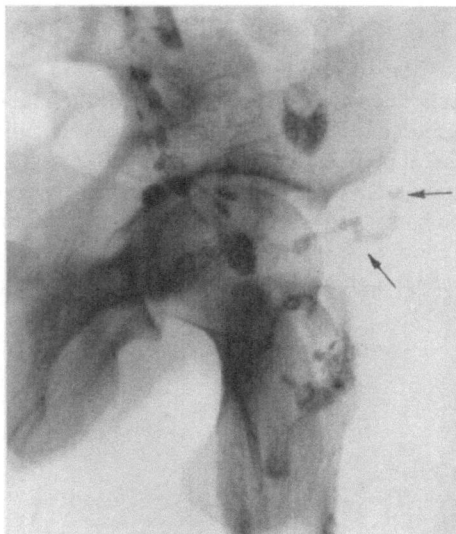

Fig. 9. Lateral superficial superior inguinal lymph nodes (→) connected by afferent lymphatics with inferior superficial inguinal lymph nodes

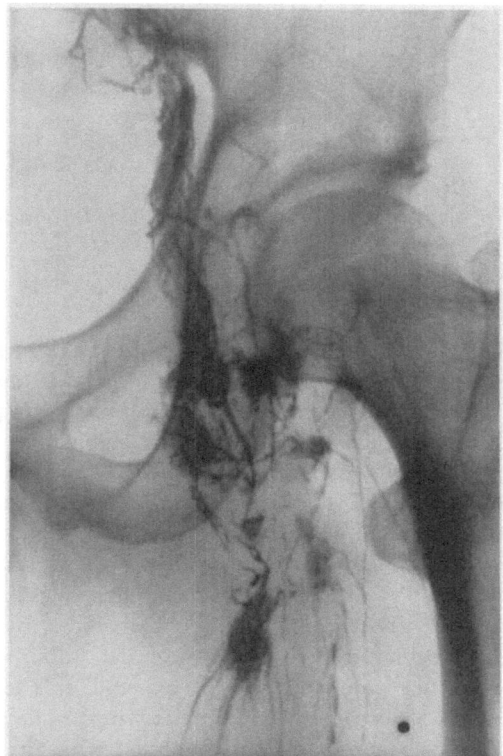

Fig. 10. *Inguinal lymph nodes.* The crural group of superior superficial inguinal lymph nodes cannot be differentiated from the deep inguinal lymph nodes

The superior superficial inguinal lymph nodes are in intimate relationship with the femoral artery and vein. They are situated cranially in the inguinal region but may not be differentiated on the lymphogram from the deep inguinal lymph nodes. The configurations of both groups are similar: round and of small size. Efferent and afferent lymphatics do not provide a distinction between the two groups. For this reason the superior superficial inguinal lymph nodes, receiving afferent lymphatics from the thigh, and the deep inguinal lymph nodes have been grouped together.

The *inferior superficial inguinal lymph nodes* (subinguinal lymph nodes) localized around the hiatus saphenus are regularly filled with contrast material because their afferent lymphatics drain the lymph from the lower extremity. Usually 1—2 large lymph nodes of this group are demonstrated by lymphography (Fig. 10). All combinations between large, medium size and small nodes are encountered. The number of nodes varies from 1 to 7 with 1 to 4 nodes most often found.

Deep Inguinal Lymph Nodes

The deep inguinal lymph nodes are situated deep to the fascia lata within the fossa iliopectinea (Barthels, Jossifow). These small sized nodes have deep afferent lymphatics which lie alongside the femoral artery and are the efferents of the superficial inguinal lymph nodes. The most cranial of the deep inguinal nodes is the largest and most constant. It is situated in the inguinal fossa close to the lacunar ligament and medial to the femoral vein in intimate relationship with the medial external iliac lymph nodes. This node is called the medial lacunar lymph node or lymphonodus anuli femoralis or lymph node of Rosenmüller, Pirogow or Cloquet.

Jossifow claims that the deep inguinal lymph nodes may be absent. Cunéo and Marcille state that they are always present. Rouvière has found 1—3, Krause 3—7, Poirier and Cunéo 1—3 nodes of this group.

As mentioned above, in the *lymphogram* the deep inguinal lymph nodes cannot be differentiated from the group of superior superficial inguinal lymph nodes receiving exclusively afferent lymphatics of the thigh (Fig. 10).

According to our investigations, this anatomically heterogeneous group of superior superficial inguinal and deep inguinal lymph nodes consists of 1—18 lymph nodes with an average of 5—7 nodes demonstrated by lymphography. The number of lymph nodes contrast-filled within the entire inguinal area ranges from 1—20 nodes with an average finding of 7—11 lymph nodes. Gerteis describes 8—12 nodes on average, Wirth 9—13 nodes with a range between 3—16.

Pelvic Region

The pelvic region is subdivided into an anterior and a posterior area, the demarcation being related to the bifurcation of the common iliac artery (Fig. 4). According to the investigations of Nilsson (1967), the bifurcation is situated as a rule 10—16 cm above the upper margin of the symphysis. The boundary line between the anterior and posterior iliac regions runs between the middle and lower third of both ilio-sacral joints. In the oblique projection it is parallel to the inguinal ligament. According to their relationship to the iliac blood vessels, the lymph nodes of the pelvic region are divided into the external, internal and common iliac node groups.

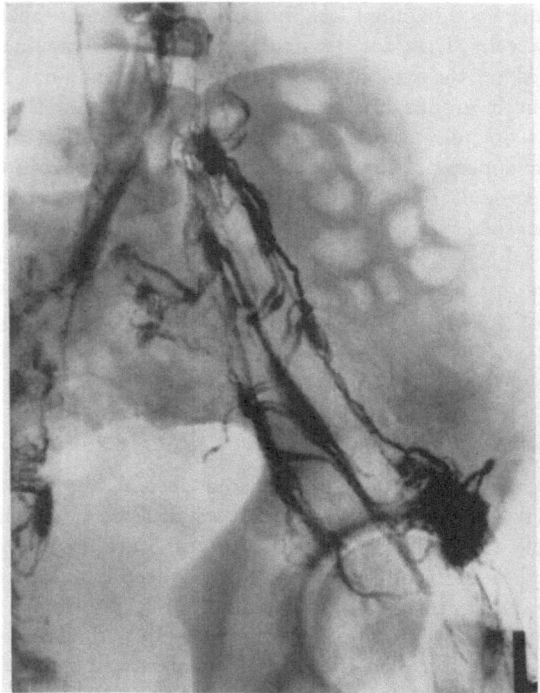

Fig. 11. The lateral, intermediate and medial external iliac lymph node chains connected by numerous lymphatics

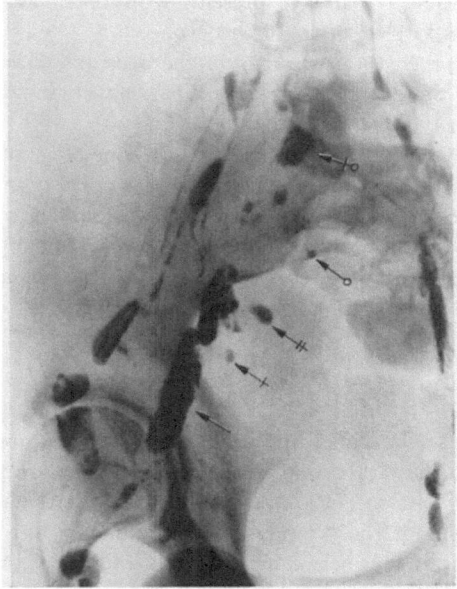

Fig. 12. Fusion of several medial external iliac lymph nodes (→). Absence of the intermediate external iliac lymph node group. Superior gluteal lymph nodes (+→), inferior gluteal lymph nodes (+→), lateral sacral lymph nodes (○→). Medial common iliac lymph nodes (○+→)

External Iliac Lymph Nodes

The external iliac lymph nodes are situated along the external iliac artery and vein and are continuous with the inguinal lymph nodes. They are subdivided into the lateral, intermedial and medial external iliac node groups which are connected by numerous lymphatics (Fig. 11).

Lateral External Iliac Lymph Nodes

The lateral external iliac node chain is localized along the lateral aspect of the external iliac artery within a cleft which the artery forms with the psoas muscle (BARTHELS and ROUVIÈRE). CUNÉO and MARCILLE state that the position of the lymph nodes along the blood vessels is variable. The most common finding is a large distal node which is situated behind the inguinal ligament in the lacuna vasorum (lateral lacunar lymph node). CUNÉO and MARCILLE count 3—4 nodes in this group, ROUVIÈRE 2—4 lymph nodes.

In the *lymphogram* 1—4 lymph nodes are common but as many as 9 have been seen (Figs. 12, 13, 14) (GERTEIS 1—3, WIRTH 3—4 nodes).

Intermediate External Iliac Lymph Nodes

The intermediate external iliac lymph node chain is situated in the cleft between the external iliac artery and vein, slightly anterior to the vein, and consists of 2—3 nodes (CUNÉO and MARCILLE, ROUVIÈRE). The most distally positioned node, the inter-mediate lacunar lymph node is often absent. The constant, most proximal lymph node is situated at the bifurcation of the common iliac artery in close relationship to the ureter (CUNÉO and MARCILLE).

In the *lymphogram* distinction of this node group from the lateral and medial external iliac groups is not difficult (Fig. 11). The most proximally situated node of this chain is well recognized because of its large size. It was found in 58% of the author's case studies. Because of its position at the bifurcation of the common iliac artery, this member of the intermediate group is called the inter-iliac lymph node. Occasionally a large lymph node of the medial external iliac group is found at the same level of the arterial bifurcation (Fig. 14). This node is also called the inter-iliac lymph node, because a corresponding node of the medial external iliac lymph node group is not present. According to our investigations, the average number of lymph nodes of this group demonstrated by lymphography is 1—4, ranging from 1—11 nodes (GERTEIS and WIRTH 2—3 nodes).

Medial External Iliac Lymph Nodes

The medial external iliac lymph node group is situated medial and dorsal to the external iliac vein, close to the pelvic wall between the external iliac artery and the obturator nerve. The most distal node of this group is called the medial lacunar lymph node, and it is positioned directly dorsal to the inguinal ligament, immediately above the Rosenmüller lymph node of the deep inguinal node group (CUNÉO and MARCILLE, ROUVIÈRE). The entire chain of lymph nodes may be reduced to 2 nodes or to a single large node. ROUVIÈRE occasionally found single nodes extending from the inguinal ligament to the internal iliac artery. CUNÉO and MARCILLE described 3—4, ROUVIÈRE 1—4 nodes of this group.

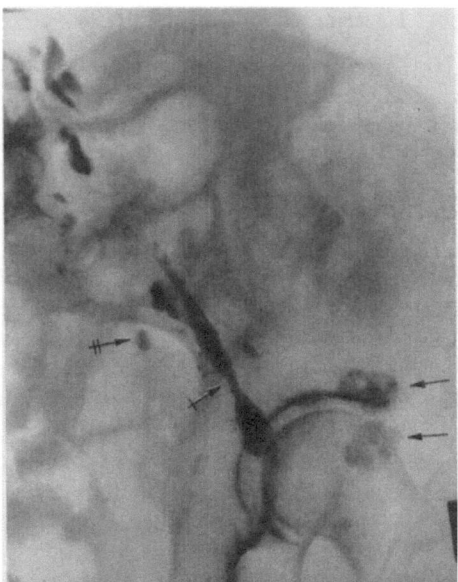

Fig. 13. Contrast-filling of two large distal lateral external iliac lymph nodes (→), fusion of several medial external iliac nodes (+→). Superior gluteal lymph node (#→)

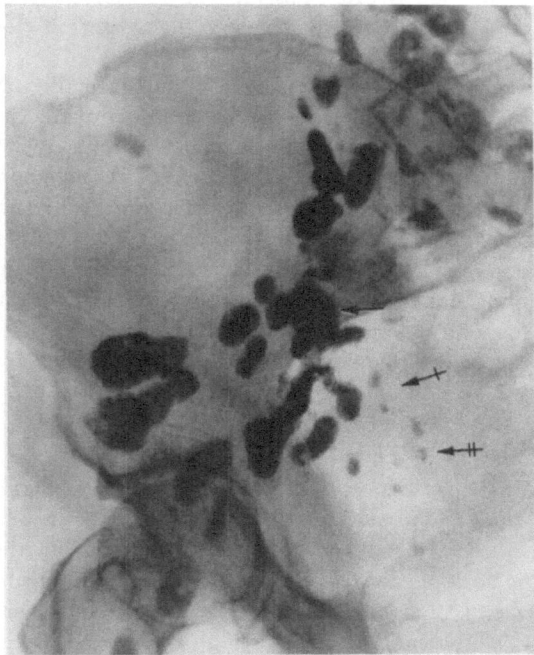

Fig. 14. Multiple rounded external and common iliac lymph nodes of the lateral intermediate and medial group. Large interiliac lymph node (→). Small superior (+→) and inferior (#→) gluteal lymph nodes

The *lymphogram* usually demonstrates one large distal lymph node, called the medial lacunar lymph node, which may be fused with the Rosenmüller node (Fig. 12). When fusiform, the lymph node is generally situated in a slightly more cranial position. The nodes of this group are generally oval (Figs. 12, 13). The lymph node of this group, situated at the bifurcation of the common iliac artery, is enlarged and may be called the inter-iliac lymph node if the corresponding intermediate external iliac lymph node is absent. In the author's material the number of nodes of this group ranged between 1—18 with an average of 6—12 nodes (GERTEIS 2—4, WIRTH 3—4 nodes). The discrepancies in the various results may be explained by the fact that the author counted nodes which were fused, but incompletely, as 2 nodes. In addition, all inter-iliac lymph nodes were attributed to the medial external iliac lymph node group.

REIFFENSTUHL (1956, 1967) considers all lymph nodes situated between the external iliac, internal iliac and obturator arteries as inter-iliac lymph nodes. This nomenclature, although anatomically correct, cannot be applied to roentgen anatomy because the intermediate and medial external iliac lymph nodes which form the main part of this group are normally visualized by lymphography, whereas contrast filling of the obturator lymph nodes is inconstant. Therefore, the term inter-iliac lymph node should be reserved for the single large node situated at the bifurcation of the common iliac artery and belonging to the medial or intermediate external lymph node group only.

Common Iliac Lymph Nodes

The boundary line between the common iliac and aortic areas is situated normally at the level of L 4 but varies according to the height of the aortic bifurcation and the configuration of the sacro-lumbar region. The common iliac lymph nodes are situated along the common iliac vessels and are a direct continuation of the lateral, intermediate and medial node groups of the external iliac area. The shape of the lymph nodes is mainly oval. Most of the lateral and intermediate common iliac nodes are of medium size; the medial common iliac lymph nodes are somewhat smaller. The 3 lymph node groups are connected by numerous lymphatics.

Lateral Common Iliac Lymph Nodes

The lateral common iliac lymph nodes are situated at the lateral aspect of the common iliac artery and on the inner margin of the psoas muscle. Their afferent lymphatics arise from the lateral external iliac lymph nodes. The efferent lymphatics reach lateral aortic lymph nodes on the corresponding side. CUNÉO and MARCILLE described 2, ROUVIÈRE 1—3 nodes belonging to this group.

In the *lymphogram* the lateral common iliac lymph nodes are recognized by their lateral position and may be easily differentiated from the intermediate common iliac lymph nodes (Figs. 12, 15). The distinction in a cranial direction from the lateral aortic lymph node group is more difficult because of the great variability of the bifurcation of the abdominal aorta. In the author's case material the maximum number of nodes filled with contrast medium was 11, with an average number of 1—3 nodes (GERTEIS 1—3, WIRTH 2—3 lymph nodes).

Intermediate Common Iliac Lymph Nodes

This chain of lymph nodes is situated on the posterior aspect of the common iliac artery and vein and is continuous with the intermediate external iliac lymph node group. Cunéo and Marcille describe 3—4, Rouvière 1—4 nodes.

Differentiation of this node group from the medial common iliac nodes in the *lymphogram* may occasionally be difficult, since the lymph vessels of this group are connected to the lateral and medial common iliac lymph nodes by a rete of lymphatics (Fig. 15). Lymphography demonstrated 1—14 nodes of this group with an average number of 2—5 nodes (Fig. 14). In 8 of the author's cases no nodes of this group were contrast-filled (Fig. 12) (Gerteis 1—2 nodes).

Medial Common Iliac Lymph Nodes

The medial common iliac lymph nodes are localized on the medial aspect of the common iliac artery and vein. The lymphatics and nodes of both sides form a triangular arrangement. Cunéo, Marcille and Rouvière state that this node group is situated at the lumbo-sacral junction. According to Cunéo and Marcille, these nodes receive afferent lymphatics from the external iliac region, the lateral sacral area and particularly from visceral lymph nodes of the prostate, urinary bladder, uterus and vagina. Cunéo and Marcille describe 2, Rouvière 2—4 nodes belonging to this group.

For *lymphographic* localization of the medial common iliac lymph nodes several facts have to be considered. The position of the nodes varies according to the site of the aortic bifurcation. Lymph nodes situated within the lumbo-sacral region are difficult to separate from lateral sacral and superior gluteal lymph nodes. Differentiation of the medial common iliac lymph nodes, superior gluteal and lateral sacral nodes is not always possible according to the position of the lymph vessels because afferent lymphatics are often poorly visualized (Figs. 12, 13). Nodes attributed to the medial common iliac lymph nodes are those which are contrast-filled by efferent lymphatics of the common and external iliac lymph nodes and which are situated on the medial aspect of the common iliac artery and vein.

The shape of the lymph nodes of this groups is oval or rounded. In the author's case studies a maximum of 15 nodes but an average of 1—4 nodes were visualized by lymphography. In 11% no lymph nodes were demonstrated. Gerteis and Wirth found an average filling of 1—2 lymph nodes.

Internal Iliac Lymph Nodes

The internal iliac lymph nodes, also called hypogastric lymph nodes, comprise all lymph nodes situated within the region of supply of the internal iliac artery and its branches. According to their relation to parietal and visceral arterial branches, they are divided into parietal or visceral lymph node groups. The parietal lymph node group is composed of the superior and inferior gluteal lymph nodes, the lateral sacral and obturator lymph nodes. The visceral lymph nodes are only partially connected with the visceral arterial branches. Most of these nodes are situated close to the related organs. The visceral group of lymph nodes is composed of the vesical, rectal and para-uterine lymph node groups. The internal iliac lymph nodes receive lymph from the joints and muscles of the pelvis and from the organs situated in the pelvic region, the upper third of the vagina, uterus, ovaries, prostate, seminal vesicles, urinary bladder and from areas of the penis and the rectum (JOSSIFOW). The internal iliac lymph nodes are in close connection with the common iliac and aortic node groups by efferent lymphatics. According to BARTHELS and JOSSIFOW the number of nodes of the internal iliac group is 9—13; ROUVIÈRE counts 4—8.

Parietal Internal Iliac Lymph Nodes

Superior Gluteal Lymph Nodes

The superior gluteal lymph nodes are situated at the point of origin of the superior gluteal artery from the internal iliac artery. Its lymph nodes are situated along the first part of the main trunk of the artery or vein or lie slightly cranially or

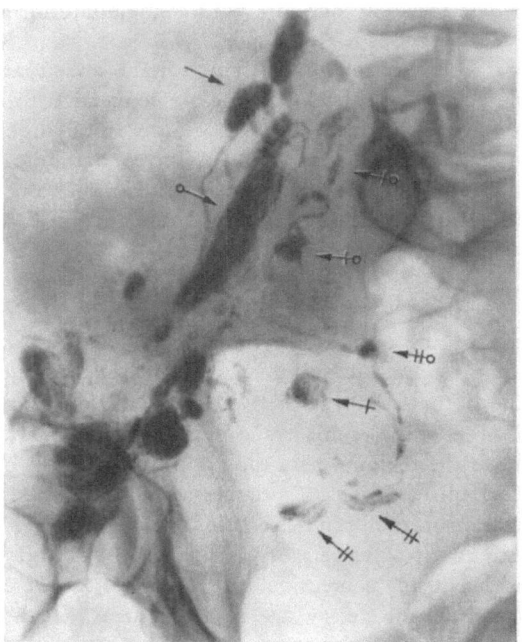

Fig. 15. Contrast-filling of multiple parietal internal iliac lymph nodes, superior (↦) and inferior (⧺→), gluteal nodes. Lateral sacral nodes (○⧺→). Fusion of the intermediate common iliac nodes (○→), medial common iliac lymph nodes (○+→), lateral common iliac lymph nodes (→)

caudally on the medial aspect of the internal iliac artery. BOURGERY and JACOB found 3—4 nodes attributed to this group. PARSONS and KEITH observed that of a series of 123 observations a single superior gluteal lymph node was present in 34 cases: 23 cases on the right and 11 cases on the left side. Otherwise lymph nodes were absent on the right side in 45 cases and on the left side in 33. Only in 2 cases were there only 2 lymph nodes present.

In the *lymphogram* the superior gluteal lymph nodes may be differentiated from medial external iliac lymph nodes by the special course of the afferent lymphatics and by their slightly more medial position (Figs. 12, 14, 15). In the a-p projection the boundary line with the inferior gluteal lymph nodes is a horizontal through the acetabular roof of both hip joints. In 62.5% of the author's cases the superior gluteal lymph nodes were demonstrated by lymphography. The range was 1—8 nodes, with an average number of 1—3. GERTEIS describes contrast-filling of this node group in 48.5% with an average number of 2—3 nodes visualized.

Inferior Gluteal Lymph Nodes

The inferior gluteal lymph nodes are situated along the common trunk of the inferior gluteal and internal pudendal arteries. According to the investigations of PARSONS and KEITH, a single lymph node of this group was found in 23 of 123 observations on the right, and in 11 on the left side. Only twice were 2 lymph nodes observed. BARTHELS describes only one case with a single inferior gluteal lymph node in his entire study.

In the *lymphogram* the inferior gluteal lymph nodes are situated below the horizontal boundary line (Figs. 14, 15). Nodes in close connection to the superior aspect of the symphysis must be distinguished from the obturator lymph nodes. The course of the afferent lymphatics is important for correct topographic evaluation. In the author's series, this group of lymph nodes was found in 5.2% of all cases with the group composed of 1—4 nodes. GERTEIS observed this node in 12%.

Obturator Lymph Nodes

The nomenclature of the obturator lymph nodes has been the subject of great controversy. According to BARTHELS and KRAUSE this node group is situated at the inner opening of the obturator foramen, within the region of the branches of the obturator artery. GERTEIS (1966) considers as obturator nodes an isolated node group situated 2—3 cm above the region where the obturator artery penetrates the obturator foramen. REIFFENSTUHL (1957, 1967) names as obturator nodes all lymph nodes localized in close relation to the branches of the obturator artery. The terminology is further complicated by the great variety of positions of the obturator artery (NILSSON, 1967). Investigations led to the conclusion that the nodes connected with the peripheral branches of the obturator artery are rarely contrast-filled by lymphography, because their afferent lymphatics belong to the internal iliac lymph vessels. The most central obturator lymph nodes are those situated close to the origin of the obturator artery, receiving afferent lymphatics which are contrast-filled from the lower extremity. They are visualized by foot lymphography and must be grouped with the medial external iliacs. Considering these facts we classify as obturator nodes only those lymph nodes situated close to the peripheral branches of the obturator artery. Those localized around the first part of the obturator artery are called medial external iliac nodes.

In the *lymphogram* these nodes are situated 1—2 cm medial to the hip joints at the level of the medial lacunar lymph nodes to which they are connected by lymphatics. They are best demonstrated in oblique projection (Fig. 16).

In the author's lymphographic studies the obturator lymph nodes were demonstrated in 2.9% of the cases. In no instance were several nodes present. GERTEIS describes the frequency of contrast-filling as 3.5%.

Lateral Sacral Lymph Nodes

Lateral sacral lymph nodes are divided into superior and inferior groups (KRAUSE). The small inferior nodes are situated behind the rectum at the anterior aspect of the sacrum, as well as at the outer wall of the rectum close to the superior

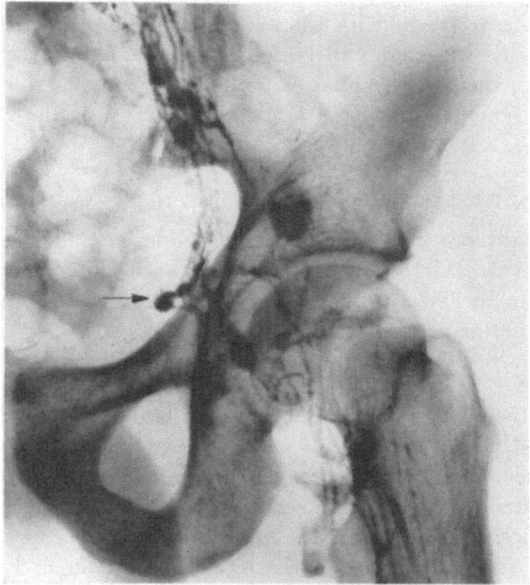

Fig. 16. Obturator lymph node (→) connected by lymphatics of the medial external iliac lymph node chain

haemorrhoidal artery and vein and close to the muscular sheet. They number 2—8 but are inconstant in number and size. The 4—5 larger superior nodes are localized close to the promontorium between the sheets of the mesorectum. According to BARTHELS, the lateral sacral lymph nodes are positioned directly anterior to the sacrum in close connection to the sacral vessels. CUNÉO and MARCILLE found 2—3 nodes, WALDEYER 5—6.

In the *lymphogram* the lateral sacral lymph nodes are projected onto the lateral margin of the sacrum or the lateral sacral foramina (Figs. 12, 15). Only lymph nodes in this topographic position may be attributed to this node group. The difficulties in differentiation from the superior gluteal and promontorium nodes are evident. The course of the afferent and efferent lymphatics is essential for evaluation. In case studies of the author visualization of the lateral sacral lymph nodes was present in 36.8% of the cases. The number of lymph nodes demonstrated ranges between 1—3. The frequency of contrast-filling of this group reported by GERTEIS is 9%.

Promontorial (Subaortic) Lymph Nodes

The lymph nodes situated distally to the aortic bifurcation on the anterior aspect of the 5th lumbar vertebra, the promontorium and the upper part of the sacrum are called promontorial (subaortic) lymph nodes. This group is very inconsistant because it includes lymph nodes of the medial common iliac group and the lateral sacral group as nodes which cannot be correctly identified. The number of nodes within this group described by Krause is 4—5, by Barthels 1—3.

In the *lymphogram* this group of nodes comprises all contrast-filled lymph nodes situated within the subaortic region. This area is demarcated cranially by the aortic bifurcation and caudally by a horizontal line connecting the bifurcations of the common iliac arteries. In correlation with the anatomic findings described above, it is very inconsistant, because it includes all lymph nodes situated on the promontorium but not attributable to the common iliac, lateral sacral and superior gluteal lymph nodes. The subaortic lymph nodes were visualized in 25% of the author's studies. Gerteis reports 42.5%.

Visceral Internal Iliac Lymph Nodes

Under normal conditions the visceral lymph nodes are not demonstrated by lymphography. However, their efferent lymphatics are in close connection with the internal iliac and common iliac lymph node groups. The visceral lymph nodes comprise the rectal, para-uterine and vesical lymph nodes.

Rectal Lymph Nodes

The rectal lymph nodes are situated close to the branches of the superior rectal artery. They are found within the inferior part of the pelvic section of the rectum in the fatty tissue between the muscular sheet and the fascia, usually within the angles formed by the branches of the superior rectal artery (Barthels, Jossifow). Their afferent lymphatics receive lymph from the mucosa of the upper and lower parts of the rectum and from the musculature of the rectum. The efferent lymphatics reach the inferior group of the lateral sacral lymph nodes. Gerota observed 2—3 in some preparations, in other preparations 6—8 nodes. Jossifow reports 2—8 lymph nodes of this group.

Para-Uterine Lymph Nodes

The para-uterine lymph nodes are situated within the broad ligament close to the cervix and the branches of the uterine and vaginal arteries. Afferent lymphatics arise from the uterine cervix; the efferents go into the medial external iliac and common iliac lymph nodes. According to investigations of Bruhns, Gerota, Sappey, Poirier, Cunéo and Marcille, para-uterine lymph nodes are found with a frequency of only 15%. The largest of these nodes is situated where the ureter and the uterine artery cross.

Vesical Lymph Nodes

The vesical lymph nodes are divided into lateral and anterior groups, with a third posterior group, described by Barthels and Jossifow, and Rouvière.

The *anterior vesical lymph nodes* are situated behind the pubic symphysis in the prevesical connective tissue. The number of nodes ranges between 7 and 10 on each side (BARTHELS, JOSSIFOW). According to ROUVIÈRE, the number of nodes varies on each side between 1 and 4.

The *posterior vesical lymph nodes* are localized on the posterior aspect of the urinary bladder and receive their afferent lymphatics from the superior part. According to ROUVIÈRE this node group is rather frequently observed.

The efferent lymphatics of the vesical lymph nodes drain into the medial external iliac and the medial common iliac node groups.

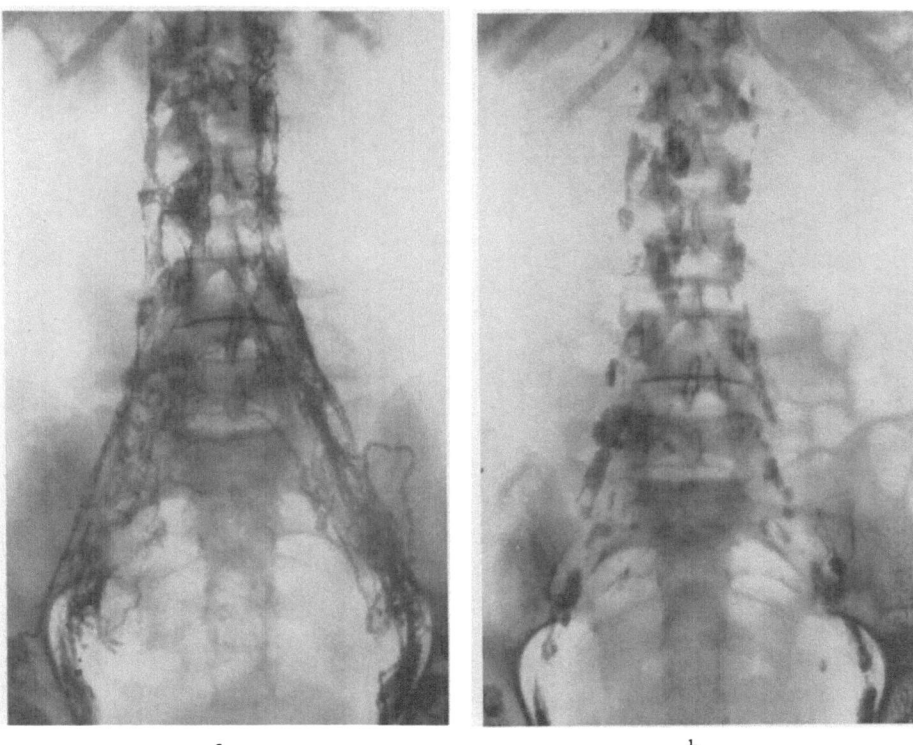

a   b

Fig. 17. *Aortic lymph nodes.* Equal development of the three aortic lymph node chains.
a Filling phase. b Storage phase

According to CUNÉO and MARCILLE, the total number of external, internal and common iliac lymph nodes is 16—20 nodes on one side. ROUVIÈRE counts 9—20 nodes. In the author's case material the sum of contrast-filled iliac lymph nodes of one side varies between 9 and 45 nodes with an average number between 18—26 lymph nodes. WIRTH describes between 7 and 31 nodes with an average number of 11 to 20 nodes.

Aortic Region

The abdominal aortic lymph nodes (BARTHELS) or abdomino-aortic lymph nodes (POIRIER and CUNÉO) are situated on the anterior aspect of the lumbar vertebrae, around the abdominal aorta and the inferior vena cava. Anatomically they are

divided into 4 main groups: the pre-aortic, retro-aortic, right aortic and left
aortic node groups (Fig. 4). In the *lymphogram* only 1 intermediate and 2 lateral
lymph node chains are discernable, because the exact positions of the pre-
aortic node groups (Fig. 4). In the *lymphogram* only 1 intermediate and 2 lateral

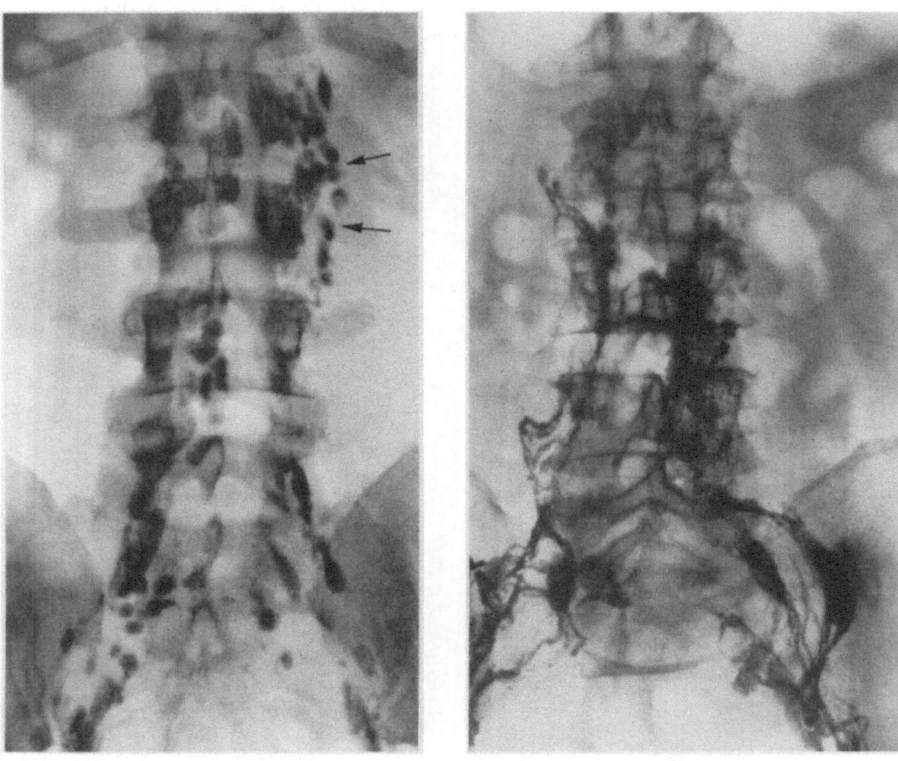

Fig. 18   Fig. 19

Fig. 18. Contrast-filling of a large number of nodes situated at the level of the left renal blood
vessels (→). Non-filling of the right aortic nodes above L 4

Fig. 19. Dislocation of the iliac and aortic lymph vessels by arterio-sclerotic pelvic arteries
and the abdominal aorta

determined on roentgenograms without using stereoscopic techniques (Fig. 17). Unilateral injection of contrast material leads to a retrograde contrast-filling of common
iliac lymph nodes of the contralateral side in about half of the cases and therefore
may not be interpreted as a pathologic finding (Figs. 20, 21). Visualization of aortic
lymph nodes at the level of L 4/5 by anastomosing lymphatics is also observed in
about 50% of normal lymphograms (Fig. 21). Contrast-filling of the left aortic
nodes was encountered more frequently than visualization of the right aortic
lymph nodes. The site of the boundary line between the aortic and the iliac regions
varies according to the height of the aortic bifurcation and the lumbo-sacral configuration with the line being situated in the a-p projection, at the level of the pelvic

crest and the 4th lumbar vertebra. In the oblique projection the demarcation parallels the boundary line between the anterior and posterior iliac regions through the 4th lumbar vertebra, 1 cm above the pelvic crest. The cranial limit of the aortic region is the aortic opening of the diaphragma at about the level of L 1.

Right Aortic Lymph Nodes

The lymph nodes situated on the right side of the abdominal aorta are grouped according to their relations to the inferior vena cava into the pre-caval, interaortico-caval, retro-caval and latero-caval nodes (ROUVIÈRE). The *interaortico-caval lymph nodes* are found in the cleft between the abdominal aorta and inferior vena cava, dispersed from the origin of the inferior vena cava to the right renal vein. The *pre-caval lymph nodes* are concentrated at the aortic bifurcation and immediately below the entrance of the right renal vein into the inferior vena cava. The number of nodes of this group is considerably larger than of those situated on the right lateral aspect of the inferior vena cava. One of those nodes is normally positioned in the angle formed by the right renal vein with the inferior vena cava. The *retro-caval lymph nodes* are found on the posterior aspect of the inferior vena cava, close to the psoas muscle and the right part of the diaphragm.

The afferent lymphatics of the right aortic lymph nodes arise from the common iliac lymph nodes, the deep lymph nodes of the abdominal wall, the kidney capsule and kidney, suprarenal gland, liver, testis, ovary, fallopian tube and the upper part of the uterus. Anatomically the right aor-

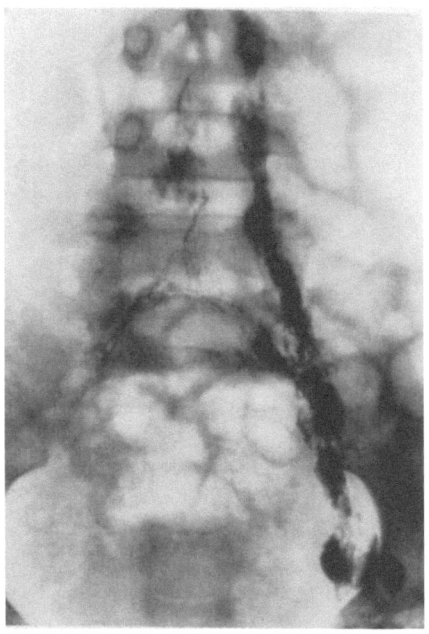

Fig. 20. Contrast-filling of right medial common lymph nodes from the contra-lateral side

tic lymph node group comprises the largest number of nodes of the four aortic lymph node chains (KUBIK et al., 1967).

In the *lymphogram* the right aortic lymph nodes are projected upon the right lateral aspect of the vertebral bodies and up to 2 cm further laterally (Figs. 17, 18). GREGL et al. (1968) studied the position of the aortic lymph nodes relative to the lumbar spine. They describe as normal a distance of 3—4 cm from the midline in 50% and 4—5 cm in 25%. In the lateral projection the distance from the ventral surface of the third lumbar vertebral body measured 2—3 cm. Varying localizations are functions of the inconstant positions of the abdominal aorta and inferior vena cava (Fig. 19). Cavography and abdominal aortography must therefore be performed in many cases in order to localize particular lymph node groups. The distinction of aortic lymph nodes into pre-caval, retro-caval, latero-caval and inter-aortico-caval groups is not possible by lymphography because of their superposition-

ing. All these node groups are called right aortic lymph nodes. The contrast-
filled efferent lymphatics of the right aortic lymph nodes arise exclusively from
the right common iliac lymph nodes and from aortic lymph nodes of the other
2 chains. Lymphography demonstrates that some lymph nodes are by-passed in all
3 aortic lymph node chains. Continuous contrast-filling of a chain of nodes is seldom
encountered. The number of right aortic lymph nodes contrast-filled by lymphography is considerably smaller than that of the two other aortic node chains (Fig. 18).
This is in contrast to anatomical findings, which show the right aortic lymph node

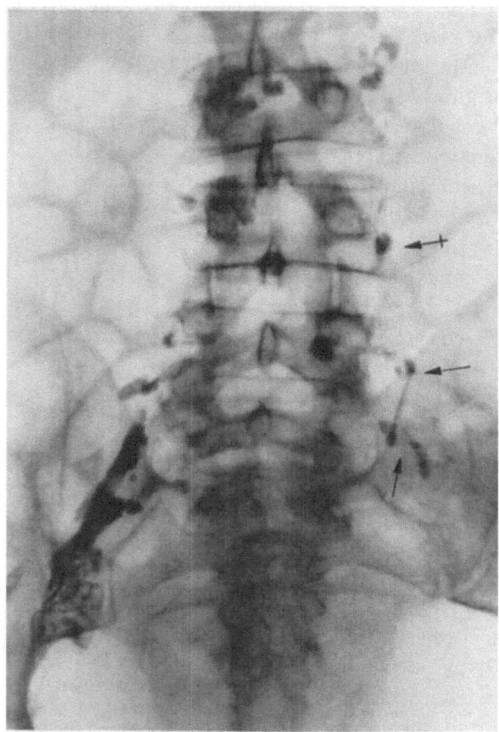

Fig. 21. Contrast-filling of left medial common iliac (→) and left aortic (+→) lymph nodes
from the contralateral side

group comprising the greatest number of nodes. In the author's studies 0—18 lymph
nodes of this group were demonstrated by lymphography with an average number of
8 nodes. In 5 lymphograms no lymph nodes were filled.

In 40% of the cases the upper border of the right aortic lymph node chain
was situated at or below the level of L 3. In 19.6% it was situated at the level of L 2
and in only 11.2% as high as L 1.

Intermediate Aortic Lymph Nodes (Pre- and Retro-Aortic Lymph Nodes

The *pre-aortic lymph nodes* are situated on the anterior aspect of the abdominal
aorta and can be divided into two groups, one close to the inferior mesenteric artery,
the other close to the renal arteries (ROUVIÈRE). The *retro-aortic lymph nodes* are

localized on the dorsal side of the abdominal aorta next to the left aortic lymph nodes. If the left aortic lymph node chain contains only a few nodes, the number of nodes of the retro-aortic lymph node group is correspondingly increased. The pre-aortic lymph nodes receive afferent lymphatics from the supply area of the inferior mesenteric artery, promontorial lymph nodes and nodes of the right and left aortic node groups. In rare instances they are connected with lymphatics from the renal capsule and the testicles. The retro-aortic lymph nodes receive lymph from the intermediate common iliac lymph nodes and the two lateral aortic node chains.

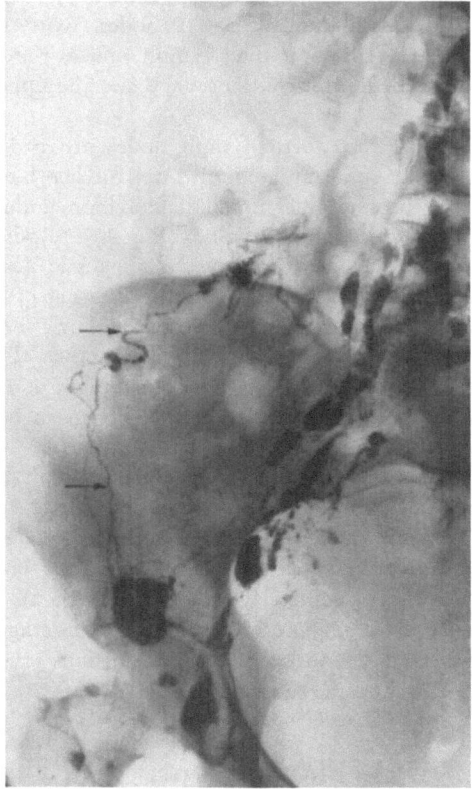

Fig. 22. Unilateral contrast-filling of right lumbar lymph vessels and nodes (→). Extensive visualization of the right aortic lymph chain

In *lymphography* the pre- and retro-aortic lymph nodes are projected onto the vertebral bodies of the lumbar spine (Fig. 17). Differentiation of pre- from retro-aortic nodes is possible by lymphography because of superpositioning of different node groups. Both chains are therefore consolidated into the intermediate aortic lymph node group. The afferent lymphatics to the intermediate lymph nodes filled with contrast material arise from the common iliac and promontoric lymph node groups. Interconnections between the different aortic lymph nodes are regularly found at the level of L 3/4, where the inferior mesenteric artery branches from the abdominal aorta. Clustering of lymph nodes is frequently found at this level also.

Contrast-filling of the intermediate aortic lymph nodes is considerably more frequent than found with the right aortic lymph node group. The whole group of lymph nodes contains 4—39 nodes with an average of 7—16 lymph nodes. Only in 2 of the examined cases was this group completely absent. In more than 21% of all lymphograms, the intermediate aortic group reached the level of L 1, in 35% L 2 and in only 7% was the upper border of this chain situated at or below L 3.

Left Aortic Lymph Nodes

The left aortic lymph node group lies in relation to the psoas muscle and the abdominal aorta. It forms a chain of 5—10 nodes (ROUVIÈRE), receiving lymphatics from the left lateral common iliac lymph nodes, the kidney capsule, the kidney, the suprarenal gland, the testicle, the ovary and the upper part of the uterus of the left side.

On the *lymphogram* the left aortic lymph nodes are projected onto the left lateral aspect of the lumbar spine and up to 2 cm further laterally. They receive afferent lymphatics from the lateral common iliac lymph nodes and have connections with other aortic lymph node chains (Fig. 17). Radiologically, the left aortic lymph node group is the most constant of all aortic node groups and comprises the largest number of contrast-filled nodes. Clustering of lymph nodes is seen below the left renal artery and vein (Fig. 18). In the author's studies this node group was demonstrated by lymphography in all but one instance. The number of nodes visualized ranges between 5 and 44 with an average number of 10—20 lymph nodes. The left aortic lymph node group reached the level of L 1 in 30.8% of the studies, L 2 in 29.4% and the level of L 3 in only 9.8%.

Contrast-filling of lumbar lymphatics and lumbar lymph nodes on the dorsal aspect of the lumbar fossa is observed as a rare variation (Fig. 22).

The total number of lymph nodes within the entire aortic region is estimated by KRAUSE as 36—45 and by ROUVIÈRE as 40—50 lymph nodes. The author's investigations encountered 8—78 contrast-filled lymph nodes with an average number of 20—45. WIRTH observed between 20 and 75 nodes with an average of 40 lymph nodes.

The efferent lymphatics of the aortic lymph node groups form the lumbar trunks which enter the cisterna chyli and the thoracic duct.

Thoracic Duct

The anatomy of the thoracic duct has been the subject of detailed anatomical studies by JOSSIFOW (1906), VAN PERNIS (1959) and JDANOV (1959). MALEK et al. (1960), ARNULF and BOELY (1961), RÜTTIMANN and DEL BUONO (1962), ARVAY and PICARD (1963), WEISSLEDER (1964), NUSSBAUM et al. (1964), FUCHS (1965) and LAMEER (1966) have described roentgen anatomic aspects of the thoracic duct based upon the observations of a few cases. HIDDEN and FLORANT (1966) give a detailed, but non-comprehensive study of the roentgen anatomy of the thoracic duct in 40 lymphograms. In a recent investigation, the roentgen anatomy of the thoracic duct has been evaluated in 336 lymphograms by FUCHS and GALEAZZI (1969).

On the basis of its embryologic development the thoracic duct is subdivided into abdominal, thoracic and cervical sections.

Abdominal Section of the Thoracic Duct

Topographic Anatomy

The abdominal section of the thoracic duct is formed by the union of the two lumbar trunks originating from the efferent lymphatics of the upper aortic lymph nodes and the intestinal trunk, which collects the lymph from the gastrointestinal tract. According to JDANOV the intestinal trunk is not a constant finding because the efferent lymphatics of the abdominal organs usually unite to form a few larger lymph vessels, which enter the thoracic duct or one of the lumbar trunks directly. According

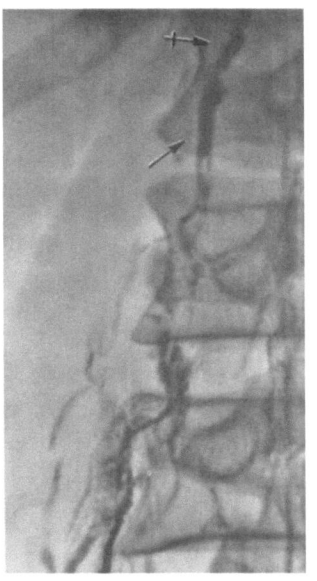
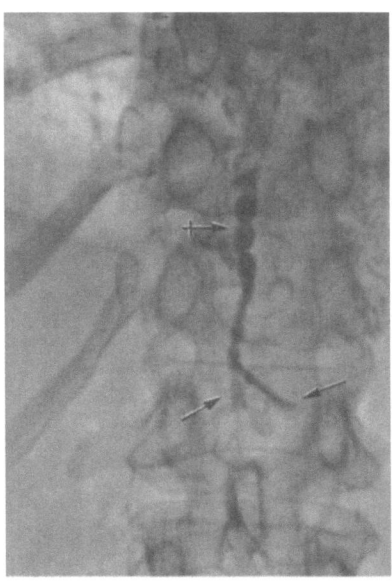

Fig. 23   Fig. 24

Fig. 23. Solitary lumbar trunk (→) in continuous connection with the fusiform cisterna chyli (+→)

Fig. 24. Two lumbar trunks (→) entering the bead-like cisterna chyli (+→)

to the anatomical studies of JOSSIFOW, extensive variations of the abdominal section of the thoracic duct are encountered. The entry of trunks into the thoracic duct is most frequently localized between Th 12 and L 2, but it may be situated between Th 11 or L 3/4. The cisterna chyli, an ampullaceous enlargement of the thoracic duct at its origin was observed by JOSSIFOW with a frequency of 20%, being found mainly when the origin of the thoracic duct was low. Large reticular lymph trunks, but no cisterna chyli, were observed in 40—50%, corresponding particularly when the origin of the thoracic duct was close to Th 11. Rare configurations are ampullaceous dilatation of the lumbar trunks and numerous anastomosing small lymphatics. A bead-like appearance of the lower thoracic duct was found by JOSSIFOW in 10%, especially in cases of low origin. According to JDANOV the cisterna chyli is present in 47% and absent in 42%. In 11% the cisterna chyli was connected with severely dilatated lumbar trunks. The configuration of the cisterna chyli may be conical, ampullaceous, fusiform or moniliform.

Roentgen Anatomy

The author's study demonstrated lumbar trunk visualization in 85 of 336 lymphograms (25.3%). In the lymphogram, lumbar trunks are demonstrated as large oblique lymph vessels with medially directed courses originating from several small efferent lymphatics. Topographic localization and configuration of the lumbar trunks are

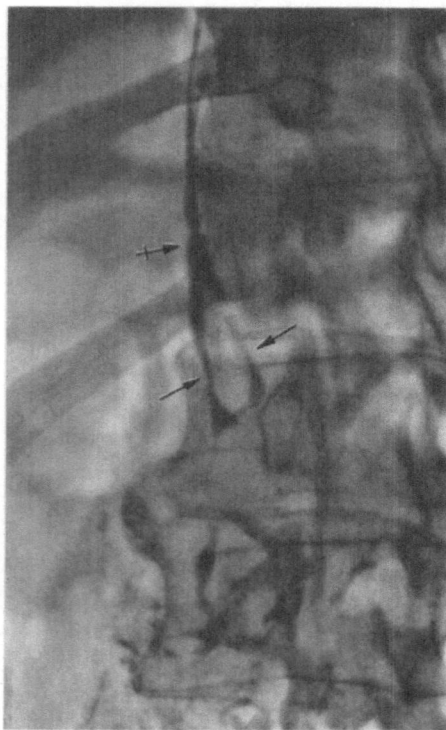

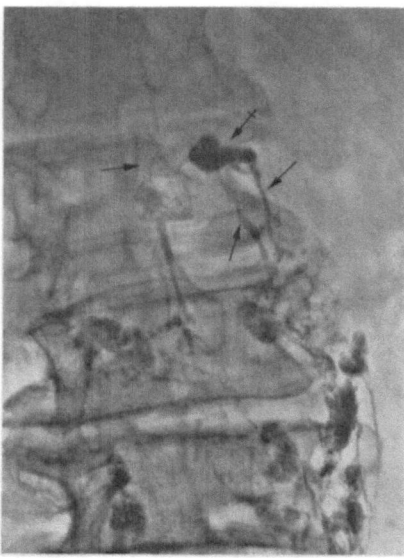

Fig. 26. Three lumbar trunks (→ entering the ampullaceous cisterna chyli (+→)

Fig. 25. Two lumbar trunks (→) in connection with the conical cisterna chyli (+→)

variable because of partial contrast-filling. A single lumbar trunk was found in 35% (Fig. 23), two lumbar trunks in 50% (Figs. 24, 25) and three lumbar trunks in 9% (Fig. 26). A reticular configuration of the lumbar trunks was observed in 5%. In 30% the lumbar trunks were situated at L 1, in 39% at L 2 and in 15% at L 3. In a few cases the beginning of the thoracic duct was found to be above Th 12 or below L 4. The diameter of the lumbar trunks varies between 1 to 6 mm with an average of 2 mm.

On the *lymphogram* the cisterna chyli is recognized as a large lymph trunk situated between Th 12 and L 3, formed by the union of the lumbar trunks from which the thoracic duct originates. Its size is definitely larger than that of all the surrounding vessels. In 30% of the authors's cases the cisterna chyli was visualized by lymphography. In 13% it was situated at the level of Th 12, in 47% at L 1, in 36% at L 2 and in 4% at L 3. The cisterna chyli was situated at the right lateral border of

the vertebral column in 9% and at the left lateral border in 13%. In 78% it was projected over the vertebral bodies. The configuration of the cisterna chyli was reticular in 27%, ampullaceous in 27% (Fig. 26), conical in 19% (Fig. 25), fusiform in 14% (Fig. 23). In 13% its appearance could not be evaluated. The diameter of the cisterna chyli ranged between 2 and 16 mm with an average of 4—6 mm.

Contrast-filling of lymph nodes connected with the abdominal part of the thoracic duct was frequently observed. In 28% the lymph nodes were situated at the level of Th 12, in 29% at L 1 and in 3% at L 2 (Fig. 27).

Thoracic Section of the Thoracic Duct

Topographic Anatomy

The variations of the topographic anatomy of this part of the thoracic duct have been especially investigated by BARTHELS and JDANOV. After passage through the diaphragm at the aortic opening, the first part of the thoracic section of the thoracic duct is situated in 60% of the cases in the posterior mediastinum on the right side of the aorta. Continuing at about the level of Th 5/6 the thoracic duct crosses obliquely to the left, dorsal to the thoracic aorta (JDANOV). It leaves the thoracic cavity between the left subclavian artery and the esophagus.

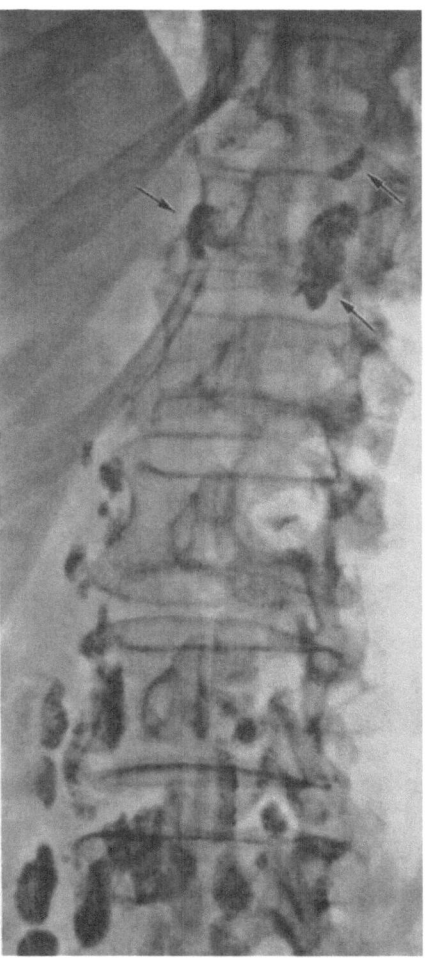

Fig. 27. Contrast-filling of several lymph nodes situated at the level of Th 10/11 (→)

The presence of a hemithoracic duct situated on the left side of the main trunk of the thoracic duct is rather frequent. Numerous narrow lymphatic channels which course away from the main trunk for short distances, often to nodes alongside, and which then return to the thoracic duct are occasionally observed (DJNOV). Duplication of the thoracic duct with one duct situated on each side of the thoracic aorta, is another rare anatomic variation. Cranially both trunks may join together. The thoracic section of the thoracic duct is frequently connected with posterior mediastinal lymph nodes. The bidirectional lymph flow within the afferent and efferent lymph vessels is demonstrated by injection of dye into the lymph nodes or into the thoracic duct. Efferent lymph vessels of the thoracic wall, the heart and the mediastinum enter the thoracic section of the thoracic duct.

Roentgen Anatomy

In 265 of 336 lymphograms the thoracic section of the thoracic duct was filled with contrast material. The upper part of the thoracic duct was visualized most frequently, and the entire thoracic duct was demonstrated in only 7⁰/₀ of the cases.

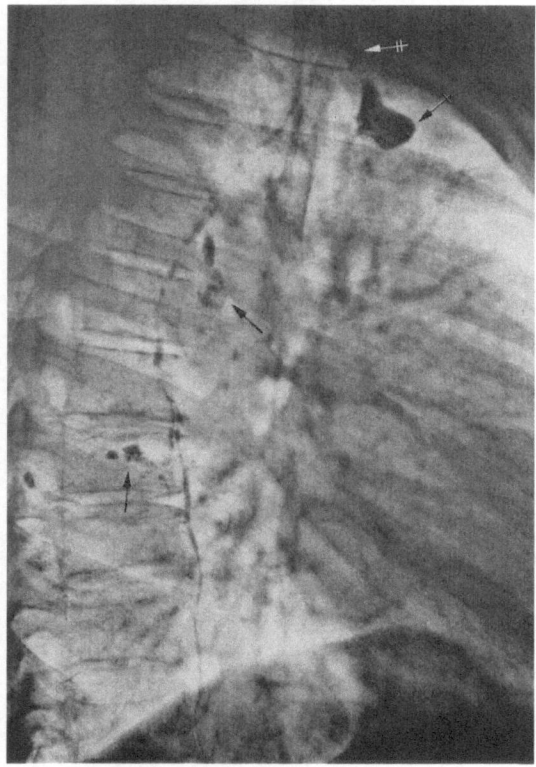

Fig. 28. Contrast-filling of the entire thoracic section of the thoracic duct and of supradiaphragmatic lymph nodes at Th 9, Th 6/7 (→) in the posterior mediastinum. Large ampullaceous configuration of the terminal part of the thoracic duct (⊢→). Supraclavicular lymph nodes (╫→)

On the *lymphogram*, the thoracic section of the thoracic duct may divide into a caudal subsection, situated between the diaphragm and Th 3 and a cranial subsection reaching the supraclavicular region. This subdivision is important because the thoracic duct is projected onto the vertebral bodies up to the region of Th 3. In nearly 70⁰/₀ of the cases the lower subsection of the thoracic duct was situated to the left of the midline (Fig. 32). In 28⁰/₀ its position was median (Figs. 31, 33) and in 3⁰/₀ it was projected to the right of the midline. The upper subsection of the thoracic duct above

Th 3 was localized on the left side in 98%. Duplication of the thoracic duct was
present in one case out of ten (Fig. 29), but in only 3% of all 340 cases was the entire
length of both trunks contrast-filled by lymhography. In 1%, both lymph trunks
were situated to the left of the midline, and in 2% separate trunks on each side of the
midline were recognized. When present, partial duplication of the thoracic duct was
observed predominantly in the lower thoracic section of the thoracic duct (Figs. 28,

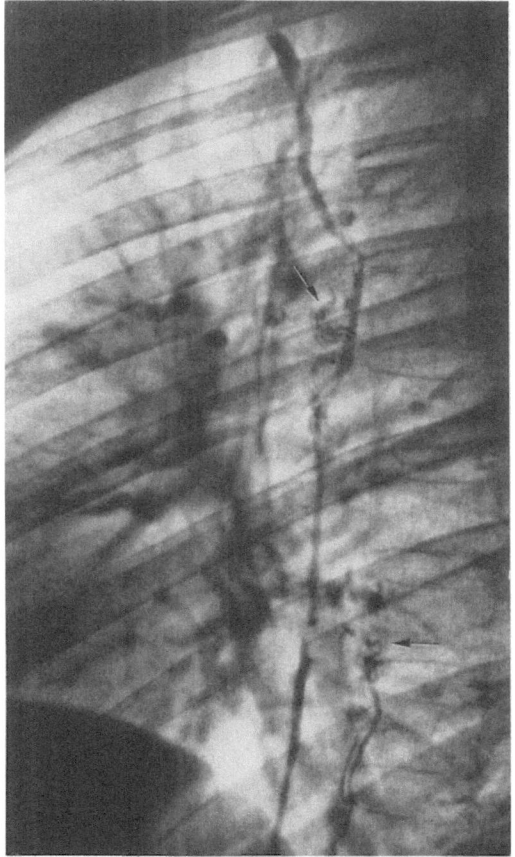

Fig. 29. Contrast-filling of the entire thoracic section of the thoracic duct and several small
concomitant lymph trunks and posterior mediastinal lymph nodes (→)

29). A reticular configuration of the thoracic duct was present in 22% (Fig. 33), but
in only 2 cases was the entire thoracic section reticular. The reticular configuration
was observed mostly in the middle (5.3%) and lower thirds (5.6%) of the thoracic
duct. In 87% the largest diameter of the thoracic section of the thoracic duct was
measured at the level of Th 2. In 60% the maximum diameter ranged between 4 and
6 mm, in 30% between 2 and 4 mm. In 10% the diameter was larger than 6 mm.
Posterior mediastinal lymph nodes connected with the thoracic duct could be demonstrated in 15% of the cases at the level of Th 4—Th 8 (Figs. 28, 29). In 4% of the

cases, retro-sternal lymph nodes situated in the anterior mediastinum, arising from the thoracic duct with netlike lymphatics were contrast-filled by lymphography (Fig. 30). In 4⁰/₀ of the cases, lymph nodes of the hilar region of the lungs were demonstrated, and in 6⁰/₀ para-tracheal lymph nodes were visualized.

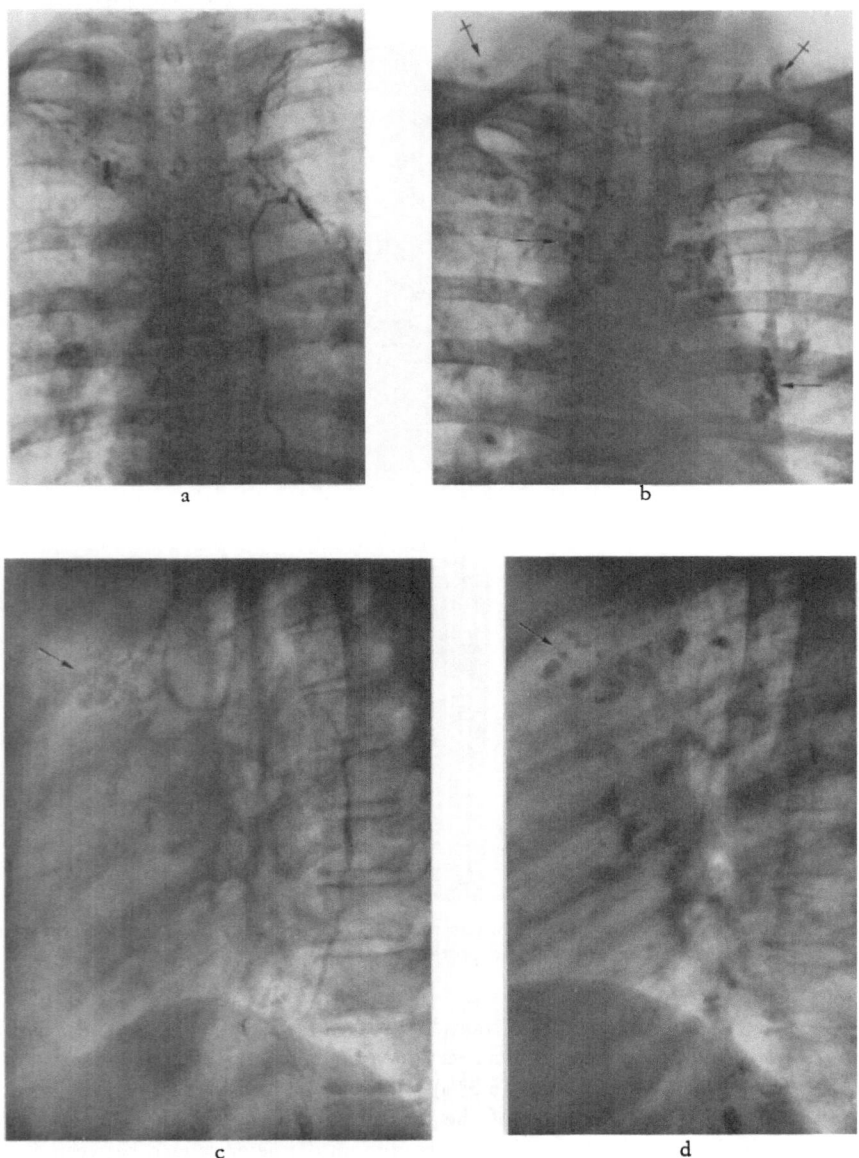

Fig. 30. Net-like configuration of the thoracic duct. Bilateral contrast-filling of hilar (→), para-tracheal (+→), retro-sternal (#→) and supraclavicular (o→) lymph nodes. a, c Filling phase. b, d Storage phase

Cervical Section of the Thoracic Duct

Topographic Anatomy

The arched cervical section of the thoracic duct runs through the left upper thoracic aperture toward the subclavian triangle to enter into the veins. In only one fourth of the cases is a single channel present. In half of the cases a double channel is observed—with 32% re-uniting again before entering the veins and 18% entering separately. Also multiple branching, accompanied by multiple entry points, may be

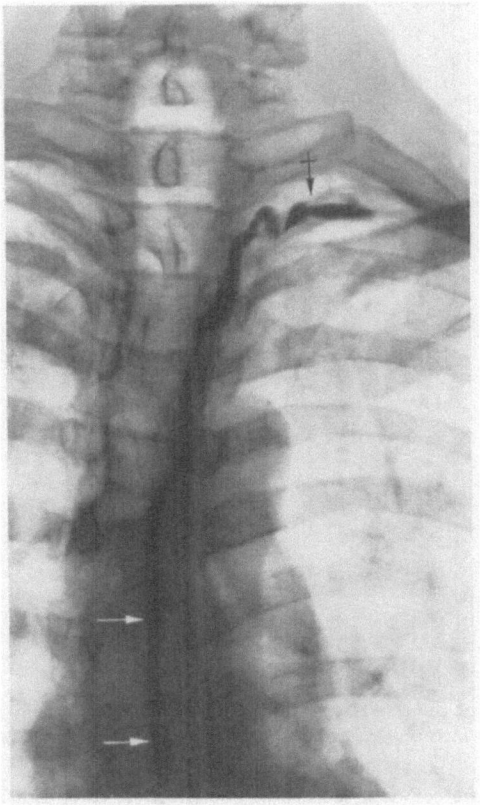

Fig. 31. Median position of the thoracic section of the thoracic duct (→). Ampullaceous cervical section containing several valves (+→)

seen. The thoracic duct may enter the internal jugular vein, the venous angle, the subclavian or the innominate vein. An ampullaceous dilatation of the terminal part of the thoracic duct containing one or two valves is observed in 50% by JDANOV. The cervical part of the thoracic duct is connected frequently with cervical and supra-clavicular lymph nodes by numerous small lymphatics with a bidirectional flow. The left subclavian and left mediastinal trunks—collecting the lymph from the left thorax the left arm and the cervical region—enter the cervical section of the thoracic duct. On the right side identical lymphatic trunks are in direct connection with the venous system or in rare cases with a right lymphatic duct.

Roentgen Anatomy

The cervical section of the thoracic duct was demonstrated in 220 out of 336 lymphograms (62%). In 202 cases (92%) it entered the venous system on the left side (Figs. 31, 32), in 6 cases (2.7%) on the right side (Fig. 33), and in 12 cases (5.3%) bilaterally (Fig. 34). In 52% there was only one lymph trunk present (Figs. 31, 33).

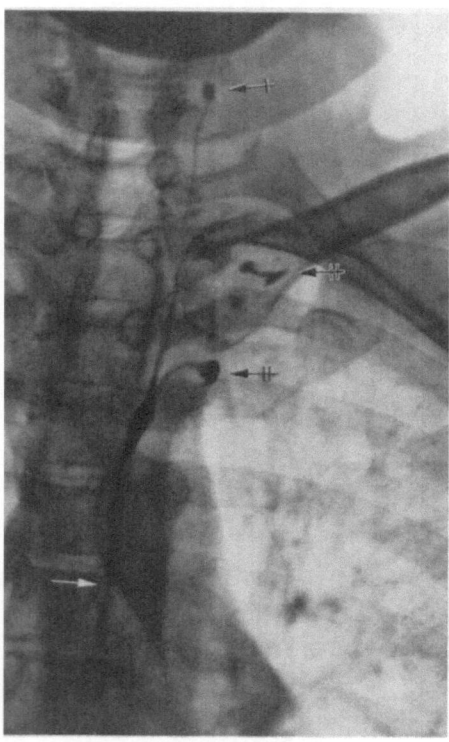

Fig. 32. Left lateral position of the thoracic section of the thoracic duct (→). Triple entering of the cervical section into the external jugular (↔) and subclavian vein (⊬→)

In 22% two branches of the cervical section of the thoracic duct and in 26% three or more lymphatic vessels were encountered. An ampullaceous configuration at the terminus of the thoracic duct was observed in 166 cases (49.5%) (Figs. 31, 33). In 112 cases there was only a single ampullaceous trunk, whereas in 14 cases 2 or 3 ampullaceous trunks were present (Fig. 32). Supraclavicular lymph nodes were visualized in 147 (44%) of 336 lymphograms. In 135 cases (40.3%) they were situated on the left side (Fig. 35) and in 19 cases (5.7%) on the right side (Fig. 36). In 7 cases (2%) lymph nodes were demonstrated within both the left and right supraclavicular regions (Fig. 37). Of the 135 lymphograms with visualization of left supraclavicular lymph nodes, 45 had only 1 lymph node, 85 had more than 2 lymph nodes, and 5 had more than 20 lymph nodes filled with contrast media. In the 19 cases with contrast-filling of right supraclavicular lymph nodes, 8 showed only 1 lymph node and 11 two or more lymph nodes. In 2.4% of the entire study (i. e. 8 of 336)

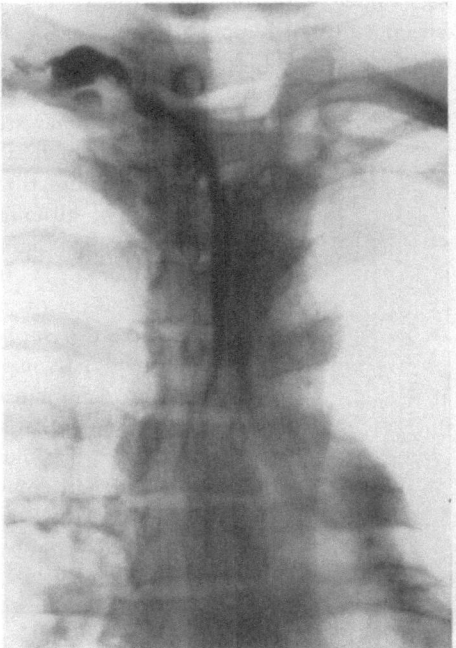

Fig. 33. Median position of the thoracic section of the thoracic duct. Right-sided
ampullaceous terminal cervical section

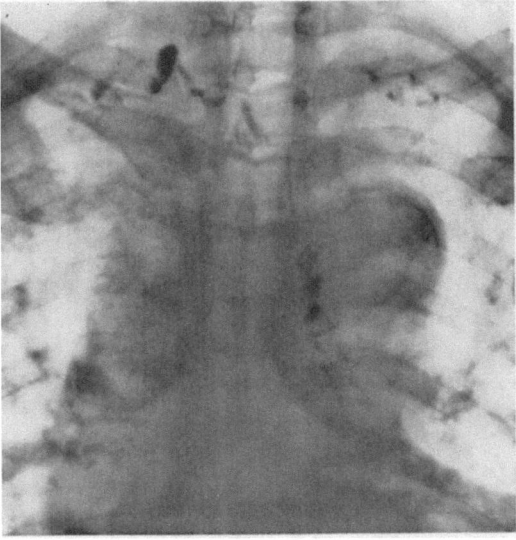

Fig. 34. Bilateral entering of the cervical section of the thoracic duct

were left axillary lymph nodes filled with contrast material (Fig. 37). Left cervical lymph nodes were visualized on 10 (3%) lymphograms (Fig. 38). In 1 case, a single right cervical lymph node was demonstrated by lymphography.

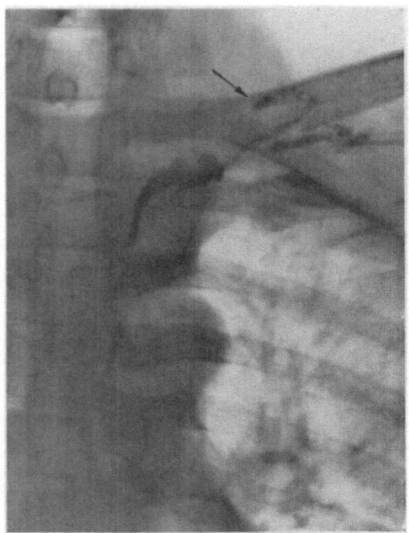

Fig. 35. Contrast-filling of left supra-clavicular lymph nodes (→) connected by numerous lymphatics with the ampulla-ceous terminal cervical section of the thoracic duct

Comparison of the results of topographic and roentgen anatomic studies shows considerable similarity of findings. Anterograde lymphography enables the careful study of roentgen anatomy, although contrast-filling of the thoracic duct, the cisterna chyli and the lumbar trunks is fairly inconstant. However, evaluation of the thoracic duct and the connected lymphatics and lymph nodes as a functional unit is achieved only by this method. Anatomical dissection leads to an exact demonstration of the topographic anatomy but not the functional connection of the different structures.

Contrast-filling of the supraclavicular, cervical, axillary, paravertebral, mediastinal and pulmonary hilar lymph nodes is of great clinical significance. Visualization of these lymph nodes is not a definitive sign of collateral circulation and is therefore not always a sign of a pathologic condition. All these nodes, which are closely connected with the thoracic duct, are necessarily demonstrated by lymphography when they are the last regional lymph nodes of the system draining the abdominal and retroperitoneal organs and the lower extremities. In cases of malignant

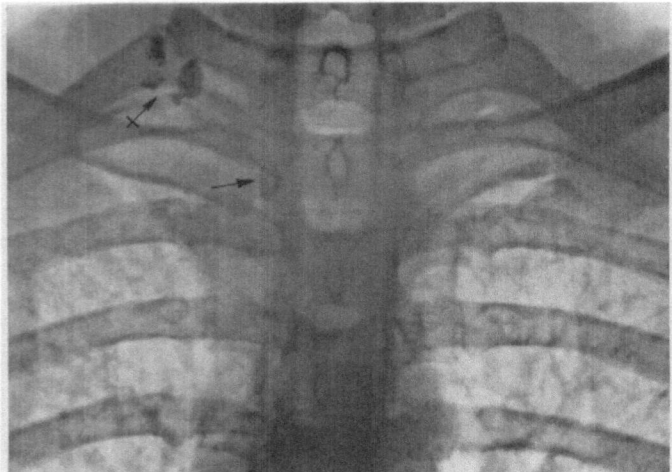

Fig. 36. Right unilateral contrast-filling of infraclavicular (→) and supraclavicular (↔) lymph nodes

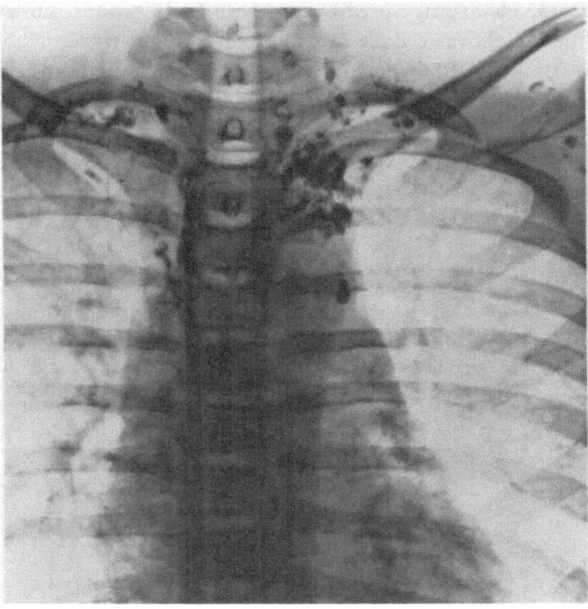

Fig. 37. Contrast-filling of bilateral supraclavicular, infraclavicular, retro-sternal and left axillary lymph nodes

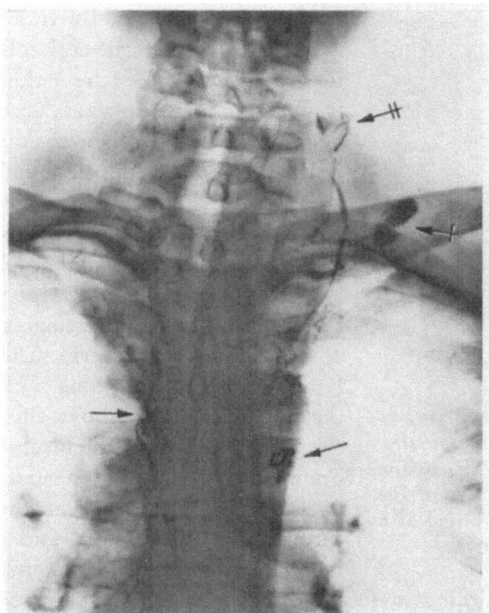

Fig. 38. Net-like configuration of the cervical section of the thoracic duct and contrast-filling of left supraclavicular (↔) and inferior cervical (#→) lymph nodes, para-tracheal (→) and retro-sternal lymph nodes

tumors in these areas, metastatic spread into these node groups must be considered. Cancer cells within the thoracic duct are relatively frequent according to the post-mortem studies of YOUNG (1956) and BRUNNER (1960). Malignant cells are likely to migrate into these lymph node groups connected with the thoracic duct. Cancer metastases in the supraclavicular lymph nodes, which are frequently demonstrated by lymphography, are therefore rather common (ZEIDMAN, 1955; BRUNNER, 1960; WALLER, 1964). In the author's experience cancer metastases in para-vertebral, tracheobronchial and anterior media-stinal lymph nodes occur occasionally (BURGENER and FUCHS, 1969) in the later stages of the disease, Consequently, the practice of prophylactic radia-tion therapy of these distant lymph node groups demonstrated by lymphography has to be re-evaluated.

Upper Extremity

The digital lymphatic plexuses are drained by vessels which run along the outer margin of the fingers to reach the web. At this point they receive vessels from the distal palm and pass posteriorly towards the dorsal surface of the hand. The rest of the palm is drained by vessels which pass proxi-mally to the wrist. Several collecting vessels from the central part of the palmar plexus unite to form a trunk which winds around the metacarpal bone of the index finger to join the dorsal vessels of the same finger and the thumb.

In the forearm and arm the *subcutaneous lym-phatics* are divided into a medial ulnar (basilic) group and a lateral radial (cephalic) group.

The *ulnar group of lymphatics* drains primar-ily the 3rd, 4th and 5th fingers and the ulnar side of the hand and forearm. The majority of these lymph channels runs along with the basilic vein to the cubital region. Above this point they follow the medial border of the biceps muscle to reach the prefascial axillary lymph nodes (Fig. 39). One or two lymphatics may accompany the basilic vein through the deep fascia and join the deep sub-fascial lymph vessels of the upper arm. The *radial group of lymphatics* drains the first and second digits and the radial side of the hand and forearm. They are situated on the lateral side of the wrist and join the cephalic vein in the forearm. They follow the vein to the level of the olecranon, where most of them curve medially to enter the lateral group of axillary lymph nodes. A few

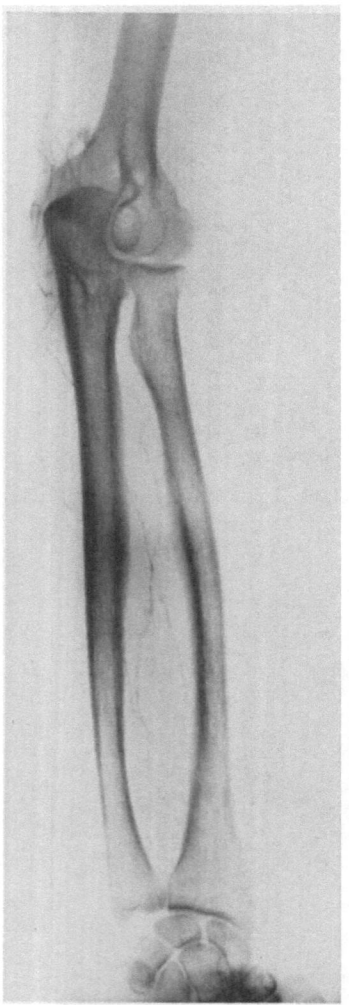

Fig. 39. *Ulnar group of lymphatics.* Lymph channels follow the basilic vein and the medial border of the biceps muscle. Contrast-filling of a cubital lymph node

lymphatics continue with the cephalic vein to reach the infraclavicular lymph nodes.

The collecting lymphatics from the deltoid region pass over the anterior and posterior axillary folds to end in axillary lymph nodes. The skin of the scapular region is drained by lymph vessels which end in the subscapular groups of axillary nodes or follow the transverse cervical vessels to the inferior deep cervical lymph nodes.

The deep lymph channels of the arm follow the muscles, vessels and nerves and end at the lateral axillary lymph nodes. They are less numerous than the superficial vessels with which they communicate at intervals. A few deep lymph nodes are connected with the deep lymphatic system.

Axillary Region

The axillary lymph nodes are the first regional nodes of the whole upper limb. Their number varies from 20—30 nodes, and they are divided into 5 groups (Fig. 40).

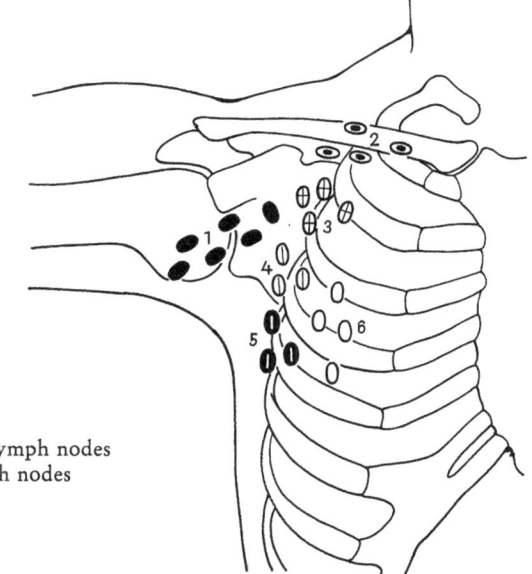

1 Lateral axillary lymph nodes
2 Supraclavicular lymph nodes
3 Apical axillary lymph nodes
4 Central axillary lymph nodes
5 Posterior or subscapular axillary lymph nodes
6 Anterior or pectoral axillary lymph nodes

Fig. 40. *Topographic roentgen anatomy of the axillary lymph nodes*

The *lateral axillary group* of 4—6 lymph nodes is situated medial and posterior to the axillary vein. The afferent lymphatics of this group drain the lymph of the entire upper extremity, except for the regions drained by radial subcutaneous vessels following the cephalic vein. The efferent vessels join the central and apical axillary lymph nodes or the inferior deep cervical lymph nodes.

The *anterior or pectoral group* of axillary lymph nodes comprises 4—5 lymph nodes which are localized along the inferior border of the lesser pectoral muscle, close to the lateral thoracic vessels. Their afferent lymphatics drain the skin and muscles of the anterior and lateral walls of the thorax, the abdominal wall above the umbilicus and the central and lateral areas of the mammary gland. Their efferent lymph vessels enter the central and apical axillary node groups.

The *posterior or subscapular axillary lymph nodes* consist of 6—7 nodes placed along the lower margin of the posterior wall of the axilla close to the axillary vessels. The afferent lymphatics of this group drain the skin and muscles of the lower part of the neck and of the dorsal aspect of the body as far inferior as the iliac crests. Their efferent lymphatics enter the apical and central groups of axillary lymph nodes.

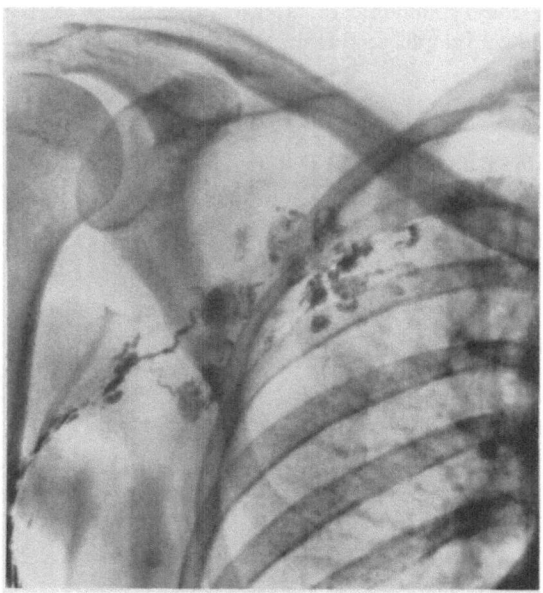

Fig. 41. *Axillary lymphogram.* Contrast-filling of lateral central and apical axillary lymph nodes, supraclavicular lymph nodes

The *central axillary lymph node group* of 3—4 large lymph nodes is situated near the base of the axilla. The group has no drainage area of its own, but receives afferent lymphatics from most of the other axillary lymph node groups. The efferent lymphatics of the group enter the apical axillary lymph nodes.

The 6—12 *apical axillary lymph nodes* are situated within the apex of the axilla, medial to the axillary vein, dorsal to the superior portion of the lesser pectoral muscle and cranial to the superior margins of the pectoral muscles. The only direct territorial afferents of this group are those which accompany the cephalic vein. The nodes receive the efferents from all the other axillary lymph node groups. The efferent vessels of the apical axillary group unite to form the subclavian trunk which opens either directly into the junction of the internal jugular and subclavian veins or into the jugular lymphatic trunk. On the left side, the subclavian trunk may enter the thoracic duct directly. A few efferents of the apical axillary lymph nodes are usually connected with inferior deep cervical nodes.

Lymphography by injection of contrast material into a lymph vessel of the radial or ulnar group of lymphatics in the forearm demonstrates only a few lymph nodes of the lateral axillary group (Fig. 41). Complete contrast-filling of all lateral axillary lymph nodes is not achieved, because each lymphatic of the forearm may enter a different node. The efferent lymphatics of the contrast-filled lateral axillary lymph nodes drain into a few nodes of the central and apical groups of axillary nodes. From the apical axillary node group, efferent lymphatics are demonstrated uniting to form the subclavian trunk. Occasionally some supraclavicular and deep cervical lymph nodes are filled with contrast material.

Cervical Lymphatic System

The topographic anatomy of lymph vessels and lymph nodes of the cervical region is based mainly upon the classical studies of ROUVIÈRE (1938) and TAILLENS (1960, 1962). The following classification of the cervical lymph node groups has been proposed by TAILLENS (1966) (Fig. 42): the triple jugular lymph node group com-

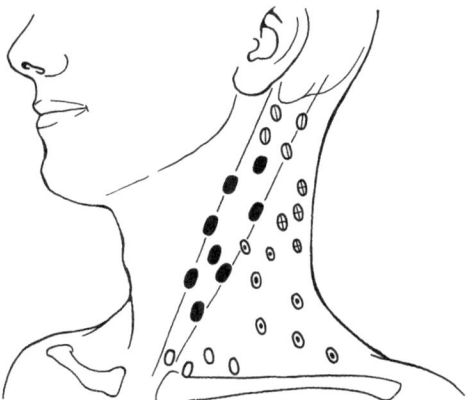

   0   Junctional lymph nodes
   ⊕   Jugular lymph node group
   ●   Supraclavicular or transverse cervical lymph node group
   ⊘   Spinal lymph nodes
   0   Nuchal lymph nodes

Fig. 42. *Lymph nodes of the deep cervical region* (according to the classification of ROUVIÈRE, TAILLENS and FISCH)

prising the prejugular, retrojugular and subjugular chains; the junctional lymph nodes; the spinal group; the supraclavicular or transverse cervical group; the nuchal lymph nodes.

Cervical lymphography systematically developed by FISCH has permitted investigation of the lymphatic system of the neck. Direct injection of oily contrast material into a deep retroauricular lymph vessel visualizes lymph nodes belonging to the deep lateral cervical lymphatic system, which consists of the jugular, spinal, supraclavicular or transverse cervical and the nuchal lymph nodes (Fig. 43). Jugular, spinal and supra-clavicular nodes are visualized in the a-p projection, the nuchal nodes in the lateral projection. In addition to the classical chains of deep lateral cervical lymph nodes, another group is constantly demonstrated by lymphography. These lymph nodes are situated in the superior aspect of the lateral triangle of the neck at the junction of the

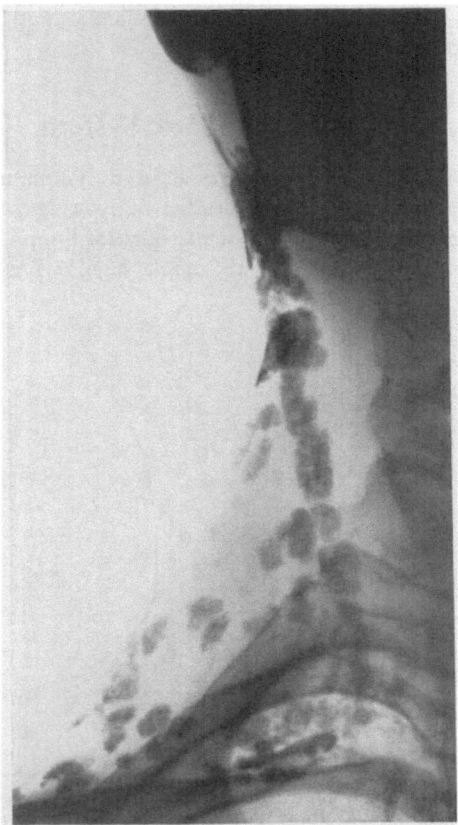

Fig. 43. *Normal right cervical lymphogram* 24 hours after injection of contrast material. a-p projection. (By Courtesy of U. Fisch, M.D., Zurich)

jugular and spinal chains. They play an important functional role in the distribution of lymph in the deep lateral region of the neck, a fact which is clearly demonstrated by cervical lymphography. Direct connections from these nodes join with the jugular and supraclavicular lymph node chains. According to the lymphographic investigations of Fisch, the deep lateral lymph nodes of the neck are functionally divided into the junctional, jugular, spinal, supraclavicular and nuchal groups. The junctional groups comprise an average number of 9 nodes, the jugular 11, the spinal 19, the supraclavicular 9 lymph nodes. The total number of cervical lymph nodes demonstrated by lymphography ranges between 44 and 64 with an average number of 48 (Fisch, 1966).

Structural Roentgen Anatomy

The basic topographic anatomy of lymph vessels and lymph nodes in the inguinal, pelvic, lumbar and axillary regions is constant, but considerable variation is encountered in size, shape, number and structure of the lymph nodes.

The description of the normal histology of the lymph nodes is based mainly upon the studies of HILLMANN (1943), JOFFEY and COURTICE (1956), MARSHALL (1956), LEIBER (1961), COTTIER (1963) and TJERNBERG (1966). The special roentgen anatomy of normal lymph nodes has been analysed by TJERNBERG (1956, 1962, 1966), FUCHS and BÖÖK-HEDERSTRÖM (1961, 1964), FISCHER et al. (1962), DITCHEK et al. (1963), ARVAY and PICARD (1963), RÜTTIMANN and DEL BUONO (1964) and WIRTH (1966).

Normal Anatomy of Lymph Nodes

Normal lymph nodes vary in size and shape. Their size—between 1 mm and 30 mm in diameter—depends on functional load, constitutional elements and age. They may be round, oval, elongated or bean-shaped with slight indentation of the hilar region. Lymph nodes consist of lymphatic tissue which is connected with the lymphatic circulation by afferent and efferent lymphatics. The lymphatic tissue is formed by a net-like stroma of reticular fibers and both free and fixed reticulo-histiocytic, lymphatic and plasma cells. Furthermore, myeloid and mast cells are present. *Loose lymphatic tissue,* consisting of a meshwork of reticular fibers and reticulo-histiocytic cells, fills the sinuses which are the main channels for lymph circulation. The diffuse lymphatic tissue of nodes is formed by a dense network of reticular fibers and uniformly distributed cells of the lymphatic group. The *nodular lymphatic tissue* of the lymph nodes includes follicles, which are rounded, dense accumulations of predominantly lymphatic cells embedded in a very loose reticular stroma.

The sinus system of the lymph nodes includes the marginal sinus, situated close to the lymph node capsule of fibrous tissue, and extensions of the marginal sinus, called the intermediate sinus, which converge towards the hilus where they unite to form the terminal sinuses. The diffuse lymphatic tissue is arranged into a cortex and a medulla, the cortex being compact and the medulla consisting of a coarse network of medullary cords.

The cortex is divided into lymphatic lobules by trabeculae of dense connective tissue arising from the capsule. The lymph follicles, which are not permanent structures, are localized predominantly in the cortex but also may be found in the medullary cords. The function of the nodules is lymph filtration and cell production, chiefly of lymphatics and plasma cells. According to the functional state of the lymph node, primary and secondary nodules may be present. These differ in that the primary follicle has a more uniform structure, whereas the secondary follicle contains a so-called germinal center. Large spherical or ovoid agglomerations of lymphatic tissue within the cortex but not manifesting germinal centers may be called tertiary follicles. They consist of tightly packed cells belonging to the lymphatic cell group.

The filling phase of lymphography immediately after injection of a contrast medium demonstrates both lymph vessels and lymph nodes. Contrast medium enters a node through the numerous afferent lymphatics that join its marginal lymph sinus, passes through the medullary sinuses in streaks and leaves the lymph node by way of efferent lymphatics from the hilus. Generally there are more afferent than efferent lymphatics. The contrast medium often passes first directly from the afferent to the efferent lymph vessels of a lymph node without demonstration of the entire sinus system. Then gradually, as more contrast dye enters the node, the whole sinus system is visualized.

Direct connections between efferent lymphatics of a lymph node and afferent lymphatics of other nodes are observed rather frequently (OTTAVIANI).

Both water-soluble and oily contrast media produce a similar lymphographic filling phase. At a later stage, however, the water-soluble contrast medium diffuses through the compact lymphatic tissue and may obscure structural changes of the node. Serial roentgenograms must be taken during the whole course of the contrast injection. On the other hand, oily contrast media and thorotrast penetrate only slightly into the diffuse and nodular lymphatic tissue. Consequently the structural pattern of the lymph node stands out clearly in the roentgenogram.

During the *storage phase*, 3—24 hours after injection, the contrast fluid has left the lymph vessels and has accumulated in the lymph nodes. Contrast-filling of the lymph vessels for more than 24 hours must be regarded generally as a sign of impaired lymphatic circulation. The oily contrast agent is retained as drops in the lymph nodes by the network of fibrous and reticulo-histiocytic cells. Intracellular deposits of contrast medium are rare, as resorption of the oily fluid takes place very slowly. The major portion of the contrast material remains embedded in the mesh-work of the reticulum cells, which are phagocytizing it, for about 5—9 months. The marginal sinus of the nodes and the peripheral parts of the intermediate sinuses are most densely filled with contrast fluid. Small structural changes in the lymph nodes may be obscured by an excessive amount of contrast medium within the sinuses. The follicular lymphatic tissue of the nodes is not penetrated by oily contrast agent. Small round filling defects of varied sizes corresponding to the different lymph follicles lead to a fine homogeneous reticular appearance. However, in the medullary parts without nodules, the distribution may appear irregular.

The size of lymph nodes and vessels as determined by lymphography tends to decrease in old age, but size is more dependent upon functional state than on age. With the same qualification, it is generally found that children and young women have fine and delicate lymphatics. A study of 100 normal lymphograms by FUCHS and PFAMMATTER (1969) showed no significant differences in lymph node size between a group aged 15—60 years and a 61—77 year group. Patients older than 70 years did show a trend towards generally smaller than normal nodes.

Regional Variations of Lymph Nodes

Consistant variations in form, size and structure of certain lymph node groups are seen. The *superficial inguinal lymph nodes*, because they are the regional lymph nodes of the lower limb, are affected frequently by inflammatory changes. The central parts of the nodes are often totally replaced by fibrosis and fatty infiltration called fibro-lipomatosis (FUCHS et al., 1960; FISCHER et al., 1962; DITCHEK et al., 1963). Lym-phatic tissue is left only in the periphery of the nodes as an incomplete cortical margin. Lymphography results in a large central filling defect, because only the reticular meshwork of the lymph node is able to retain contrast substance. All these changes are manifestations of the normal physiologic involution of the lymphatic system.

The size of the superficial inguinal lymph nodes varies from 1.5 cm to 3 cm. They are round or oval, rarely elongated.

Deep inguinal lymph nodes are usually small and rounded with the exception of the Rosenmüller node, which is large and often fused with the internal lacunar node.

The *iliac lymph nodes* are oval and elongated except for the lacunar nodes. The lateral lacunar node is usually large and shows extensive filling defects due to fibrolipomatosis. The size of the other external and common iliac lymph nodes varies up to a diameter of 3 cm. Smaller nodes are round or oval. Rounded filling defects of varying size due to fibrolipomatosis are not as common as in the inguinal and lacunar nodes.

The *aortic lymph nodes* are mainly oval and elongated. Generally they measure up to 2 cm in diameter, but a length of 4 cm is not uncommon. Peripheral and intermediary sinuses are well developed and large, leading to a reticular lymphographic pattern. Fibrolipomatosis of the aortic lymph nodes is a rare finding except for the nodes within the region L 2/3. These nodes are the regional lymph nodes of the testicle or the upper part of the uterus and are therefore subjected to reactive changes.

The *axillary lymph nodes* are of various sizes and their structural pattern is also variable. Because they are the regional lymph nodes of the upper extremity, fibrolipomatous alterations are very common.

Conglomeration of several small lymph nodes may sometimes hardly be differentiated from a single large inguinal node. Efferent lymphatics may sometimes simulate small filling defects in the hilar region of the nodes during the filling phase. Superposition of lymph nodes and conglomeration of several small nodes may also simulate filling defects. Roentgenograms in different projections and tomography will lead to correct interpretation.

References

ABBES, M. E., V. MARTIN et A. PASCHETTA: La lymphographie en cancérologie. Paris: L'expansion scientifique Française 1964.

ARNULF, M. G., et C. BOELY: Physiopathologie des lymphatiques et du canal thoracique. Presse méd. 69, 2381, 2505 (1961).

ARVAY, N., et J. D. PICARD: La lymphographie. Etude radiologique des voies lymphatiques normales et pathologiques. Paris: Masson & Cie 1963.

BARTHELS, P.: Das Lymphgefäßsystem. In: v. BARDELEBEN, Handb. d. Anat. d. Menschen. Jena: G. Fischer 1909, Bd. III (1909).

BOURGERY, J. M.: Anatomie déscriptive ou physiologique. Paris 1851.

—, u. JACOB: In: WALDEYER: Das Becken. Bonn 1899.

BRUHNS, C.: Ueber die Lymphgefäße der weiblichen Genitalien nebst einigen Bemerkungen über die Topographie der Leistendrüsen. Arch. Anat. Phys. Anat. Abt. 57 (1898).

— Ueber die Lymphgefäße der äußeren männlichen Genitalien und die Zuflüsse der Leistendrüsen. Arch. Anat. Phys. Anat. Abt. 291 (1900).

— Untersuchungen über die Lymphgefäße und Lymphdrüsen der Prostata beim Menschen. Arch. Anat. Phys. Anat. Abt. 330 (1904).

BRUNNER, U.: Die Bedeutung des Ductus thoracicus als Metastasierungsweg abdomineller Geschwülste. Schweiz. med. Wschr. 90, 554 (1960).

BRZEK, V., V. KREN u. V. BARTOS: Retrograde Lymphographie des Ductus thoracicus. Fortschr. Röntgenstr. 102, 125 (1965).

CHIAPPA, S., G. GALLI, S. BARBAINI, G. RAVASI et G. BAGLIANI: La lymphographie peropératoire dans les tumeurs du testicule. J. Radiol. 44, 613 (1963).

COLLETTE, J. M.: Envahissements ganglionnaires inguino-iliopelviens par lymphographie. Acta radiol. (Stockh.) 49, 1954 (1958).

COTTIER, H.: Morphologische Orthologie der immunologisch aktiven Gewebe. In: Die Plasmaproteine in der klinischen Medizin von W. H. HITZIG. Berlin-Göttingen-Heidelberg: Springer 1963.

CRUISHANK, W.: The anatomy of the absorbing vessels of the human body. London 1782.

CUNÉO, B.: Note sur les lymphatiques du testicule. Bull. Soc. Anat. (Paris) 105 (1901).

—, et M. MARCILLE: Topographies des ganglions iliopelviens. Bull. Soc. Anat. (Paris) 653 (1901).

— Note sur les lymphatiques de la vessie. Bull. Soc. Anat. (Paris) 649 (1901).

DITCHEK, T., R. J. BLAHUT, and A. C. KITTLESON: Lymphadenography in normal subjects. Radiology 80, 175 (1963).

FISCH, U.: Lymphographische Untersuchungen über das zervikale Lymphsystem. Basel-New York: Karger 1966.

FISCHER, H. W., M. S. LAWRENCE, and J. R. THORNBURY: Lymphography of the normal adult male. Radiology 78, 399 (1962).

FRAIMOW, W., S. WALLACE, P. LEWIS, R. R. GREENING, and R. T. LATHCART: Changes in pulmonary function due to lymphangiography. Radiology 85, 231 (1965).

FUCHS, W. A.: Lymphographie und Tumordiagnostik. Berlin-Heidelberg-New York: Springer 1965.

— Tumordiagnostik durch Lymphographie. Radiol. Clin. 31, 277 (1962).

— Discussion note: Visualization of hypogastric lymph nodes. Progress in Lymphology, p. 65. Stuttgart: G. Thieme 1967.

—, A. RÜTTIMANN u. M. S. DEL BUONO: Zur Lymphographie bei chronisch-sekundären Lymphoedemen. Fortschr. Röntgenstr. 92, 608 (1960).

—, and G. BÖÖK-HEDERSTRÖM: Inguinal and pelvic lymphography. Acta radiol. (Stockh.) 56, 340 (1961).

— — Lymphography in the diagnosis of metastases with special reference to the carcinoma of the uterine cervix. Acta radiol. (Stockh.) Diagnosis 2 (1964).

—, R. PREISIG, and H. BUCHER: Liver function after Lymphography. Proc. 2. Int. Symp. Lymphology, Miami 1968.

—, u. R. GALEAZZI: Die Röntgenanatomie des Ductus thoracicus. Radiologe 1969 (in print).

—, u. TH. PFAMMATTER: Die topographische Röntgenanatomie der inguinalen und retroperitonealen Lymphknoten. Radiologe 1969 (in print).

—, u. M. A. HOPF: Die Lymphographie, Cavographie und Urographie als Kombinationsuntersuchung. Radiologe 1969 (in print).

—, u. F. BURGENER: Die Bedeutung der Lymphographie in der Diagnostik und Therapie maligner Hodentumoren. Schweiz. med. Wschr. 99, 764 (1969).

GEROTA, D.: Der anorectale Lymphapparat. Sitz.-Ber. Preuss. Akad. d. Wiss. 253 (1895).

— Die Lymphgefäße des Rectums und des Anus. Arch. Anat. Phys., Anat. Abt. 240 (1895).

— Über die Lymphgefäße und die Lymphdrüsen der Nabelgegend und der Harnblase. Anat. Anz. 151 (1896).

— Bemerkungen über die Lymphgefäße der Harnblase. Anat. Anz. 13, 605 (1897).

— Sur les ganglions prévésicaux. Bull. Soc. Chir. Paris, N.S.T. 28, 537 (1902).

GERTEIS, W.: Lymphographie und topographische Anatomie des Beckenlymphsystems. Beilageheft zur Zeitschrift für Geburtshilfe Bd. 165. Stuttgart: Ferdinand Enke 1966.

GINSBERG, V. V.: Some anatomical data about the lymph nodes of the lower extremities for clinical need. Progress in Lymphology, p. 80. Stuttgart: G. Thieme 1967.

GOFFRINI, P.: L'injection radio-opaque du canal thoracique. Observations, morphologiques et fonctionelles sur la circulation lymphatique lors des blocages néoplastique des ganglions lymphatiques sous-diaphragmatiques et médiastineaux. Presse méd. 70, 2751 (1962).

GREGL, A., M. EYDT, E. FERNANDEZ-REDO, U. KRACK, J. KIENLE u. D. YU: Die lymphographische Anatomie des Retroperitonealraumes. Fortschr. Röntgenstr. 109, 5 (1968).

HALLER, A. v.: Observationes de Ductu thoracico in Theatro Gottingensi factae. Gott. (1741). In Hallers Disp. anat. Tl, 793.
— Disputationes anatomicae selectae. Gott. (1746), Vol. I.
— Elementa corporis humani. Lausanne (1757).
HERMAN, P. G., D. L. BENNINGHOFF, J. H. NELSON, and H. Z. MELLINS: Roentgen anatomy of the ilio-pelvic-aortic-lymphatic system. Radiology 80, 182 (1963).
HIDDEN, G., et J. FLORANT: Etude radio-anatomique du canal thoracique opacifié par lymphographie pédieuse. J. Chir. (Paris) 91, 373 (1966).
HELLMANN, T. J.: Lymphgefäße. Lymphknötchen und Lymphknoten. In: Handbuch der mikroskopischen Anatomie des Menschen, Bd. 6: 4., S. 174. Hrsg. W. VON MÖLLENDORFF. Berlin: Springer 1943.
HUNTER, W.: Medical commentaries. Part I, London (1762) (Chapt. 2: Of the origin and use of the lymphatic vessels) 5.
—, u. W. CRUISHANK: In: BARTHELS, P.: Das Lymphgefäßsystem. 1909.
JACOBSSON, S., and S. JOHANSSON: Normal roentgen anatomy of the lymph vessels of the upper and lower extremities. Acta radiol. (Stockh.) 51, 321 (1962).
JDANOV, D. A.: Anatomie du canal thoracique et des principaux collecteurs lymphatiques du tronc chez l'homme. Acta anat. 37, 20 (1959).
JOSSIFOW, G. M.: Der Anfang des Ductus thoracicus und dessen Erweiterung. Arch. Anat. Phys., anat. Abt. 68 (1906).
— Das Lymphgefäßsystem des Menschen. Jena: G. Fischer 1930.
KAINDL, F., u. B. THURNHER: Lymphangiographie und Lymphadenographie am Menschen. Fortschr. Röntgenstr. 100, 557 (1964).
KAMPEIER, O. F.: Ursprung und Entwicklungsgeschichte des Ductus thoracicus nebst Saccus lymphaticus jugularis und Cisterna chyli beim Menschen. Morph. Jb. 67, 157 (1931).
KOWALSKY, H. J.: Topographische Räume. Basel: Birkhäuser 1961.
KRAUSE, W.: Handbuch der Anatomie des Menschen. Leipzig 1903.
KUBIK, S., G. RÖNDURY, A. RÜTTIMANN, and W. WIRTH: Nomenclature of the lymph nodes of the Retroperitoneum, the Pelvis and the lower Extremity. Progress in Lymphology, p. 52. Stuttgart: G. Thieme 1967.
LAMEER, C.: Röntgenonderzoekvan de ductus thoracicus bij de mens. Nederl. T. Geneesk. 110, 1900 (1966).
LEIBER, B.: Der menschliche Lymphknoten. München: Urban und Schwarzenberg 1961.
LÉGER, L., M. PRÉMONT et G. HUGON: Lymphographie du canal thoracique dans les cancers oesophagiens. Gaz. méd. France 69, 2801 (1962).
MALEK, P., A. BELAN u. J. KOLC: Der Ductus thoracicus in der Röntgenkinematographie. Fortschr. Röntgenstr. 93, 723 (1960).
MARSHALL, A. H. E.: An outline of the cytology and pathology of the reticular tissue. Edinburgh and London: Olivier and Boyd 1956.
MASCAGNI, P.: Vasorum lymphaticorum corporis humani. Historia et ichonographia. Senis Edig. Siena: Carlo Pazzini 1787.
McCLURE, C. F. W., and C. F. SILVESTER: A comparative study of the lymphaticovenous communications in adult mammels. Anat. Rec. 3, 534 (1909).
MOST, A.: Chirurgie der Lymphgefäße und Lymphdrüsen. Neue Deutsche Chirurgie. Stuttgart: Enke 1917.
NELSON, J. H., J. G. MASTERSON, P. G. HERMAN, and D. L. BENNINGHOFF: Anatomy of the female pelvic and aortic systems demonstrated by lymphangiography. Amer. J. Obst. Gynec. 88, 460 (1964).
NILSSON, J.: Angiography in tumours of the urinary bladder. Acta radiol. (Stockh.) suppl. 263 (1967).
NUSSBAUM, M., S. BAUM, R. C. HEDGES, and W. S. BLAKEMORE: Roentgenographic and direct visualization of the thoracic duct. Arch. Surg. 88, 105 (1964).
PARSONS, F. G., and A. KEITH: The arrangement of the lymphatic glands accompanying the common external iliac artery. J. Anat. Phys. 172 (1897).
PELLEGRINI, P., F. MARGIOTTA, L. ABLEROTANZA et N. DI CAGNO: Tentativi di Visualizzazione Radiologica dei Collettori Linfatici del Testicolo e delle Linfogliandole lumbo-aortiche. Gazz. inter. med. chir. 63, 1 (1957).

Pernis, P. A. van: Variations of the thoracic duct. Surgery 26, 806 (1949).

Poirier, P.: Traité d'anatomie humaine. Paris: Masson & Cie. 1898.

— Note sur les ganglions lymphatiques de la vessie. Bull. Soc. Chir. (Paris) 559 (1902).

—, et B. Cunéo: Etude spéciale des lymphatiques des différentes parties du corps. In: Poirier et Charpey: Traité d'anatomie humaine, II, 4. Paris: Masson & Cie. 1902.

Reiffenstuhl, G.: Das Lymphsystem des weiblichen Genitale. München-Berlin-Wien: Urban und Schwarzenberg 1957.

— Das Lymphknotenproblem beim Carcinoma colli uteri und die Lymphirradiatio pelvis. München-Berlin-Wien: Urban und Schwarzenberg 1967.

— Nomenclature and anatomy of the pelvic lymph nodes. Progress in Lymphology, p. 56. Stuttgart: G. Thieme 1967.

Rouvière, H.: Anatomie des lymphatiques de l'homme. Paris: Masson & Cie. 1932.

Rüttimann, A.: Die Lymphographie. In: Lehrbuch der Röntgendiagnostik, Band I. Schinz-Baensch-Frommhold-Glauner-Uehlinger-Wellauer. 6. Auflage (1965).

—, and M. S. Del Buono: Die Lymphographie mit öligem Kontrastmittel. Fortschr. Röntgenstr. 97, 552 (1962).

— Die Lymphographie. In: Ergebnisse der medizinischen Strahlenforschung. Neue Folge. Band I. Hrsg. Schinz-Glauner-Rüttimann. Stuttgart: G. Thieme 1964.

Sappey, P.: Traité d'anatomie déscriptive. Vol. II. Paris: Masson & Cie. 1888.

Tagliafferro, A., P. Falcidieno ed I. Donini: Technica di incannulamento e visualizzazione radiografica del dotto thoracico. Minerva chir. 14, 1439 (1959).

Taillens, J. P.: Etude anatomo-clinique des chaines ganglionnaires lymphatiques du cou et de leurs ganglions satellites bucco-linguopharyngés. Pract. oto-rhino-laryng. (Basel) 22, 44 (1960).

— Les ganglions tuberculeux du cou. Paris: Masson 1962.

— Anatomical and clinical studies of the cervical lymph node chains. Progress in Lymphology, p. 275. Stuttgart: G. Thieme 1967.

Tjernberg, B.: Lymphography as an aid to examination of lymph nodes. Acta Soc. Med. upsalien. 61, 207 (1956).

— Lymphography, an animal study on the diagnosis of V×2 carcinoma and inflammation. Acta radiol. (Stockh.) Suppl., 214 (1962).

Waller, H.: Zur Tumormetastasierung in die beiderseitigen supraklavikulären Lymphknoten. Med. Klin. 59, 645 (1964).

Waldeyer, W.: Das Becken. Bonn 1899.

Waerden, B. L. van der: Mathematische Statistik. Berlin: Springer 1957.

Weissleder, H.: Röntgenkinematographische Untersuchungen des Ductus thoracicus. Fortschr. Röntgenstr. 100, 435 (1964).

— Das pathologische Lymphangiogramm des Ductus thoracicus. Fortschr. Röntgenstr. 101, 573 (1964).

Winslow, J. B.: Exposition anatomique de la structure du corps humain. Traité de la poitrine. Paris 1732.

Wirth, W.: Zur Röntgenanatomie des Lymphsystems der inguinalen, pelvinen und aortalen Region. Röntgenstr. 105 (1966).

—, N. Ganzoni u. A. Rüttimann: Die Bedeutung der Lymphographie in der Chirurgie der Leistengegend. Helv. Chir. Acta 32, 14 (1965).

Young, J. M.: Amer. J. Path. 32, 253 (1956).

Zeidmann, I., and J. M. Buss: Experimental studies on the spread of cancer in the lymphatic system. J. Cancer Res. 14, 403 (1954).

Chapter 6

Benign Lymph Node Disease

W. A. Fuchs

With 12 Figures

Involutive Changes

Fibrolipomatosis is considered to be a manifestation of the normal physiologic involution of the lymphatic system and is characterized by the complete replacement of the central parts of lymph nodes by connective and fatty tissue. Lymphatic structures are left only in the periphery of the nodes as incomplete cortical margins, and

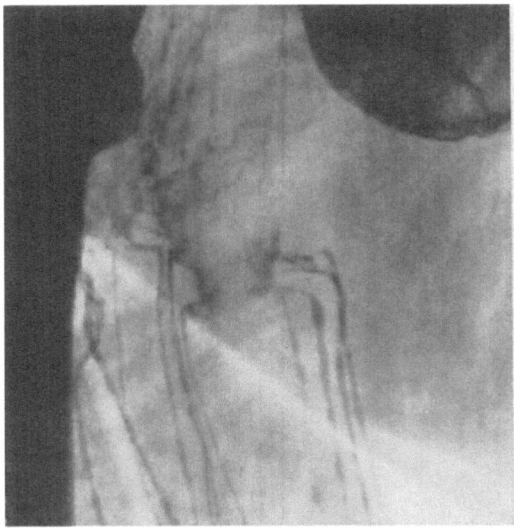

Fig. 1. *Fibrolipomatosis* of an inferior superficial inguinal lymph node. Extensive central filling defects. Marginal contrast-filled lymphatic tissue (verified by biopsy)

because of this the lymphographic appearance of such nodes is characterized by large central filling defects (FUCHS et al., 1960; FISCHER et al., 1962; DITCHEK et al., 1963). Fibrolipomatosis is most common in inguinal and axillary lymph nodes because they are the primary regional node groups of the extremities, and therefore are most often affected by inflammatory lesions (Fig. 1). The external iliac and the aortic node

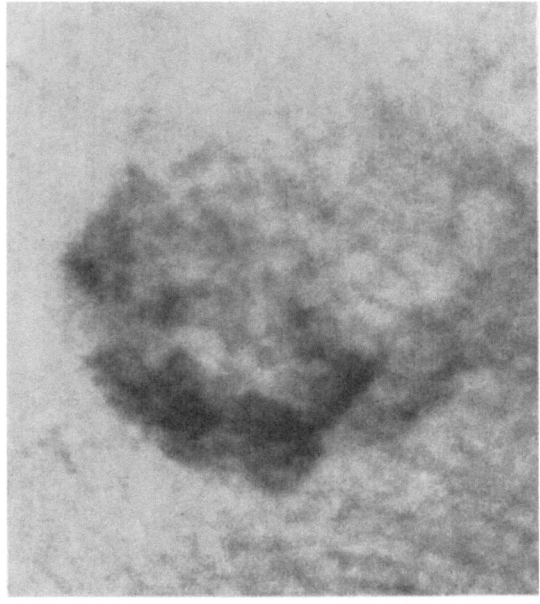

a

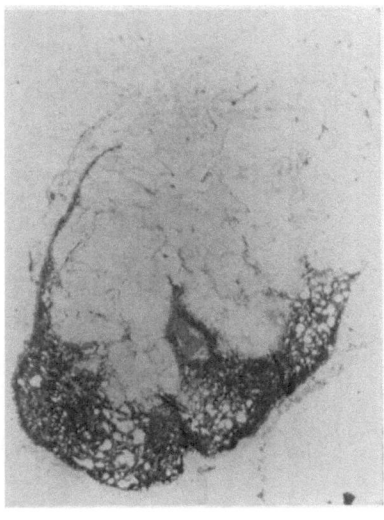

b   c

Fig. 2. *Fibrolipomatosis* of a lateral external iliac lymph node. a Central and marginal filling defects in the lymphogram. b Roentgenogram of the excised lymph node. c Histologic preparation (10× enlargement). The lymphatic tissue of the central parts of the node is replaced by connective and fatty tissue. Lymphatic structures are left only in the periphery of the node

groups at the level of L1/2 manifest similar but less extensive involutive changes (Figs. 2, 3). Fibrolipomatosis is more pronounced in patients of the middle and older age groups.

Inflammatory Disease

Classification of inflammatory reactions of lymph nodes ist best made on the basis of morphological change and not on the basis of etiology. The cellular reactions are not specific even though they might be characteristic for a certain group of agents (RÜTTNER, 1966). In lymphography, the observed patterns are necessarily less specific.

The morphologic alterations distinguished are hyperplastic inflammatory changes, granulomatous epitheloid cell changes and abscess-forming necrotizing changes.

Hyperplastic Inflammatory Changes

Inflammatory reaction of lymph nodes has been investigated by TJERNBERG (1956, 1959, 1962) by comparing lymphographic and histologic findings in animal experiments. The characteristic histologic changes were generalized hyperplasia of lymphatic

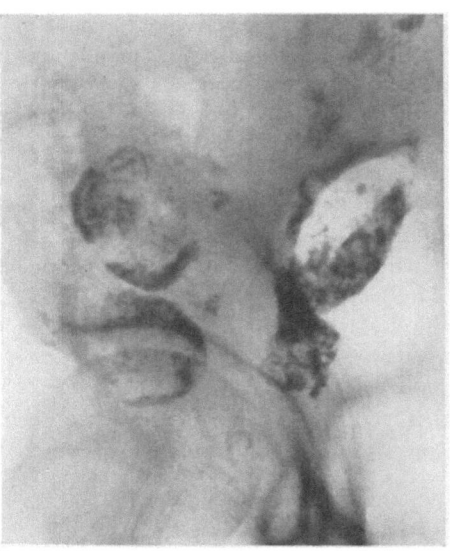 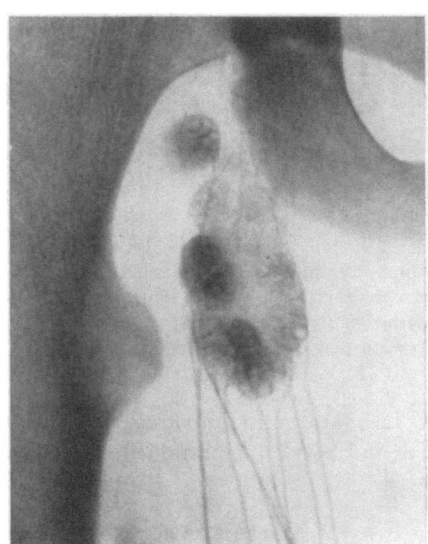

Fig. 3   Fig. 4

Fig. 3. *Fibrolipomatosis and reactive hyperplasia* in external iliac lymph nodes. Enlarged lymph nodes with extensive central filling defects due to fibrolipomatosis. Evenly distributed filling defect caused by follicular hyperplasia in the remaining lymphatic tissue (verified by biopsy)

Fig. 4. *Chronic hyperplastic inflammatory reaction* of inguinal lymph nodes. Enlarged lymph nodes with extensive filling defects caused by very large follicles (verified by biopsy)

tissue with consequent node enlargement and new lymph follicle formation. The newly formed follicles cause filling defects which alter the structural pattern seen in the lymphadenogram. The number and size of the follicles vary from node to node depending on the degree of the inflammatory reaction. Therefore, marked variations in the structural lymphographic architecture of the nodes arise.

The *lymphographic pattern* of an inflamed node resembles that of an enlarged node. However, a great variety of structural patterns in hyperplastic inflammatory disease is encountered. Large follicles and wide sinuses produce large filling defects within coarse opaque strands. An increase in follicle size will loosen up the storage pattern which, however, always presents a regular harmonious structure. In some cases extensive filling defects caused by very large follicles may dominate the lymphadenogram (Fig. 4). The storage phase of the lymph nodes is most often characterized by a reticular pattern in which contrast droplets are localized within small sinuses. When sinuses are wide, coarse droplets within them may dominate the lymphadenogram.

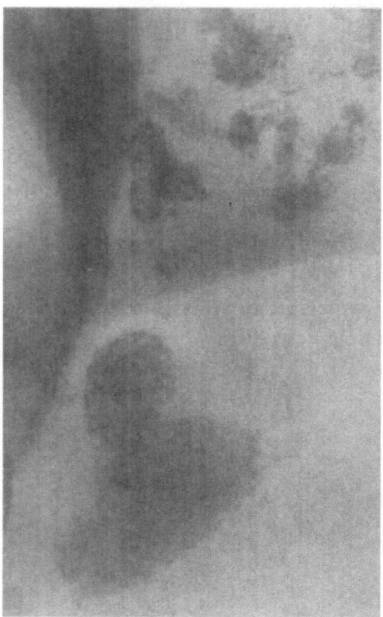

Fig. 5. *Rheumatoid arthritis*. Enlarged axillary lymph nodes with coarse reticular pattern in a patient with rheumatoid arthritis of 6 years duration (By Courtesy of M. Wiljasalo, M. D., Helsinki)

Hyperplastic inflammatory changes of lymph nodes occur as unspecific reactive phenomena in general infectious disease, infectious mononucleosis, measles, other viral infections and in both rheumatic arthritis and ankylosing spondylitis.

Wiljasalo et al. (1966) investigated 12 patients with *rheumatoid arthritis* and 12 suffering from *ankylosing spondylitis*. In rheumatoid arthritis, enlarged lymph nodes demonstrating a coarse reticular pattern were found in the node groups of the most severely affected joints (Fig. 5), and in ankylosing spondylitis, the lymph nodes in the region of the sacroiliac joints showed similar inflammatory changes (Fig. 6).

In *psoriatic arthropathy*, Viamonte et al. (1963) observed enlargement of the iliac and aortic lymph nodes as well as an increase in the size and number of lymph vessels.

Granulomatous Epitheloid Cell Inflammatory Changes

Granulomatous epitheloid cell reactions are encountered in chronic inflammatory diseases of widely varying etiology as listed below: tuberculosis, sarcoidosis, toxoplasmosis, brucellosis, lues, histoplasmosis, coccidiomycosis, blastomycosis, tularemia, leprosy, Crohn's disease and parasites.

Tuberculosis

Filling defects of various size in enlarged lymph nodes are the structural alterations of the lymphographic pattern encountered most often in tuberculosis. The multiple, well-demarcated central and marginal filling defects are due to the tuberculous granuloma. The pathologic lymph nodes are slightly enlarged and mainly situated within the aortic area. These changes are non-specific and may resemble malignancy. Cases have been observed by the author, in which large central and marginal filling defects in nodes that are only slightly enlarged or of normal size were found, thus making a conclusive diagnosis impossible prior to lymph node biopsy (Fig. 7). Case reports of lymphographic findings in tuberculosis of lymph nodes have been published by SCHAFFER et al. (1963), RÜTTIMANN (1964), BUSSAT

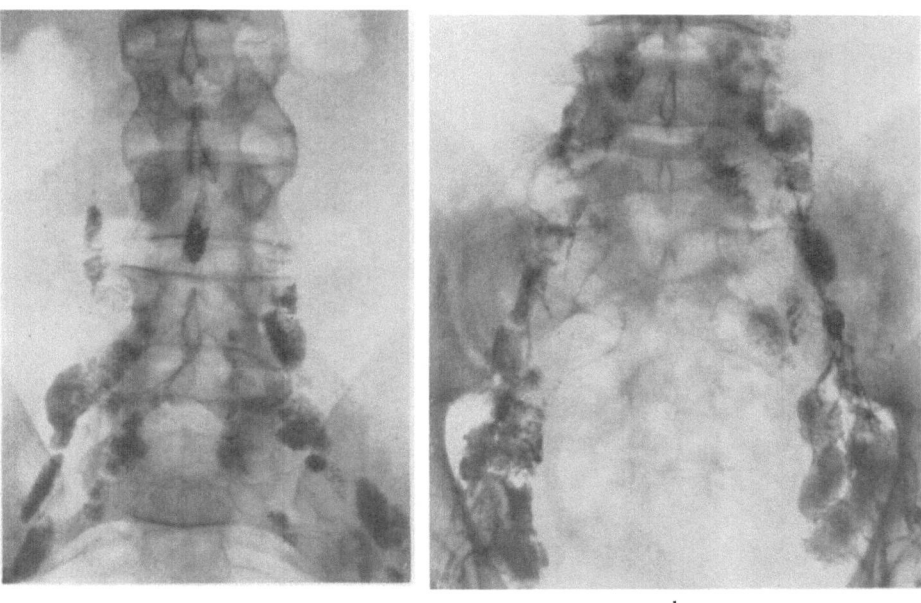

a   b

Fig. 6. *Ankylosing spondylitis.* a Enlarged aortic lymph nodes demonstrating a coarse reticular pattern due to follicular enlargement. Characteristic skeletal changes in the lumbar spine. b Coarse reticular pattern of the external and common iliac lymph nodes. Arthritis of the ileo-sacral joints (By Courtesy of M. WILJASALO, M. D., Helsinki)

et al. (1966). VIAMONTE et al. (1963) reported 3 positive lymphographic findings in 6 cases investigated by lymphography and stated that tuberculous adenitis may closely resemble metastatic carcinoma. Similar observations were made by BABEAU and FOURIER (1965) and DESPREZ-CURELY (1966).

ALBRECHT et al. (1967) investigated 15 patients with histologically verified tuberculosis of cervical lymph nodes. In 6 cases they were able to demonstrate slight enlargement of aortic nodes with multiple well-demarcated marginal and central filling defects. They observed similar lymph node patterns in tuberculous supraclavicular and cervical lymph nodes which were contrast-filled by foot lymphography BÉTOULIÈRES et al. (1968) report 7 cases of tuberculosis of the retroperitoneal lymph nodes investigated by lymphography and verified by biopsy. Three lymphograms showed changes similar to reactive hyperplasia, and in 4 patients well-demarcated filling defects in pelvic and aortic lymph nodes were seen.

Sarcoidosis

The lymphographic pattern of sarcoidosis has been described as similar to that of malignant lymphoma (VIAMONTE, 1963, 1966). ALBRECHT et al. (1967) investigated 20 patients with sarcoidosis but without the clinical signs of general lymph node enlargement. In 11 of these cases, lymphography revealed enlarged retroperitoneal lymph nodes. The node patterns manifested structural loosening because of lacunar filling defects and drop-like deposits of contrast material (Fig. 8). Similar observa-

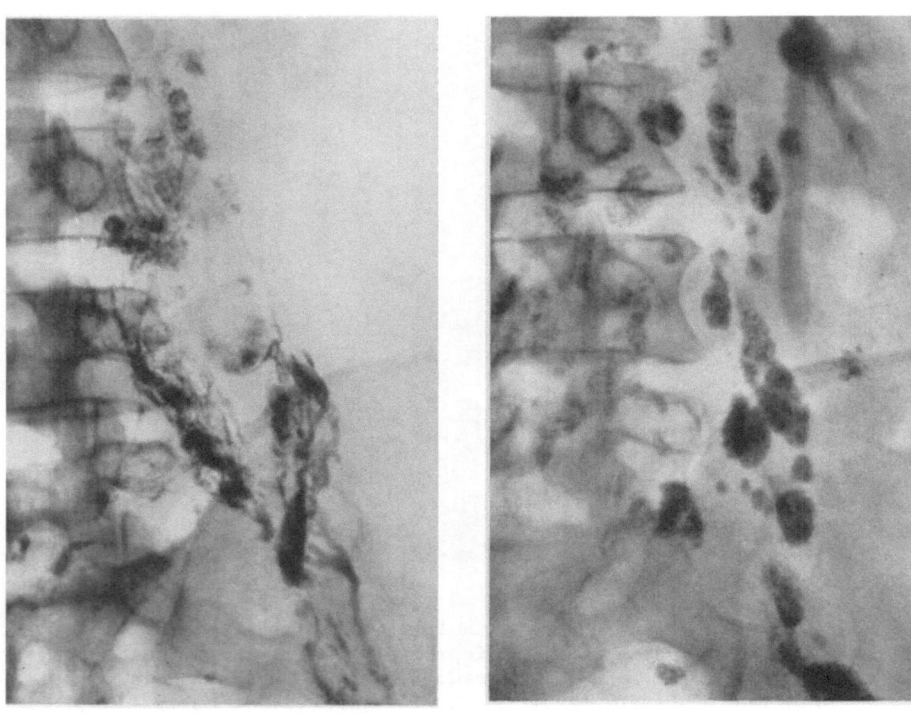

a   b

Fig. 7. *Tuberculosis* of the common iliac and aortic lymph nodes. a Enlarged lymph nodes containing large central filling defects with loosening of the storage pattern. Slight obstruction of the lymphatic circulation. b 2 months following tuberculostatic therapy: marked regression of the pathologic changes. Moderate hyperplasia of the common iliac and aortic lymph nodes

tions were made by SCHAFFER et al. (1963), RIEMANN (1965) and BASCA and MANDI (1966). STRICKSTROCK and WEISSLEDER (1968) discuss the lymphographic criteria in 4 patients with sarcoidosis of which 3 had a pathologic lymphadenogram of the retroperitoneal lymph nodes. The authors state that differentiation from malignant lymphoma is extremely difficult. They do not recommend routine lymphography in cases with histologically verified diagnosis of pulmonary sarcoidosis, since the demonstration of retroperitoneal lymph node disease is of no therapeutic consequence. The high frequency of involvement of retroperitoneal node groups is an interesting fact and is to be expected when considering sarcoidosis as a generalized disease. SILVER et al. (1966) report a case of sarcoidosis with retroperitoneal lymph node involvement and lymphedema of legs. Steroids produced an impressive clinical and radiologic improvement of the edema, suggesting that the extensive primary lymph node disease may be a significant factor in producing lymphedema.

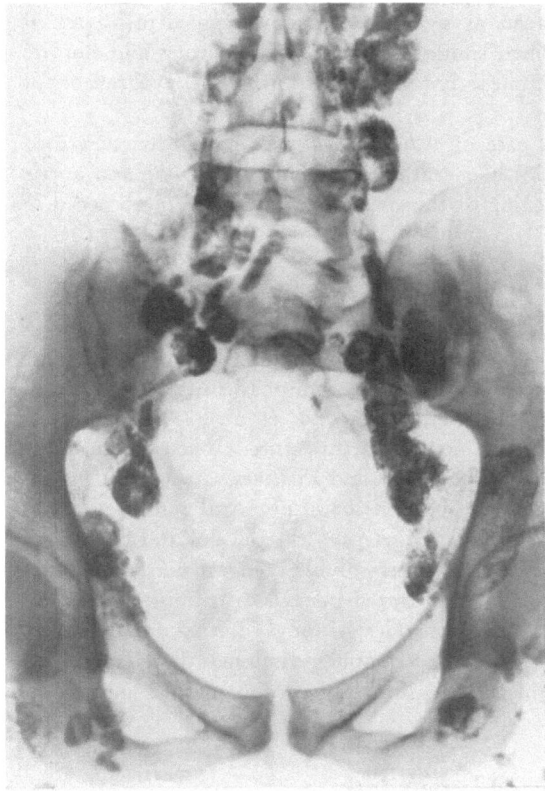
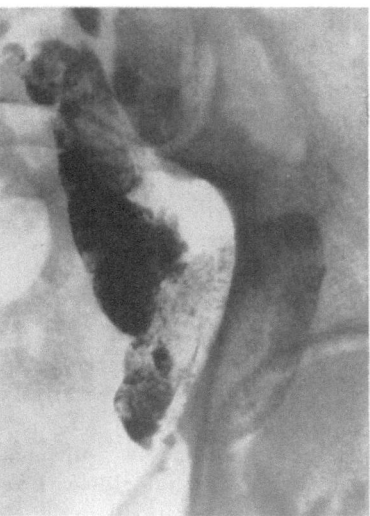

a   b

Fig. 8. *Sarcoidosis*. Enlarged iliac and aortic lymph nodes with structural loosening because of lacunar filling and drop-like deposits of contrast material (By Courtesy of V. TAENZER, M. D., and A. AL-BRECHT, M. D., Berlin)

Brucellosis, syphilis and leprosy have been seen to produce the same type of lymphographic pattern as non-specific inflammation, as concluded from the answers of a questionnaire at the First International Symposium on Lymphology in 1966. DESPREZ-CURELY (1966), however, reports a case of primary syphilis with invasion of a pelvic lymph node, which demonstrated irregular marginal filling defects similar to those of cancer metastases.

Histoplasmosis is claimed to produce lymph node involvement which is also similar in appearance to that of malignant lymphoma. VIAMONTE (1963, 1966) has observed non-specific hyperplastic inflammatory reactions.

The lymphographic pattern of *toxoplasmosis* is also that of a non-specific hyperplastic reaction.

Filariosis

In *Bancroft's filariosis* Montangerand et al. (1965) observed signs of reactive inflammatory reaction in early stages of the disease and poor filling of the lymph nodes when permanent chyluria and stasis of the lymph circulation were present due to extensive fibrosis in the final stages of filariosis. Da Rocha et al. (1965) investigated 50 patients with filariosis. The inguinal and pelvic lymph nodes were involved. Hyperplastic inflammatory changes were present in early disease; node enlargement and extensive filling defects as signs of fibrosis were seen in advanced cases. Kantekar et al. (1966) described similar reactive inflammatory and fibrotic alterations of inguinal and retroperitoneal lymph nodes during the progression of filariosis.

The lymphographic findings in a case of *Whipple's disease* have been described by Rüttimann and Del Buono (1962). General enlargement of the iliac and aortic lymph nodes, filling defects and loosening of the structural pattern were observed in some of the nodes.

Abscess Forming and Necrotizing Reactions

Abscess forming and necrotizing reactions develop in inguinal lymphogranuloma (Nicolas-Favre), cat scratch disease, abscess forming lymphadenitis. In a case of lymphadenitis secondary to cat scratch fever, Viamonte et al. (1963) described enlarged lymph nodes with maintained normal architecture. When suppuration occured, irregular filling defects were noted. Fischer and Zimmermann (1959) experimentally produced small sterile electrocautery abscesses in popliteal lymph nodes of dogs. Filling defects were observed in the lymphograms with ethiodol and thorotrast. Abscesses in lymph nodes were concealed by water-soluble contrast material due to its rapid diffusion. Malék et al. (1959) demonstrated uneven distribution of water-soluble contrast medium in popliteal lymph nodes of dogs due to inflammatory abscess formation. In a case of venereal inguinal lymphogranuloma Vessal·and Teller (1967) observed large central filling defects in enlarged subinguinal lymph nodes due to abscess formation.

Reactive Hyperplasia

Reactive hyperplasia is characterized histologically by a proliferative process in which histio-reticular and lymphocytic cells may take part. Hyperplasia may involve the medulla and cortex separately, but also medullary and follicular hyperplasia may be present simultaneously (Rüttner, 1966). The lymphographic node pattern of reactive hyperplasia is similar to that of unspecific hyperplastic inflammatory reaction. The large follicles and wide sinuses give rise to larger, evenly distributed filling defects. No impairment of the lymph circulation is present (Fig. 9).

Reactive hyperplasia is encountered in regional lymph nodes of primary tumors or of operation sites and should be regarded as a reactive change induced by inflammatory toxic products and metabolic agents of tumor cells. The presence of reactive hyperplasia in regional lymph nodes of a primary tumor implies the presence of a defense mechanism within these nodes.

Reactive hyperplasia of cervical lymph nodes differs from that of other regional lymph nodes by producing obstruction of the lymphatic flow. Investigations by FISCH (1966, 1968), showed that partial contrast-filling of a lymph node and obstruction of

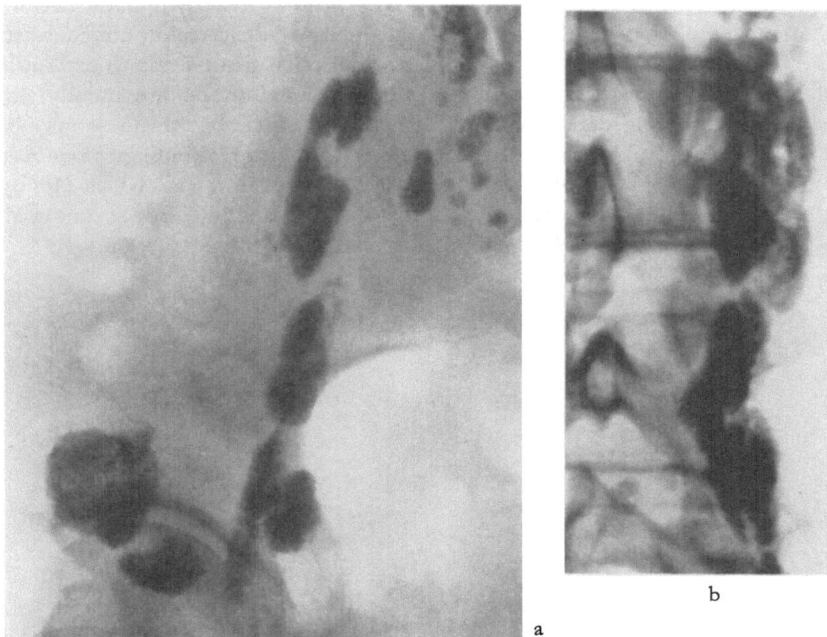

b

a

Fig. 9. *Reactive hyperplasia.* a Enlarged external iliac (lacunar) lymph nodes. Homogenous storage pattern. b Enlarged aortic lymph nodes. Lymphoma-like storage pattern (embryonal carcinoma of the right testis)

the lymph flow were caused by a compact mass of reticulum cells and fibres within the sinuses or by compression of the sinuses after follicular hyperplasia. Similar changes have been observed in inguinal, retroperitoneal and axillary lymph nodes. The reason for this important difference has not yet been clarified.

Retroperitoneal Fibrosis

Idiopathic retroperitoneal fibrosis, first described by ORMOND in 1948, is a relatively uncommon clinical entity. The etiology of this disease is still unknown, but it may be considered to be a hypersensitivity or auto-immune phenomenon. Dysfunction of cholesterin metabolism is concommitant.

Microscopic investigation reveals fibrous tissue and granulomatous fibroblastic areas containing reticulo-histiocytes, lymphocytes and plasma cells. Secondary fatty degeneration of these cells due to deposits of lipids may occur.

The clinical symptoms are non-specific and irreversible, renal damage may result before a diagnosis is made. Abdominal pain, anorexia, renal dysfunction, hypertension, anemia and dysproteinemia are suggestive diagnostic symptoms.

Conventional roentgen diagnostic methods give further information. Plain radiographs of the abdomen may demonstrate the absence of the normal contours of the psoas and lumbosacral muscles. Urography and retrograde pyelography reveal delayed excretion of contrast material, dilatation of the renal calices and renal pelvis or complete obstruction of one or both ureters. The ureters may taper gradually to the point of obstruction and deviate medially.

Lymphography reveals complete or partial obstruction of the lymphatic circulation. Collateral lymphatics within the pelvic and inferior aortic region are contrast-filled. Fibrotic induration of the retroperitoneal connective tissue leads to externisic compression of the lymphatics. The lymph vessels cranial to L4 are usually not visualized. Irregular filling defects within the iliac and aortic lymph nodes may be observed (Fig. 10). Several cases presenting these lymphographic findings have been reported by CLOUSE et al. (1964), RÜTTIMANN (1965), LEMMON and KISER (1966), HAHN (1966), SUBY et al. (1965), BELTZ and LYMBEROPOULOS (1966), BOOKSTEIN et al. (1966), VIRTAMA and HELELÄ (1967) and GREGL et al. (1967), BELTZ (1968).

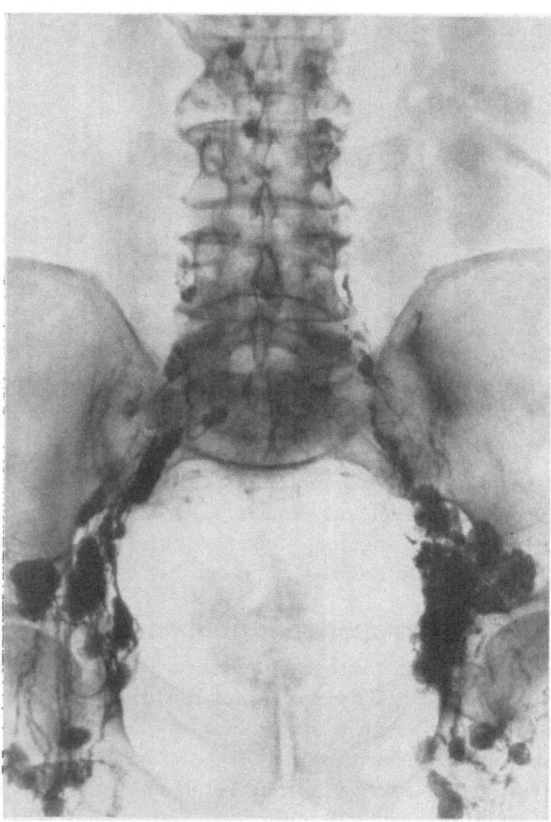

Fig. 10. *Retroperitoneal fibrosis.* Bilateral complete obstruction of the ureters. Contrast filling of the dilated left renal pelvis through nephrostomy. Partial obstruction of the lymphatic circulation. Collateral lymphatics within the pelvic and inferior aortic region. Poor visualization of lymph vessels cranical to L 4 (By Courtesy of L. BELTZ, M. D., Bonn)

Some of these authors stress the diagnostic importance of *cavography*. Dislocation, compression and complete obstruction resulting in extensive collateral circulation are the common features and are encountered most frequently at the level of L2/4.

Irradiation Fibrosis

The irradiation of lymph nodes causes the alteration and destruction of lymphocytes even when using such small doses as 50 to 800 R (COTTIER, 1966). Repopulation of the irradiated lymph nodes with lymphocytes from the circulating blood is a continuous process giving a false impression of lymph node regeneration (GOWANS, 1959). Circumscribed necrosis usually occurs when high irradiation doses are applied and additional vascular and inflammatory lesions are present. The sensitivity of lymphatics to irradiation is small. Slight changes in the lymph vessel wall occur when doses of 4000 R are applied. A high dosage of 15 000 R is necessary to significantly alter the lymphatic circulation (VAN DEN BRENK, 1957; SHERMAN and O'BRIEN, 1967). LENZI and BASSANI (1963) irradiated the uterine lymphatic system of the rabbit and found obstruction of the lymph vessels only when applying doses in the range of 25 000 R, which produced necrosis. The impairment of lymphatic circulation following irradiations is consequent mainly to scar formation in adjacent highly radio sensitive connective tissue (ZOLLINGER, 1960).

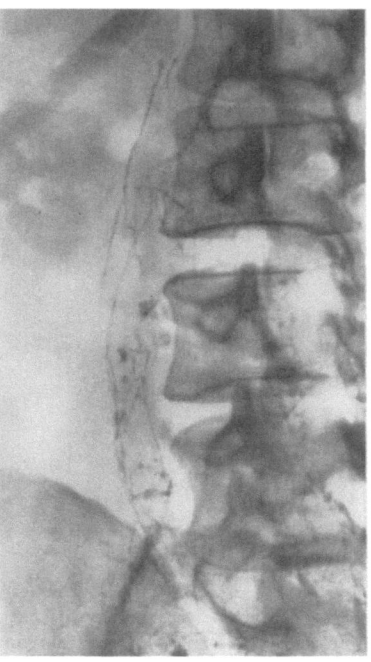

Fig. 11. *Irradiation fibrosis* of aortic lymph vessels and lymph nodes following 7500 rad. Multiple, fine lymphatics and small lymph nodes (32 year-old patient with Hodgkin's disease)

The effect of irradiation on lymph nodes has been investigated by lymphography in rats (ENGESET, 1961, 1963, 1964). The irradiated popliteal and retroperitoneal nodes were patent for more than 6 months and in a few cases even up to 22 months after irradiation with a single dose of 3000 R. One year after irradiation collateral lymph circulation by-passing the irradiated area was present because of subcutaneous scar formation. Histologic investigation of the lymph nodes on the first day after irradiation revealed a severe degeneration of lymphocytes, germinal centers and follicles. After 9—12 months the node was almost completely structureless demonstrating neither follicles nor sinuses. Simultaneously the connective tissue increased replacing lymphatic tissue of the nodes. Histologic reaction to local irradiation was uniform but secondarily a wide range of variation was still present possibly because of infection and secondary inflammation from the drainage area.

DETTMAN et al. (1966) could produce a slight decrease of the storage capacity for Au[198] in popliteal lymph nodes of dogs 6 months after 6000 R. They conclude that large doses, in the range of 10 000 R, are required to significantly alter lymphatics. AVERETTE and FERGUSON (1964) observed a significant impairment of the lymphatic circulation because of irradiation fibrosis and described extravasation of contrast material and formation of collateral circulation. LUDVIK et al. (1969) examined the effect of ionizing radiation on the lymphatic system in 47 patients by lymphography. Despite reduction in size of lymph nodes and narrowing of the lymphatics, stasis of lymph flow was seen only in the presence of radiation fibrosis of the connective tissue in the inguinal and pelvic areas.

Reviewing their clinical material, many authors (Fuchs, 1965; Rüttimann, 1965; Malina et al., 1965; Miceli et al., 1966; Wiljasalo and Perttala, 1966; Vuskanovic et al., 1966; Ariel et al., 1967; Beltz and Thurn, 1967) come to the

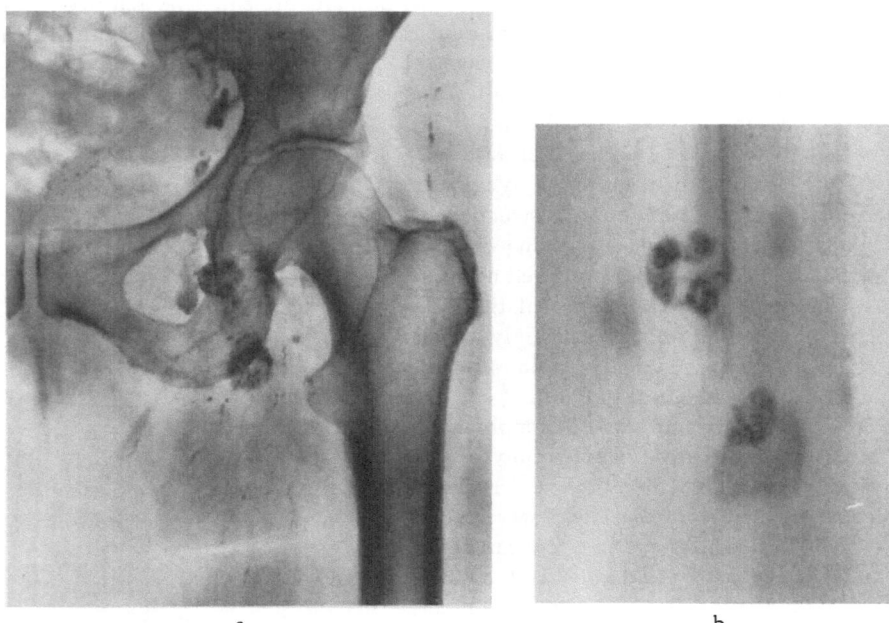

a   b

Fig. 12. *Irradiation fibrosis* of the left external iliac lymph nodes. Obstruction of the lymphatic circulation leading to collaterals. Reactive hyperplasia of deep inguinal lymph nodes confirmed by biopsy. 3 years following radiotherapy (7500 rad) of infiltrating cervical carcinoma. No symptoms of recurrence. a Filling phase. b Tomography of the deep inguinal lymph nodes (confirmed by biopsy)

same conclusion that no alterations of the lymphatic circulation occur in the normal and slightly altered lymphatic system when a therapeutic radiation dose is applied. Small delicate lymph vessels and small lymph nodes with structural patterns still intact are encountered (Fig. 11). The small irradiated lymph nodes are not able to retain large amounts of contrast material. Irradiation of lymph nodes and lymph vessels extensively infiltrated by malignant disease frequently causes partial or complete obstruction of the lymph vessels because of necrosis and secondary scar formation within the connective tissue of the pelvic region. Formation of a collateral circulation follows (Fig. 12). Complete fibrosis and replacement of the lymphatic tissue makes visualization of the lymph nodes impossible by lymphography. Secondary inflammations seem to play an important role in producing these obstructive fibrotic changes.

References

AKISADA, M., u. S. TANI: Filarial chyluria in Japan. Radiology 90, 311 (1968).

ALBRECHT, A., V. TAENZER u. H. NICKLING: Lymphographische Befunde bei Sarkoidose und Lymphknotentuberkulose. Fortschr. Röntgenstr. 106, 178 (1967).

AVERETTE, H. E., and J. H. FERGUSON: Lymphographic alterations of pelvic lymphatics after radiotherapy. J. Amer. Med. Ass. 186, 554 (1964).

ARIEL, I. M., M. I. RESNICK, and R. OROPEZA: The effects irradiation (external and internal) on lymphatic dynamics. Amer. J. Roentgenol. 99, 404 (1967).

BABEAU, P., and A. FOURIER: Rapport clinique de la lymphographie lipiodolée dans certaines formes de lymphadénite tuberculeuse. J. Belge Radiol. 48, 332 (1965).

BASCA, S., and L. MANDI: Lymphography in thoracic sarcoidosis. Orv. Hetil. 107, 1641 (1966).

BELTZ, L.: Retroperitoneale Fibrose. Radiol. Austriaca 1, 29 (1968).

—, u. S. LYMBEROPOULOS: Die retroperitoneale Fibrose. Urologe 5, 276 (1966).

—, u. P. THURN: Diagnose und Differentialdiagnose des Lymphangiogramms bei retroperitonealen Tumormetastasen. Fortschr. Röntgenstr. 107, 1 (1967).

BÉTOULIÈRES, P., J. L. LAMARQUE, J. F. GINESTIE et C. CAUBES: Etude des aspects lymphographiques de la tuberculose ganglionnaire. J. Radiol. 49, 1 (1968).

BOOKSTEIN, J. J., K. F. SCHROEDER, and J. G. BATSAKIS: Lymphangiography in the diagnosis of retroperitoneal fibrosis: Case report. J. Urol. (Baltimore) 95, 99 (1966).

BRENK, H. S. VAN DEN: Effect of ionizing radiation on mammalian lymphatics. Amer. J. Roentgenol. 78, 837 (1957).

BUSSAT, PH. L., J. M. BÉBOUX, J. PETITE, and P. WETTSTEIN: Lymphography in a patient with non-reactive tuberculosis. Amer. J. Roentgenol. 98, 436 (1966).

CLOUSE, M. E., E. E. FRALEY, and S. B. LITWIN: Lymphangiographic criteria for diagnosis of retroperitoneal fibrosis. Radiology 83, 1 (1964).

COTTIER, H.: Histopathologie der Wirkung ionisierender Strahlen auf höhere Organismen (Tier und Mensch). In: Encyclopedia of Medical Radiology II/2. Berlin-Heidelberg-New York: Springer 1966, p. 100.

DA ROCHA, R., A. DE SOURA, E. DA COSTA, and M. LEITAO: Quelques aspect lymphographiques dans la pathologie tropicale. J. Belge Radiol. 48, 275 (1965).

DESPREZ-CURELY, J. P.: Benign lymph node disease. Progress in Lymphology. p. 148. Stuttgart: G. Thieme 1967.

DETTMANN, P. M., E. R. KING, and Y. H. ZIMBERG: Evaluation of lymph node function following irradiation or surgery. Amer. J. Roentgenol. 96, 711 (1966).

DITCHEK, T., R. J. BLAHUT, and A. C. KITTLESON: Lymphadenography in normal subjects. Radiology 80, 175 (1963).

ENGESET, A.: Barrier function of lymph glands. Lancet 10, 324 (1962).

— Local röntgenbestraling av lymfeknuter. Nordisk Med. 70, 1127 (1963).

— Irradiation of lymph nodes and vessels. Acta Radiol. Suppl. 229 (1964).

FISCH, U.: Lymphography of the cervical lymphatic system. Philadelphia-London-Toronto: Saunders 1968.

FISCHER, H, W., M. S. LAWRENCE, and J. R. THORNBURY: Lymphography of the normal adult male. Radiology 78, 399 (1962).

—, and G. R. ZIMMERMANN: Roentgenographic visualization of lymph nodes and lymphatic channels. Amer. J. Roentgenol. 81, 517 (1959).

FUCHS, W. A.: Lymphographie und Tumordiagnostik. Berlin-Heidelberg-New York: Springer 1965.

—, A. RÜTTIMANN, and M. S. DEL BUONO: Zur Lymphographie bei chronischen sekundären Lymphödemen. Fortschr. Röntgenstr. 92, 608 (1960).

GOWANS, J. L.: The circulation of lymphocytes from blood to lymph in the rat. J. Physiol. (Lond.) 146, 54 (1959).

GREGL, A., F. TRUSS, F. GRABNER u. J. KIENLE: Lymphographie und Cavographie bei der idiopathischen retroperitonealen Fibrose. Fortschr. Röntgenstr. 107, 329 (1967).

HAHN, B. D.: The use of lymphangiography for the diagnosis of idiopathic retroperitoneal fibrosis. Amer. J. Obstet. Gynec. 14, 539 (1966).

Kantekar, A., S. M. Deshmukh, R. S. Pradhan, M. D. Kelkar, and P. K. Sen: Lymphographic patterns in filarial oedema of lower units. Clin. Radiol. 17, 258 (1966).

Lenzi, M., and G. Bassani: The effect of radiation on the lymph and on the lymph vessels.
Radiology 80, 814 (1963).

Lemmon, W. T., and W. S. Kiser: J. Urol. (Baltimore) 96, 658 (1966).

Ludvik, W., F. Wachtler und W. Zaunbauer: Veränderungen am Lymphogramm durch
Operation und ionisierende Strahlen. Fortschr. Röntgenstr. 110, 307 (1969).

Malék, P., J. Kolc u. J. Fischer: Veränderungen der Lymphknoten im Bilde der funktionellen zweiteiligen Lymphographie. Fortschr. Röntgenstr. 91, 1 (1959).

Malina, J., L. Brückner, F. Beška, J. Cerny u. J. Klega: Lymphographie nach durchgeführ-
ter Röntgenbestrahlung der Leisten- und Beckenlymphknoten. Radiol. Clin. Biol. (Basel)
34, 357 (1965).

Miceli, R., H. Corinaldesi e C. Rimondi: Modificazioni dei quadri linfografici iliaci e
lombo-aortici in seguito ad irradiazione. Radiol. Med. 51, 629 (1965).

Montangerand, Y., R. Huet et M. Fouques: La lymphographie dans les lymphoedemes des
membres de la filariose de Bancroft. Ann. Radiol. 8, 309 (1965).

Ormond, J. K.: J. Urol. (Baltimore) 59, 1072 (1948).

Riemann, H.: Lymphographische Befunde bei selteneren Erkrankungen. Radiologe 5, 333
(1965).

Rüttimann, A.: Die Lymphographie. In: Ergebnisse der medizinischen Strahlenforschung.
Neue Folge. Band I. Hrsg. Schinz-Glauner-Rüttimann. Stuttgart: Thieme 1964.

— u. M. S. Del Buono: Die Lymphographie mit öligem Kontrastmittel. Fortschr. Röntgenstr.
97, 552 (1962).

Rüttner, J. R.: Pathological anatomy of "benign" lymph node disease. Progress in Lymphology. pp. 98. Stuttgart: G. Thieme 1967.

Schaffer, B., P. R. Koehler, C. R. Daniel, G. T. Wohl, E. Rivera, W. A. Meyers, and
J. F. Skelley: A critical evaluation of lymphography. Radiology 80, 917 (1963).

Sherman, J. O., and P. H. O'Brien: Effect of ionizing irradiation on normal lymph vessels
and lymph nodes. Cancer 20, 1851 (1967).

Silver, H. M., N. T. Tsangaris, and D. M. Eaton: Lymphedema and lymphography in
sarcoidosis. Arch. int. Med. 117, 712 (1966).

Suby, H. J., W. S. Kerr, J. R. Graham, and E. E. Fraley: J. Urol. (Baltimore) 93, 144 (1965).

Strickstrock, K. H., u. H. Weissleder: Lymphographische Diagnose und Differentialdiagnose bei der Sarkoidose. Fortschr. Röntgenstr. 108, 576 (1968).

Tjernberg, B.: Lymphography as an aid to examination of lymph nodes. Acta Soc. Med.
upsalien. 61, 207 (1956).

— Lymphographie. Technik und diagnostische Möglichkeiten bei Entzündung und Karzinom-
metastasen. (Eine experimentelle Untersuchung.) In: IXth internal. Congr. Radiol. 1959 in
München, I. p. 404. Stuttgart: Thieme 1961.

— Lymphography. Acta Radiol. (Stockh.) Suppl. 214 (1962).

Vessel, K., u. H. Teller: Lymphographie und Lymphscintigraphie des Beckens bei Lympho-
pathia venerea im Bubonenstadium. Hautarzt 18, 256 (1967).

Virtama, P., and T. Helelä: Lymphography and cavography in retroperitoneal fibrosis.
Brit. J. Radiol. 40, 231 (1967).

Viamonte, M.: Lymphography in inflammatory conditions. Progress in Lymphology. Stuttgart: G. Thieme 1967.

—, D. Altman, R. Parks, E. Blum, M. Bevilaqua, and L. Recher: Radiographic-pathologic
correlation in the interpretation of lymphoangioadenograms. Radiology 80, 903 (1963).

Vuskanovic, M., M. Viamonte, and J. E. Martin: The place of lymphangioadenography in
the diagnosis and during the treatment of malignant diseases. Amer. J. Roentgenol. 96, 205
(1966).

Wiljasalo, M., H. Julkunen, and I. Salven: Lymphography in rheumatic diseases. Ann.
Med. int. Fenn. 55, 125 (1966).

—, and Y. Perttala: Lymphographic changes caused by radiotherapy. Ann. Med. int. Fenn.
55, 57 (1966).

Zollinger, H. U.: Radio-Histologie und Radiohistopathologie. In: F. Büchner, E. Lette-
rer und F. Roulet: Handbuch der Allgemeinen Pathologie X. Berlin: Springer 1960, S. 127.

Chapter 7

Diagnosis of Cancer Metastases in Lymph Nodes

W. A. Fuchs

With 78 Figures

Principles of Lymphographic Diagnosis

Formation of Cancer Metastases

Malignant metastatic spread in the lymphatic system has been investigated by ZEIDMAN and BUSS (1954), who injected tumor cells into afferent lymphatics of the popliteal node in rabbits, and by TJERNBERG (1956, 1959, 1962), who conducted similar experiments in rabbits and dogs using V²-carcinoma to evaluate the diagnostic possibilities of lymphography. The results of these studies indicate that lymph node metastases are formed by emboli of small groups of cancer cells which reach the marginal sinuses via afferent lymphatics. In the first stages of the disease tumor cells are deposited in a node in close proximity to the entry-points of the afferent lymph vessels and in the intermediary sinuses. With increasing growth of the malignant cell formation, irregular destruction of the marginal area of the affected lymph node is characteristic.

Further malignant infiltration of the node leads to compression of the lymphatic tissue, destruction of the capsule, and obliteration of the marginal sinus. Because malignant cells from a primary tumor reach a regional lymph node by way of numerous afferent lymphatics, multiple foci of malignant growth may implant in the periphery of the node. In advanced stages, the entire lymph node is infiltrated and the afferent lymphatics obstructed. Lymph flow is blocked, and a collateral circulation develops.

The possible pathways of malignant metastatic spread in the lymphatic system have been demonstrated by ENGESET (1959), LUDWIG (1962), STRÄULI (1962), WALLACE et al. (1964) and ARIEL et al. (1967). Metastases from a cancerous organ do not necessarily implant in the primary regional lymph nodes of the organ. Malignant infiltration may occur in only secondary and tertiary regional node groups. Primary regional lymph nodes may be by-passed via direct anastomoses between afferent and efferent lymphatics. Some of the major lymphatic channels may not be linked directly with the primary regional nodes. Also some of the intermediate sinuses in lymph nodes may be so large that they do not act as filters. Malignant metastases to non-regional lymph node groups may also occur when lymphatic vessels are obstructed. Consequent dilatation of the afferent lymphatics renders their valves incompetent and leads to retrograde flow, collateral lymph circulation and atypical metastatic spread. Lymphography has documented this process through visualization of the contrast-filled collaterals.

Lymphographic Findings

Malignant tissue is impervious to oily contrast media and only slightly pervious to water-soluble contrast agents. Consequently, tumor metastases in lymph nodes will appear as filling defects in the lymphadenogram. The form and size of metastatic foci in lymph nodes and the resulting shapes of the filling defects in the lymphadenogram vary considerably. Filling defects in lymph nodes are, however, not pathognomonic for cancer metastases. They appear in quite normal human lymph nodes, representing lymph follicles, in which case the defects are evenly round, regular and sharply demarcated. When the follicles are enlarged, as in inflammation of a node or in reactive hyperplasia, the defects appear larger on the lymphadenogram, but they retain their form and their regular distribution throughout the node. Filling defects are produced experimentally by small abscesses caused by staphylococcal toxin (MALEK et al., 1959) and by small sterile electrocautery abscesses (FISCHER and ZIMMERMANN, 1959).

Consequently, the diagnostic value of lymphography is limited from the outset. Distinction between metastatic foci and defects from other causes is difficult or even impossible in the early stage of a malignancy. Opinions on the minimum size of a cancer deposit recognizable on the lymphadenogram are basically similar: KOEHLER et al., 1964, in a survey of 22 investigatiors in the United States and Europe, reported minimum diameters of 2 to 10 mm; the International Symposium on Lymphology in Zurich in 1966 considered 5 mm the minimum size.

TJERNBERG (1962) offers the guide that tumor foci must be larger than the largest follicle in the affected node before lymphographic recognition is possible. The histopathologic investigations of GOFFRINI et al. (1961) indicate that even microradiography — with its inherent high resolution — does not enable identification of small neoplastic foci.

The size of lymph nodes affected by cancer spread is generally increased, particularly in fast growing tumors. The structure of the preserved lymphatic tissue is normal or slightly loosened because of reactive hyperplasia. However, the affected nodes may remain normal in size. WILJASALO (1965) describes an interesting analysis of lymph node measurement which he claims enables differentiation of malignant from non-malignant nodes. Those with metastases are found to be globular or cylindric, whereas normal or fibrolipomatous nodes are flat. A-p and both 45° oblique projections are made, and then the widths of the nodes are measured in each of the three projections. Normal nodes show a considerable variability in width in different projections — indicative of non-cylindric form — whereas the metastatic nodes exhibit greater uniformity. The variation is quantitated as the percentage of the minimum nodal width and is shown to exceed 20% for normal lymph nodes, and to lie below 20% for metastatic nodes. Sixty-two lymphograms showing signs of metastatic lymph node involvement were studied. Lymph node biopsy confirmed metastases in 70% of the total case material. The method was reported to be correct in identifying 97% of the normal and benign defective nodes and 92% of the metastatic nodes. In view of the results, the technique seems to be of value when malignant metastatic spread is suspected. However, the degree of malignant involvement must be considerable before the size and shape of a lymph node are altered, and other diagnostic signs such as confluent marginal filling defects, node enlargement, and statis of the afferent lymphatics may then lead to a conclusive diagnosis.

The filling defects of malignancy are best demonstrated in lymphadenograms made during the storage phase, applying tangential projections and tomography. The genesis of cancer metastases leads to their peripheral deposition in a node, hence the filling defects are commonly located peripherally and not at the hilus of the nodes. Identification of the hilar region is made through its association with the efferent lymphatics, whereas the afferents empty into the peripherally situated marginal sinus. Distinction of afferent and efferent lymphatics is facilitated by analysis of both filling-phase and storage-phase roentgenograms, and for this reason combined evaluation is of particular importance.

The filling defects of fibrolipomatosis are produced by connective and fatty tissue replacements of lymphatic tissue. The central areas of the lymph node are involved predominantly, hence the defects are seen in the hilar region. Their contours are irregular, in contrast to any metastatic foci which may happen to be centrally located. As a rule though, metastases are highly unlikely if filling defects are limited exclusively to the hilar region. On the combined evidence of localization and contour appearance, the distinction between fibrolipomatoses and cancer metastases is made reliably in most cases. However, interpretation of inguinal and axillary lymph nodes may be very difficult because involutive changes in these node groups are common findings. The technique of postlymphographic control films [1] enables the disease and its therapy to be followed. Doubtful lymphographic diagnoses may be confirmed at a later date at which time enlargement of previously normal nodes or appearance of new filling defects may be seen. The method is described in detail in Chapter 9.

Differentiation between certain histologic types of carcinoma on the basis of the topographic arrangement of filling defects caused by metastatic foci within lymph nodes seems to be impossible because the process of malignant metastatic spread into regional lymph nodes is independent of the histologic type of a malignant tumor. But the growth rate of the malignant tissue depends on its histologic structure, and a degree of differentiation on the basis of the growth rate should be possible. Measurement of the node size-doubling time yields additional information on the biologic behavior of certain types of carcinoma (MAC DONALD et al., 1968). The number of malignant cells deposited within a lymph node may be another important factor influencing the lymph node architecture and facilitating diagnosis. For example, in malignant melanoma, central filling defects within enlarged lymph nodes are frequent findings, not commonly seen in other histological types of lymph node metastases. The central position of the defects may be explained by the fact that the number of tumor cells invading the lymphatic system is particularly large. The numerous malignant cell groups are deposited not only within the marginal sinuses of a lymph node but may invade the entire node leading to large central filling defects in the lymphogram.

---

[1] "Control film" as used throughout the text is identical to "follow-up film".

Dislocation of Lymph Vessels and Lymph Nodes

In view of the great normal anatomic variation of the lymph system, dislocation of lymph vessels and lymph nodes is of limited value in the diagnosis of malignant involvement. Topographic lines of reference such as proposed by Viamonte (1967) have been established to localize certain groups of lymphatics and lymph nodes.

The diagnostic value of such boundary lines is limited, however, because of the dislocation of lymph vessels and lymph nodes associated with tortous arteries and innumerable anatomic variations.

Obstruction of the Lymphatic Circulation

The main cause of obstruction of lymph flow is malignant infiltration of lymph nodes and lymphatic vessels. Non-specific reactive hyperplasia may also lead to blockage as demonstrated by Fisch (1968) in the cervical lymph nodes. Lymphangitis and chronic inflammation of lymph nodes may cause secondary lymphedema, and retroperitoneal fibrosis is etiologic for obstruction. Surgical excision of lymph nodes, particularly if combined with wound infection or radiation therapy, may interfere with the regeneration of lymph vessels, and radiotherapy alone of areas invaded by malignant growth will also cause blockage. However, irradiation of normal lymphatic structures does not interrupt the lymphatic circulation. Consequently, differentiation between recurrent malignant disease and post-therapeutic sequelae may become extremely difficult or even impossible.

Lymph stasis is visualized on the lymphogram as dilated afferent lymphatics which remain contrast-filled 24 hours after injection. Node groups distal to the site of obstruction are not demonstrated when blockage is complete. A stenosis of the vessel just before the occlusion is also a common finding. Impeded flow results in increased intralymphatic pressure, and extravasation of contrast medium may occur during injection. In addition a collateral circulation by-passing the obstruction develops, so that lymph vessels appear which are not normally visible. The collaterals are contrast-filled by a reversed flow, consequent to the process of lymph stasis, vessel dilatation and the resulting valve insufficiencies. Collateral lymph flow in perivascular fibrous sheaths (Herman et al., 1964) and perineural sheaths (Wallace et al., 1964), is occasionally observed. However, differentiation of these conditions from simple extravasation may be difficult.

In obstruction of the lymphatic circulation direct connections between the lymphatic and venous systems are opened. These *lymphatico-venous anastomoses* serve as functionally significant collaterals, and during lymphography, contrast agent injected into the lymph vessels enters the venous system directly. Lymphatico-venous connections to the caval system lead to pulmonary oil embolism. Direct shunts to the portal system produce embolism in the small intrahepatic branches of the portal vein. Consequently, lymphography must be performed with a minimal amount of contrast agent in all cases of clinically suspected lymphatic obstruction.

Recognition of intravenous contrast material is possible on the filling-phase roentgenograms. By conglomeration of the oil droplets, their particle size becomes too large to be carried away by the venous circulation. The oil droplets are trapped within the lumens of small veins and can be recognized on the lymphogram. Differentiation of intravascular oil droplets from extravasated contrast material may be difficult.

Topographic Anatomy of Collateral Lymphatic Circulation

The type of collateral circulation is determined by the topographic-anatomic localization of lymphatic obstruction.

Blockage of a subcutaneous lymph vessel group in the *lower extremity* leads to the formation of collaterals in unaffected areas. Obstruction of the lymph vessels of the saphena magna region introduces lymphatic collaterals in the saphena parva region and vice versa. Additional cutaneous, subcutaneous, interstitial and deep collateral lymphatics are commonly filled with contrast material.

Obstruction of the lymph flow in the *inguinal region* will cause collaterals via subcutaneous lymphatics in the thigh, the outer genital organs (scrotum, vulva), across the perineum to the opposite side, and in lymphatics of the lateral and medial aspects of the anterior abdominal wall.

Interruption of the lymphatic circulation in one of the *external iliac lymph node chains* leads to collateral circulation via the remaining patent external iliac lymphatics. Lymph vessels situated medially in the pelvic region serve as collaterals to the contralateral side.

Lymph vessels of the urinary bladder, uterus and rectum may also act as collaterals. Laterally situated collateral lymphatics of the lower lumbar region are frequently observed. Extravasation of contrast agent into the abdominal cavity and the lumen of pelvic organs may occasionally be demonstrated by lymphography. In rare cases direct collaterals to the axillary region are formed. In subtotal and total blockage of the lymphatic circulation in the common iliac lymph node group, retroperitoneal lymph vessels and nodes in the parietal lumbar region act as collaterals. Aortic lymph nodes distal to the obstruction site may then be contrast-filled via these particular groups of lymphatics.

Obstruction of the *aortic lymph vessels and nodes* produces collateral circulation to lymph vessels of the contralateral side. The unaffected lymph nodes situated distal to the malignant infiltration are usually filled with contrast medium. The extent of collateral formation in the retroperitoneal and inguinal region depends mainly on the degree of obstruction of the lymph flow. In the case of circumscribed lymphatic obstruction, collaterals via slightly dilated and displaced neighboring lymph vessels and nodes of the same group are established. Anatomic variations, especially the non-filling of the right aortic node group, are of special practical interest and must be ruled out with certainty, utilizing cavography and urography. Dislocation of lymph vessels and nodes because of elongated arteriosclerotic abdominal vessels may also pose diagnostic problems. Obstruction of the *thoracic duct* leads to dilatation of the cisterna chyli and the lumbar trunks. Valvular insufficiency develops, and reflux of lymph may occur to the intestinal, pleural, peritoneal, renal and hepatic lymphatics with consequent chylothorax, chylascites and chyluria. Lymphography demonstrates extravasation of contrast material into the pleural and peritoneal cavities and to the renal pelvis. Contrast-filling of collateral intercostal lymph channels and axillary lymphatics is occasionally observed. Lymphatico-venous anastomoses to the inferior and superior vena cava and the portal venous system frequently occur. The mechanisms of collateral circulation in obstruction of the thoracic duct have been studied experimentally by ligation of the thoracic duct in dogs (TAKASHIMA and BENNINGHOFF, 1966). The results of these investigations reproduce exactly the pathophysiologic data observed in malignant obstruction of the thoracic duct and resemble those seen in congenital lymphatic malformation.

Topographic Anatomy of Regional Lymph Nodes

Exact knowledge of the topographic anatomy of the regional lymph nodes likely to be involved in the metastatic spread of a primary tumor is of great importance. Diagnostic evaluation of a lymphogram must be directed towards the closest regional lymph node group that is contrast-filled by the conventional technique of lymphography. Certain lymph node groups are not contrast-filled by lymphography and some only occasionally, because they do not receive afferent lymphatics connected with the subcutaneous lymph vessels into which contrast material is injected. In addition, because of frequent anatomic variations, failure to demonstrate certain lymph node groups cannot be taken as evidence for malignant infiltration, particularly if no signs of lymphatic obstruction are present. These particular lymph nodes are usually the primary regional nodes of an organ and are situated close to it. These node groups are commonly involved at an earlier stage in metastatic spread from carcinoma, and early diagnosis of metastases is therefore limited for anatomic reasons. However, it must be stressed that lymphography does detect early metastases which would be unsuspected clinically, because it enables demonstration of metastatic spread to contrast-filled regional lymph nodes. Suspicious changes within the nodes of these node groups should be considered carefully, and additional investigations such as tomography and control studies must be applied. Filling defects and other alterations of the node storage pattern in lymph node groups not localized within the regional lymph drainage area of the organ affected by the carcinomatous growth may be given less attention. However, rare concomittant primary malignant involvement of the lymphatic system should be considered. In contrast, all lymph node groups, whether of primary, secondary or tertiary order must be checked carefully, because metastases may occur in lymph nodes of secondary and tertiary order even if those of the primary order do not present abnormalities in the lymphogram. Metastatic spread to lymph node groups situated outside the drainage area of the particular organ affected by the malignant tumor are to be expected in the presence of lymphatic obstruction due to the altered lymphatic dynamics: tumor cells may be deposited in lymph nodes of the regions involved in the collateral circulation.

References

ARIEL, I. M., and M. I. RESNICK: Altered lymphatic dynamics caused by cancer metastases. Arch. Surg. 941, 117 (1967).

ENGESET, A.: The route of peripheral lymph to the blood stream. An X-ray study of the barrier theory. J. Anat. (Lond.) 93, 96 (1959).

FISCH, U.: Lymphography of the cervical lymphatic system. Philadelphia-London-Toronto: Saunders 1968.

FISCHER, H. W., and G. R. ZIMMERMANN: Roentgenographic visualization of lymph nodes and lymphatic channels. Amer. J. Roentgenol. 81, 517 (1959).

GOFFRINI, P., P. BOBBIO, G. PERACCHIA e F. PELLEGRINO: Presentazione di un metodo còmparativa anatomo-linfografico per lo studio della patologia del linfonodo con particolare riguardo a quella tumorale. Arch. ital. Chir. 87, 613 (1961).

HERMAN, P. G., and S. SCHWARZ: A physiologic approach to lymphflow in lymphography. Amer. J. Roentgenol. 91, 1207 (1964).

KOEHLER, R. P., G. T. WOHL, and B. SCHAFFER: Lymphangiography — a survey of its current status. Amer. J. Roentgenol. 91, 1216 (1964).

LUDWIG, J.: Über Kurzschlußwege der Lymphbahnen und ihre Beziehungen zur lymphogenen Krebsmetastasierung. Path. et Microbiol. (Basel) 25, 329 (1962).

MACDONALD, J. S., A. LANGIER, and M. SCHLIENGER: Observations on the growth of tumours in lymph nodes changing from normal to abnormal while remaining opacified after lymphography. Clin. Radiol. 19, 20 (1968).

MALEK, P., and A. BELAN: Lymphography of the deep lymphatic system of the thigh. Acta radiol. (Stockh.) 51, 442 (1959).

STRÄULI, P.: Erreichte und erstrebte Ziele der Metastasenforschung. Oncologia (Basel) 15, 123 (1962).

TAKASHIMA, T., and D. L. BENNINGHOFF: Lymphatic venous communications and lymph reflux after thoracic duct obstruction. An experimental study in the dog. Invest. Radiol. 1, 188 (1966).

— — Effects of experimental thoracic duct obstruction in the dog. II. Chylous reflux. Invest. Radiol. 1, 449 (1966).

TJERNBERG, B.: Lymphography as an aid to examination of lymph nodes. Acta Soc. Med. upsalien. 61, 207 (1956).

— Lymphography. Acta. radiol. (Stockh.) Suppl. 214 (1962).

VIAMONTE, M.: Discussion note. Progress in Lymphology. p. 69. Stuttgart: G. Thieme 1967.

WALLACE, S., L. JACKSON, G. D. DODD, and R. R. GREENING: Lymphatic dynamics in certain abnormal states. Amer. J. Roentgenol. 91, 1187 (1964).

ZEIDMAN, I., and J. M. BUSS: Experimental studies on the spread of cancer in the lymphatic system. I. Effectivness of the lymph nodes as a barrier to the passage of embolic tumor cells. Cancer Res. 14, 403 (1954).

Female Genital Organs

Carcinoma of the Uterine Cervix

Anatomy of the Regional Lymph Nodes (Fig. 1)

Numerous lymphatics arise on either side of the uterine cervix at various levels and collect into about 8—11 larger lymph channels containing numerous valves. Within the broad ligament they assemble into larger ducts leading in various directions towards the regional lymph nodes. The main lymphatics run alongside the uterine artery and anterior to the ureter towards the obturator and the external iliac lymph nodes, close to the bifurcation of the common iliac artery. Other important drainage areas of the uterine cervix are the superior and inferior gluteal lymph nodes. Some lymph vessels lead directly to the lateral and medial common iliac nodes. Wide lymphatics follow the medial margin of the parietal lymph vessels of the pelvis towards the precaval, preaortic and aortic lymph nodes below the level of the inferior mesenteric artery. Other lymph vessels run to the lateral sacral and superior rectal lymph nodes.

Lymphographic observation of the regional lymph nodes of the uterine cervix is confined to the external and common iliac and aortic lymph nodes. All other reginal groups are not demonstrated by foot lymphography.

Lymphographic Diagnosis

The main purpose of the author's investigation was to detect early malignant lymph node metastases. Therefore, two thirds of the 145 patients studied by lymphography were classified as in clinical stages I and II. The roentgenologic diagnoses in 57 patients were verified by lymph node excision, and in the remaining 88 cases the

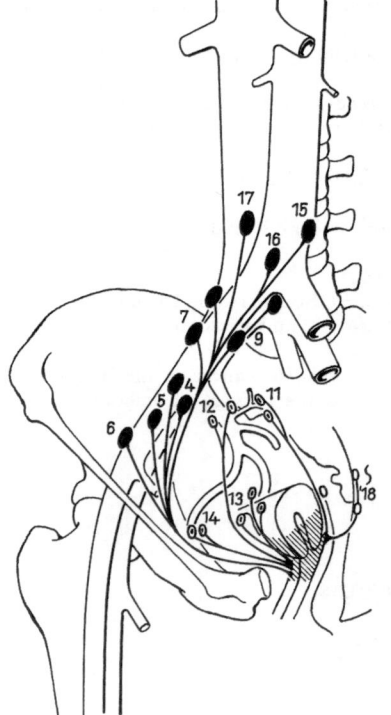

4 Medial external iliac lymph nodes
5 Intermediate external iliac lymph nodes
6 Lateral external iliac lymph nodes
7 Lateral common iliac lymph nodes
9 Medial common iliac lymph nodes
11 Lateral sacral lymph nodes
12 Superior gluteal lymph nodes
13 Inferior gluteal lymph nodes
14 Obturator lymph nodes
15 Left aortic lymph nodes
16 Pre-retroaortic lymph nodes
17 Right aortic lymph nodes
18 Superior rectal lymph nodes

● Routinely demonstratet by lymphography;
⊖ Facultatively demonstrated by lymphography; ○ Not demonstrated by lymphography

Fig. 1. *Anatomy of the regional lymph nodes of the uterine cervix*

lymphographic results were compared and evaluated with the results of cavography and with the clinical course of the disease.

In a total of 40 patients (27%) malignant lymph node metastases or direct tumor infiltration of the pelvic lymphatic system were correctly diagnosed. Eighty-three negative lymphographic findings (57%) proved to be accurate. Fourteen of the positive lymphographs, mainly in cases of clinical stage I and II, were verified histologically by extraperitoneal lymph excision or radical hysterectomy, and 26 positive results were proved correct by the subsequent fatal course of the disease or by indirect radiologic methods such as cavography and urography. Four lymphographies were diagnosed as normal, and in 3 of these cases, malignant metastases in the obturator and gluteal lymph nodes, not demonstrable by lymphography, were found at opera-

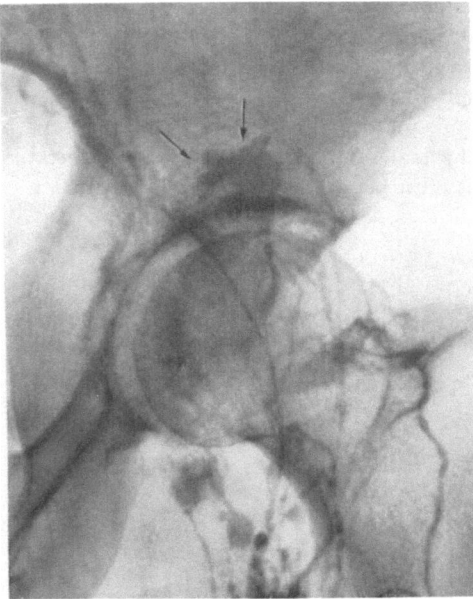

Fig. 2. *Carcinoma of the cervix, stage II*. Metastases in a lateral external iliac lymph node. Numerous marginal filling defects caused by metastatic foci (→) (verified by lymph node excision)

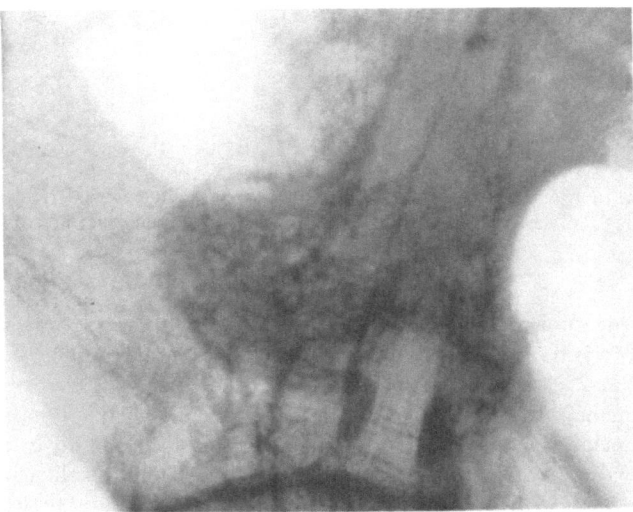

Fig. 3. *Carcinoma of the cervix, stage III*. Metastases in an enlarged lateral external iliac lymph node. Numerous small filling defects caused by metastatic foci (verified by lymph node excision)

tion. In 1 patient, histologic investigation revealed metastases of microscopic size within the external iliac lymph nodes. Malignant involvement of the external iliac lymph nodes was diagnosed in 3 cases: 1 in stage I and 2 in stage II, in which only chronic inflammatory and fibrolipomatous lesions were found at operation. Sixteen patients with clinically advanced malignant involvement of the parametria reaching the pelvic wall had a normal lymphogram, although metastatic spread to the external iliac lymph nodes must be assumed to have been present.

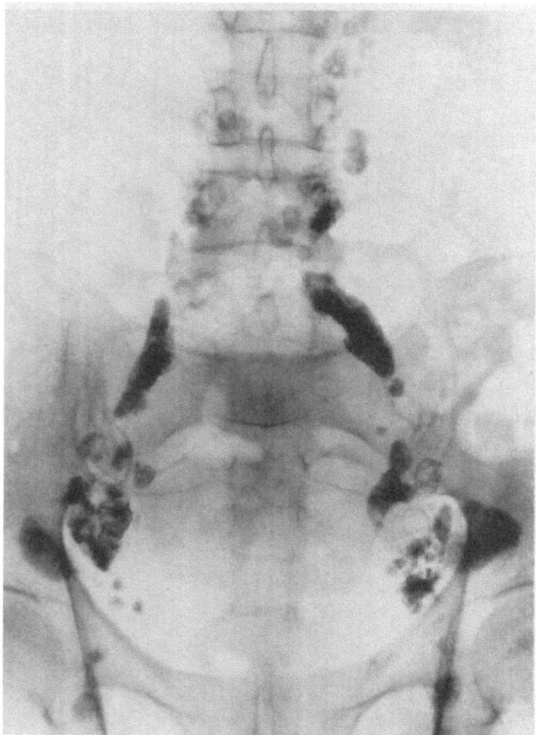

Fig. 4. *Carcinoma of the cervix, stage II*. Bilateral metastases in external iliac lymph nodes. Reactive hyperplasia of the common iliac and aortic lymph nodes (verified by lymph node excision)

In 11 cases of clinical stage I and II, metastatic malignancy was diagnosed in the absence of positive clinical findings. Positive lymphographic diagnosis was proved correct in 7 cases by histologic findings, and 4 lymphograms were characteristic of malignancy. In 2 of these latter patients, in which pelvic lymphadenectomy was performed prior to lymphography, malignant metastatic spread to aortic lymph nodes at the level of L 4 was demonstrated. The topographic localization of lymph node metastases showed the following pattern: in 22 cases unilateral (Figs. 2, 3) and in 5 cases bilateral metastatic spread to the iliac lymph nodes was observed (Fig. 4). The lower aortic lymph nodes alone were infiltrated by metastatic cancer in 5 cases (Fig. 5). Malignant involvement of both the iliac and aortic lymph node groups was found in 8 cases, all of which had progressed to stage III and IV (Fig. 6). Obstruction of the lymphatic circulation was present in 9 patients with stage III cancer and in 5 patients with stage IV cancer (Figs. 7, 8).

To summarize: in a total of 145 patients with carcinoma of the cervix, the roentgenologic diagnosis was correct in 122 cases; in 23 cases it was misleading or wrong, corresponding to a failure rate of 16%. Metastatic involvement of regional lymph nodes was revealed by lymphography in 11 of 95 patients (12.5%) with stage I and II cancer, in 16 of 33 patients (48.5%) with stage III cancer, and in 12 of 17 patients (70%) with stage IV cancer.

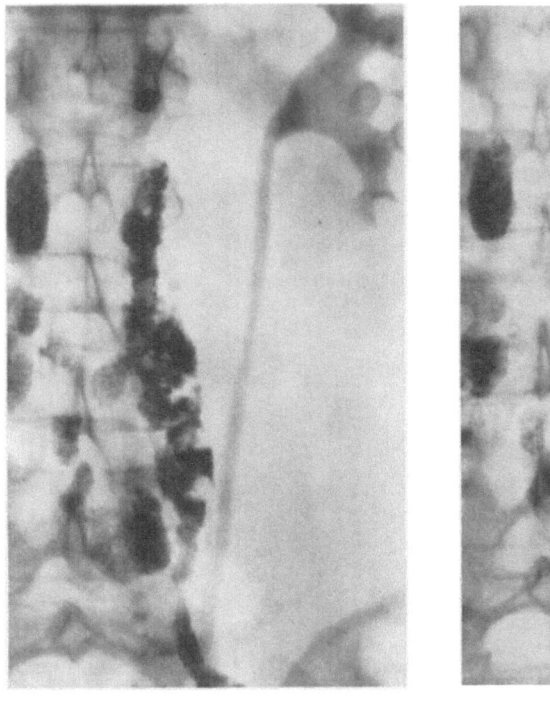 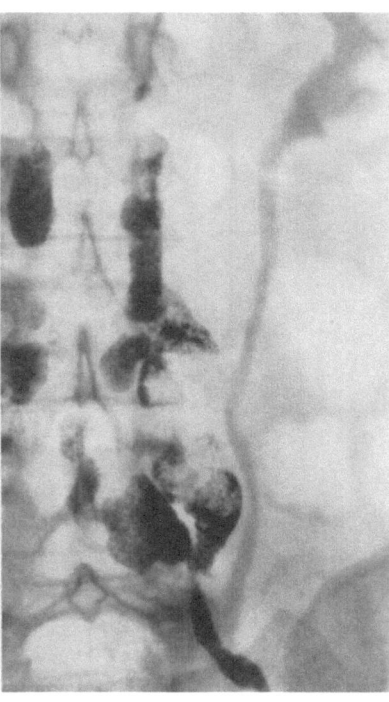

a   b

Fig. 5. *Carcinoma of the cervix, stage I.* a Metastases in left latero-aortic lymph nodes. b Increase in size of the lymph nodes caused by malignant growth during 9 months without treatment. Dislocation of the left ureter

The frequency of metastatic spread to the regional lymph nodes demonstrated by lymphography has also been studied by GERTEIS (1966). Of his 181 cases in clinical stage I, 24% showed involvement of pelvic and aortic lymph nodes and 9% of aortic lymph nodes alone. In 33% of 124 cases in clinical stage II, lymphography demonstrated metastases to the pelvic and aortic nodes and in 5% to the aortic nodes alone. Of 84 patients in clinical stage III, 56% demonstrated metastases to the pelvic and aortic lymph nodes and 21% to the aortic lymph nodes, and in 15 patients in stage IV, 80% manifested positive lymphographic findings within the pelvic and aortic node groups. Interpreting these results, one must consider that GERTEIS (1966) claims that the diagnostic accuracy of lymphography is 96% in a series of more than 3000 histologically examined lymph nodes. The high percentage of lymph node metastases (24%) seen in the first clinical stage is remarkable, and the frequency of 9% for involvement of aortic lymph nodes is particularly so. KUNITSCH and HOLSTEN (1968) investigated 293 patients with cervical carcinoma by lymphography. Lymph node metastases were found in 13 of 109 patients in stage I (12%), 36 of 86 in stage II (41%), in 20 of 31 in stage III (65%) and in 2 of 3 in stage IV. In a comparative study of lymphographic and histologic findings in 43 patients with stage I carcinoma, WOLFF et al. (1968) state that in 33 cases without metastatic

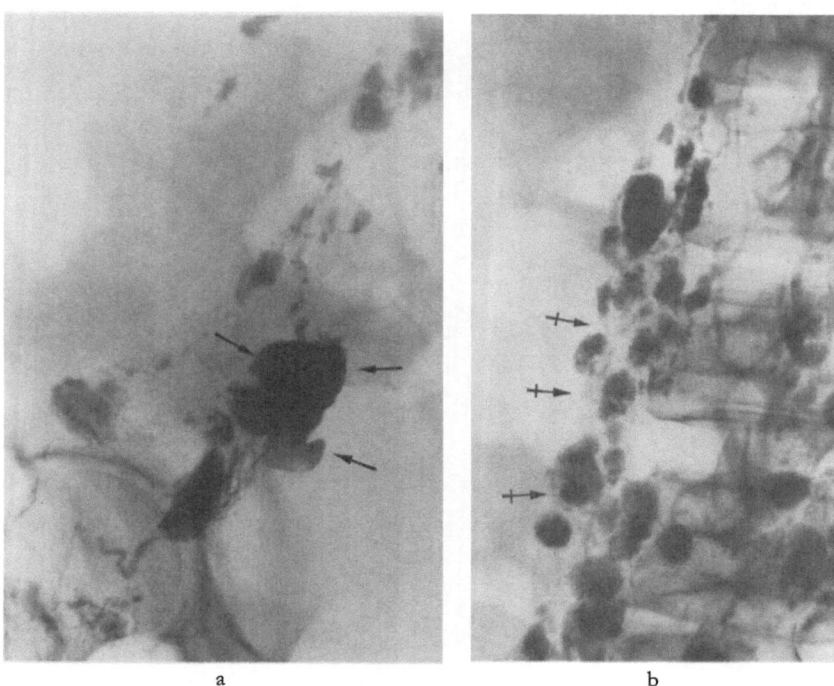

a   b

Fig. 6. *Carcinoma of the uterine cervix, stage III.* a Postoperative lymph cyst in the right external iliac region (→). b Marginal filling defects in right aortic lymph nodes indicating metastatic foci (↦)

involvement of the lymph nodes, one false positive was found, and in 6 of 10 cases with lymph node metastases the radiologic assessment was falsely negative. DARGENT (1963) reports 19 misinterpretations of the lymphographic findings in 62 cases; ABBES (1963) reports 7 in 16 cases. CHAVANNE et al. (1967) published a series of 150 cases of stage I and II cancer of the uterine cervix and found metastatic involvement of the regional lymph nodes in 19 patients. Correct lymphographic diagnoses were made in only 6 patients with 9 lymphograms falsely interpreted as positive. BACHMANN (1967) published the results of lymphography in 78 patients with carcinoma of the cervix. Of 24 cases verified by lymph node excision, 6 had positive findings. In 4 suspicious cases metastases of microscopic size were found. Two of 14 negative lymphographs proved to be false negative. JANISCH and WAGENBICHLER (1968) studied 113 patients with carcinoma of the uterine cervix by lymphography. The roentgenologic findings were verified by lymph node excision in 102 cases. In 90 cases the lymphographic diagnosis was proven correct. However, the lymphographic evaluation was falsely positive in 9 cases and falsely negative in 3 cases. REIFFENSTUHL (1967) states an accuracy of 50% based on comparative histologic and lymphographic findings in his carefully investigated material. FRISCH-BIER (1966) rates the value of lymphography as low in cases of early cervical

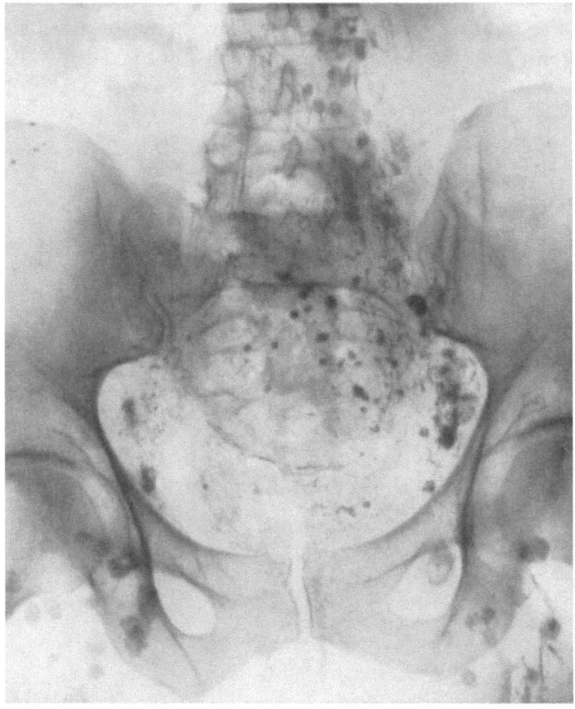

Fig. 7. *Recurrent carcinoma of the cervix.* Bilateral obstruction of the lymphatic circulation following curative radiotherapy. Enlarged external iliac lymph nodes, containing filling defects. Dislocation of aortic collaterals by malignant tissue

carcinoma, but reports that in a series of 72 patients with stage III cancer, lymphography demonstrated 13 positive findings in lymph nodes not accessible to clinical investigations. VUSKANOVIC et al. (1966) report a series of 27 patients with carcinoma of the uterine cervix, in which roentgenologic and histologic correlation was obtained. There were 6 false positive and 3 false negative studies. Of the false positives, 2 patients were seen to have histologically positive lymph nodes in a location different from that diagnosed by lymphography. Three false negative findings were proven to have malignant metastases in internal iliac lymph nodes not demonstrated by lymphography. In 2 cases histologically positive lymph nodes were overlooked at lymphography. BENNINGHOFF et al. (1966) report the results of lymphographic studies on 28 patients with gynecological tumors, predominantly of the uterine cervix. Correct correlation between the lymphogram and the histologic findings was observed in 26 cases. In 18 of these cases, both studies were negative; in 8 others both lymphogram and histology were positive. In 2 cases the lymphogram was considered to be negative, but the lymph nodes were histologically positive. For the combined groups of 86 patients with carcinoma of the cervix in stages I and II as reported by the four authors DOLAN (1964), AVERETTE et al. (1964), FISCHER and THORNBURY (1965) and FUCHS and BÖÖK-HEDERSTRÖM (1961) the rate of diagnostic error was 15%. Several investigators (MOULONGUET-DOLÉRIS et al. (1961), VIAMONTE et al. (1963), KRITTER et al. (1963), PICARD (1962) and ARVAY and PICARD (1963) have studied a large number of patients with carcinoma of the uterine cervix, and the results correspond well to the above mentioned findings.

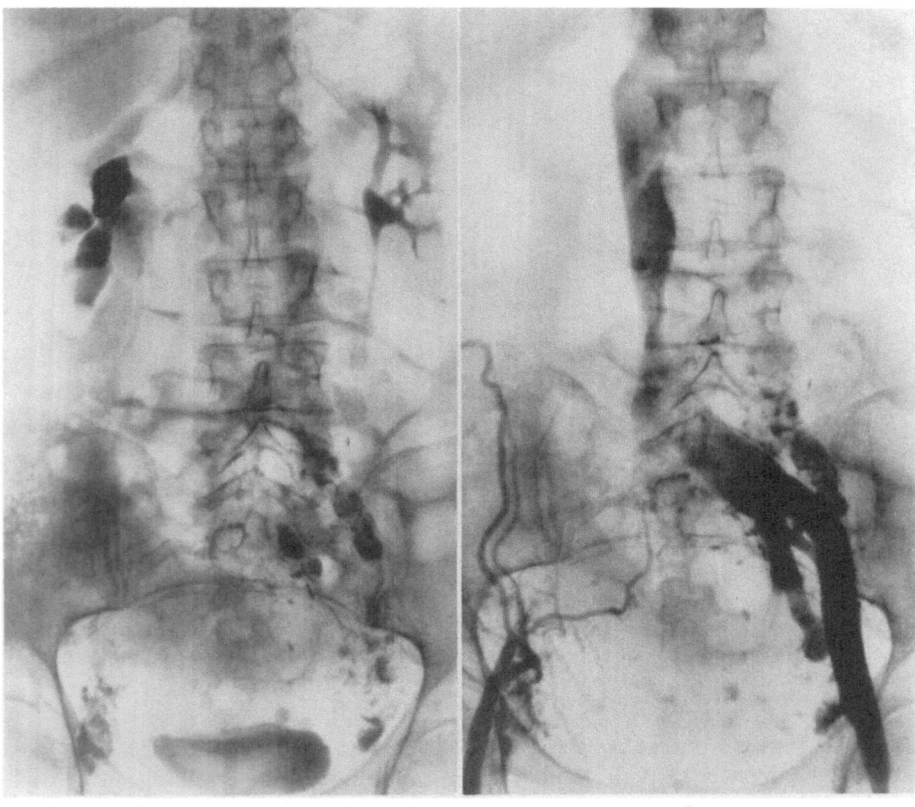

a   b

Fig. 8. *Recurrent carcinoma of the cervix.* Metastases in bilateral iliac and aortic lymph nodes. Complete bilateral obstruction of the lymphatic circulation. Collateral circulation. Constriction of the right common iliac vein and inferior vena cava. Obstruction of the right ureter

A review of the results of the lymphographic studies indicates that lymphography is of great value, even in cases of stage I and II, because it is the only clinical method capable of demonstrating metastatic spread to the iliac and aortic lymph nodes. The 15% rate of diagnostic error reported by the author in an earlier study

(FUCHS and BÖÖK-HEDERSTRÖM, 1964) is still valid for most groups of investigators. False negative interpretations of lymphographic findings occur in metastases of microscopic size and in malignant disease limited to all the internal iliac lymph node groups not demonstratable by lymphography. A false positive diagnosis is less frequent because fibrolipomatous changes can usually be differentiated from malignant deposits.

Diagnosis of *recurrent carcinoma* is greatly improved by lymphography. Clinical differentiation of the sequelae of surgical and radiation therapy and recurrent neoplasm is difficult. Edematous and, in later stages, scarred infiltrations of the parametria occasionally may simulate malignant recurrence. Lymphography yields great diagnostic information, but interpretation may occasionally be difficult. Small collateral lymphatics and pseudocysts develop following lymphadenectomy, whereas prophylactic irradiation of lymph vessels and nodes with doses of 5000—6000 R does not impair the lymph flow. Irradiation therapy of lymphatic structures invaded by malignant tissue results in partial and complete obstruction of the lymphatic circulation. Numerous lymphatics, forming a dense network of collaterals, tend to bypass the fibrotic area. In case of malignant infiltration, obstruction of the lymphatic circulation is even more prominent. Dislocation of lymphatics and non-visualization of lymph vessels in certain areas are strong indications of malignant infiltration (Fig. 7). Pelvic venography and cavography is an indispensable supplemental method where indentations and stenoses of the veins caused by enlarged malignant lymph nodes and direct malignant infiltration are diagnostic for malignancy (Fig. 8). In case of complete venous obstruction the type of venous collateral circulation may give certain indicative signs to establish a correct diagnosis. Malignant tumor invasion within an irradiated area occludes venous collaterals, whereas fibrotic tissue does not affect the venous systems to the same degree. The diagnostic value of lymphography in the clinically suspected recurrence of cervix carcinoma has been studied by FRISCHBIER (1967), SIEBER (1967) and GERTEIS (1967) in large series of patients. FRISCHBIER (1967) states that in 25% of 105 patients, the lymphographic findings were more extensive than the findings at clinical examination. SIEBER (1967) reports that in a series of 50 patients there were 10 lymphograms which revealed malignant recurrence where definite clinical signs were absent. In 9 patients with recurrent malignancy in the inferior gluteal lymph nodes diagnosed by rectal palpation, the lymphographic findings were of course negative. In 7 out of 10 patients with normal clinical examinations, suspicious signs of recurrency were seen on lymphadenograms. In 2 of these 7 cases, recurrency was evident despite additional radio therapy. GERTEIS reports a 21% incidence of recurrency in 34 cases manifesting no definite signs of malignancy, a 36% incidence in 28 patients with histologically verified, limited, local recurrence, a 28% incidence in 50 cases with clinical suspicion of recurrent tumor within the parametria, and a 62% incidence in 24 patients whose gynecological investigations were positive. KUNITSCH and HOLSTEN (1968) revealed lymph node metastases by lymphography in 39 (62%) of 63 patients, with a relapse of cervical carcinoma clinically evident or suspected.

The diagnostic accuracy of lymphography in recurrent carcinoma of the uterine cervix, as reported by the above investigators, correlates well with the author's experience. Lymphography is of primary importance in determining the presence of malignant recurrence. It enables precise localization of the malignant processes occurring in the pelvic and aortic area. Also, malignancy may be ruled out, and the dangers of unnecessary irradiation therapy can be avoided. On the other hand it should be remembered that interpretational difficulties may occur and conclusive evaluation may be impossible.

The main clinical indication for lymphography in carcinoma of the uterine cervix is the need to determine accurately the stage of malignant disease. The planning of surgical and radiation therapy in any case depends predominantly upon the extent of lymph node metastasis. Because lymphography demonstrates the precise locations of the regional lymph noaes, the radiation dose for each node group may be more readily calculated. Moreover, surgical lymph node excision is more thorough when use is made of lymphography as a guide to identify and locate different node groups. Particular attention should be given to the aortic lymph nodes because of their high incidence of involvement in malignant metastatic disease. The prolonged retention of contrast material facilitates the careful evaluation of therapeutic results. The effectiveness of radio therapy and surgery may be assessed directly. Control films during an operative procedure insure thorough excision all contrast-filled nodes; the change in size of nodes after radio therapy is also observable and important for prescribing subsequent treatment.

Carcinoma of the Corpus Uteri

Anatomy of the Regional Lymph Nodes (Fig. 9)

The lymph from the uterine corpus drains predominantly through 2—3 lymphatic channels which follow the uterine artery and join the lymphatics of the subovarian plexus coursing from the ovaries. These lymph vessels then follow the subovarian blood vessels and empty into the aortic lymph nodes at the level of L2/3. A few small uterine lymphatics extend along the utero-inguinal ligament and enter the superficial inguinal lymph nodes. Other lymph vessels join the lymphatics of the uterine cervix in the broad ligament which lead to the external iliac and to the medial common lymph nodes, situated at the bifurcation of the common iliac artery.

Foot lymphography demonstrates the medial external iliac nodes and most of the aortic lymph nodes. The ureteute-uterine lymph nodes, situated at the crossing of the uterine artery with the ureter, are not contrast-filled by this investigative technique, and some aortic lymph nodes cannot be visualized because their afferent lymphatics have not arisen from the iliac node groups.

Lymphographic Diagnosis

The author investigated 49 patients with carcinoma of the uterine corpus by lymphography. Twenty-three cases were classified as in clinical stage I, 9 cases as in stage II, 8 cases in stage III and 9 cases in stage IV. The radiologic diagnosis was checked by lymph node excision in 20 cases, and in the 29 remaining cases, the lymphographic findings were compared and evaluated with the results of cavography and with the clinical course of the disease. In 16 patients (33%), tumor metastases within the regional lymph nodes were correctly diagnosed. In 30 patients (61%) the lymphadenograms were negative in good correlation with later verification.

Three diagnoses were false negatives: the lymph node excision of a patient in stage I revealed bilateral metastases in the external iliac node groups, and 2 patients were clinically advanced with malignant infiltration of the parametria reaching the pelvic wall. In 2 patients lymphograms gave indications of primary malignant lymphoma, however, reactive hyperplasia with considerable enlargement of the lymph nodes simulating malignant lymphoma was observed histologically and

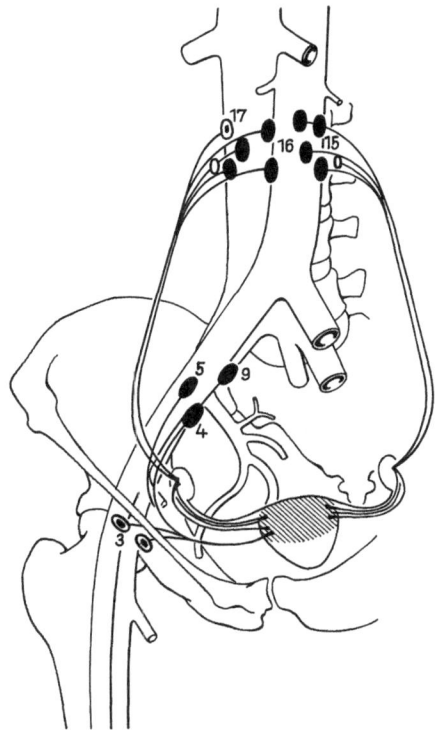

3 Superior superficial inguinal lymph nodes
   (genital group)
4 Medial external iliac lymph nodes
5 Intermediate external iliac lymph nodes
9 Medial common iliac lymph nodes
15 Left aortic lymph nodes
16 Pre-retroaortic lymph nodes
17 Right aortic lymph nodes

● Routinely demonstrated by lymphography;
⊖ Facultatively demonstrated by lymphography; ○ Not demonstrated by lymphography

Fig. 9. *Anatomy of the regional lymph nodes of the corpus uteri*

proved to be benign. The frequency of malignant metastases to the regional lymph nodes diagnosed by lymphography in the 32 cases of stage I and II was 16%, in the 17 cases of stage III and IV, 65%. Involvement of the iliac lymph nodes was most common (8 cases) (Fig. 10). Metastases in the aortic node groups alone were encountered in 3 cases of stage I and II (Fig. 11), whereas both the aortic and iliac groups were infiltrated in 4 cases of clinical stage IV (Fig. 12). Malignant metastatic spread to the common iliac and aortic lymph nodes was demonstrated in a patient with a large solitary uterine metastasis of a breast carcinoma (Fig. 13).

GERTEIS (1967) states that the frequency of metastatic invasion of the regional lymph nodes as diagnosed by lymphography in 101 cases was 20% in clinical stage I, 44% in stage II, 50% in stage III and 86% in stage IV. FRISCHBIER (1966) was able to demonstrate metastases in aortic lymph nodes in 2 of 15 patients, VIAMONTE et al. (1963) in 3 of 5 patients and DOLAN (1964) in 4 of 6 patients.

Lymphography is of considerable value in evaluating *malignant recurrency* (Figs. 12, 14). Although the percentage of malignant lymph node metastases revealed by lymphography varies with the investigator, it may be concluded that the incidence of malignant lymphatic involvement is by no means as small as is often believed.

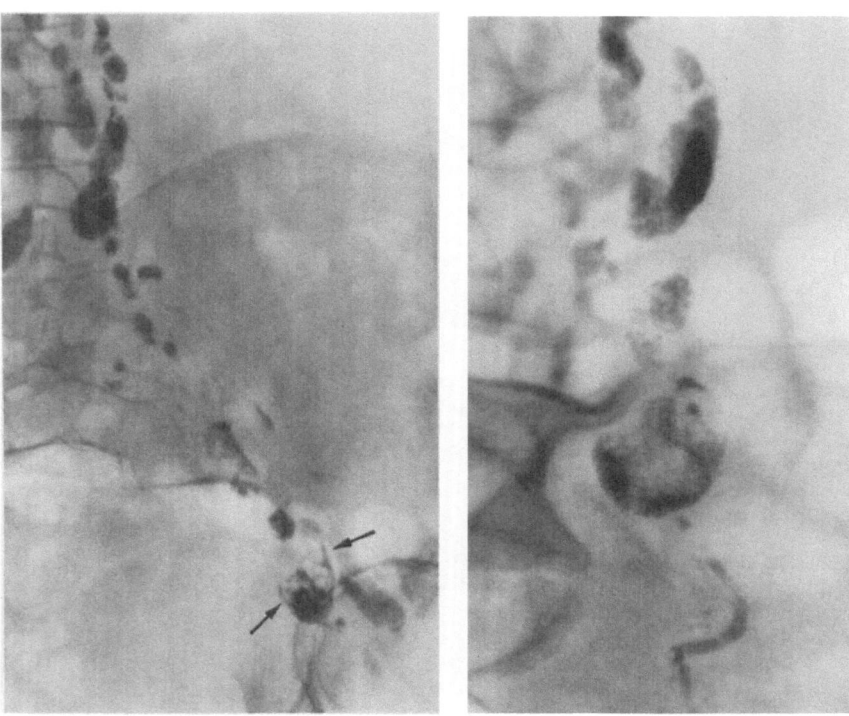

Fig. 10   Fig. 11

Fig. 10. *Carcinoma of the corpus uteri, stage II.* Metastases in medial external iliac lymph nodes (→). Extensive central filling defects caused by malignant tissue. Small-sized external and common iliac lymph nodes. Reactive hyperplasia of the aortic lymph nodes

Fig. 11. *Carcinoma of the corpus uteri, stage II.* Extensive metastases in enlarged left aortic lymph nodes containing massive filling defects caused by metastatic foci

FRISCHBIER (1967) observed a frequency of aortic metastasis in recurrent carcinoma of 65% in 20 patients.

Consequently, lymphography plays an important role in the staging, therapy planning and therefore in the prognosis of carcinoma of the uterine corpus. Lymph node metastases in iliac and aortic lymph nodes are detectable only by this method. Furthermore, follow-up observation of the lymph nodes demonstrated by contrast material, using control roentgenograms at a later date is particularly important.

Any observed change in the originally visualized nodes within a period of six to nine months is indicative of progressive metastatic disease. Observation at a later date requires a repeat lymphography study, a so-called "second-look" procedure.

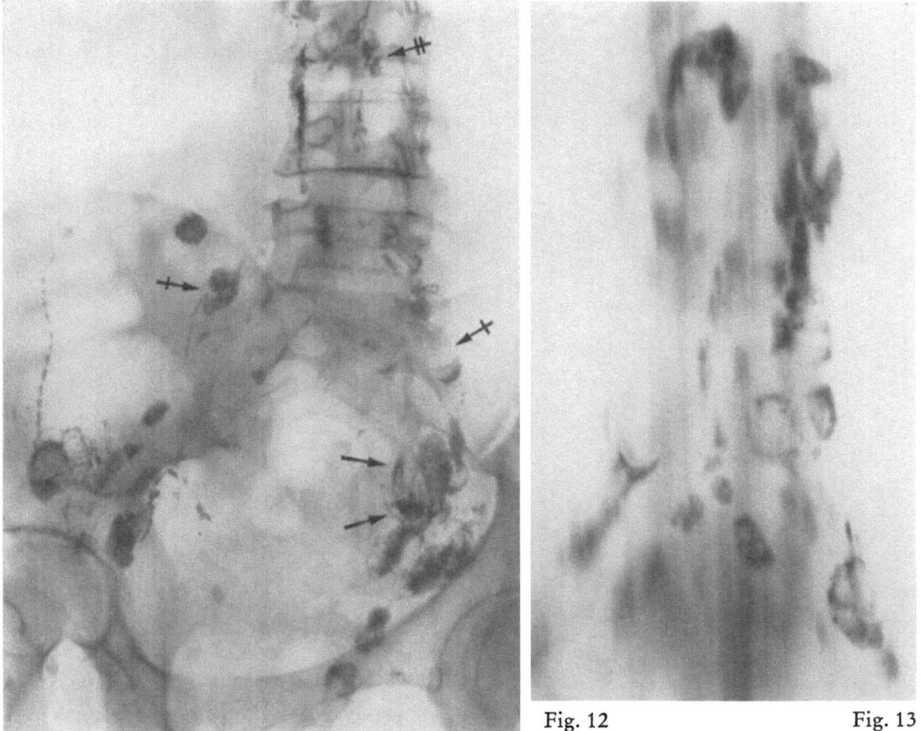

Fig. 12   Fig. 13

Fig. 12. *Recurrent carcinoma of the corpus uteri.* Disseminated metastases in bilateral external (→) and common (↦) iliac and some aortic (-ǀ→) lymph nodes presenting marginal and central filling defects. Scarce demonstration of the aortic lymph nodes

Fig. 13. *Scirrhous carcinoma of the breast.* Disseminated metastases to the common iliac and aortic lymph nodes of a solitary metastasis localized in the uterine corpus

Malignant Tumors of the Ovary

Anatomy of the Regional Lymph Nodes (Fig. 15)

The efferent lymphatics of the ovaries constitute the main part of the subovarian lymphatic plexus. They follow the ovarian arteries and veins without interposition of lymph nodes to end in the aortic lymph nodes at the level of L1/2: the latero-caval and intraaortico-caval on the right side and the pre- and lateroaortic nodes on the left side. With a frequency of occurrence of 50%, lymph vessels of the ovaries are directly connected with external iliac lymph nodes. With a frequency of approximately 15%, efferents of the fallopian tube run into one of

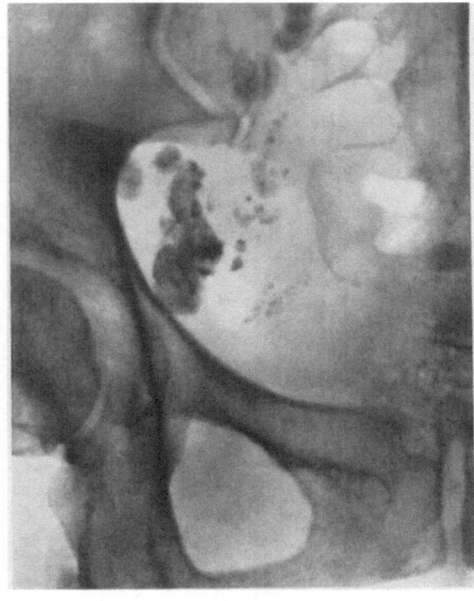

a

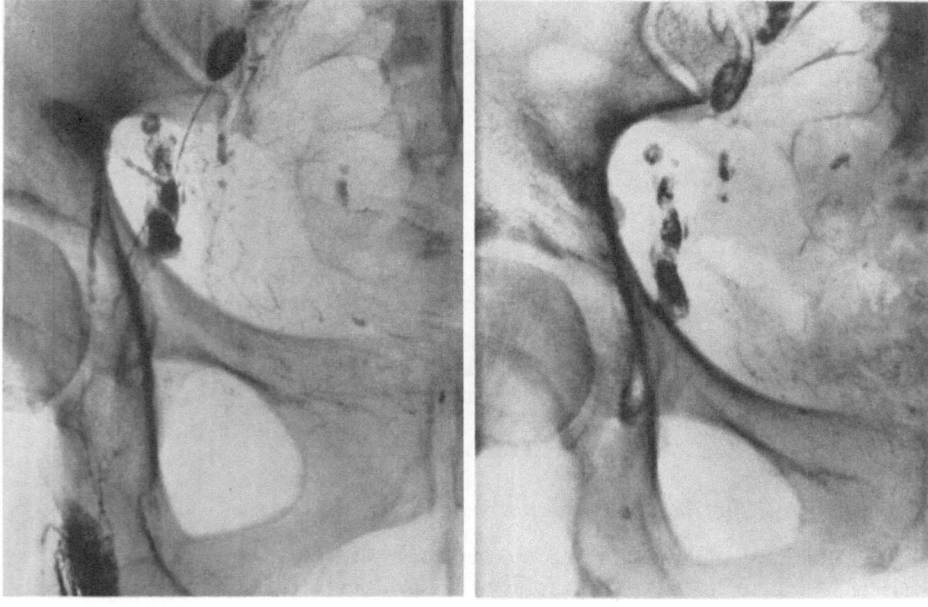

b   c

Fig. 14. *Suspected recurrency of a carcinoma of the corpus uteri.* a Metastases in slightly
enlarged medial external iliac lymph nodes. b Partial obstruction of the lymphatic circulation. Collaterals within the pelvic area 12 months following radiotherapy (6000 rad.).
c Small-sized medial external iliac lymph nodes. No signs of recurrent malignancy

the internal iliac nodes. Aortic lymph nodes which are supplied exclusively by ovarian lymphatics are not demonstrated by routine foot lymphography. Contrast-filling of aortic lymph nodes at the level of L1/2, particularly on the right side, is inconstant.

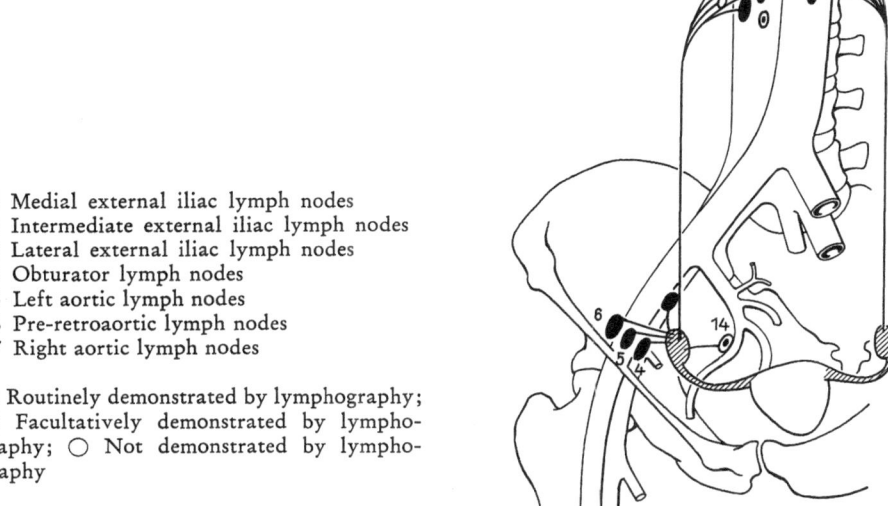

 4 Medial external iliac lymph nodes
 5 Intermediate external iliac lymph nodes
 6 Lateral external iliac lymph nodes
14 Obturator lymph nodes
15 Left aortic lymph nodes
16 Pre-retroaortic lymph nodes
17 Right aortic lymph nodes

● Routinely demonstrated by lymphography;
⊖ Facultatively demonstrated by lympho-graphy; ○ Not demonstrated by lympho-graphy

Fig. 15. *Anatomy of the regional lymph nodes of the ovaries*

Lymphographic Diagnosis

The author's series of lymphographic investigations consisted of 39 patients with malignant ovarian tumors. In 19 cases (48%), lymph node metastases were demonstrated by lymphography, 6 of which were verified by operation. In 9 of the remaining 13 cases not operated on, cavography and urography supported the positive lymphographic diagnoses. The frequency of lymph node metastases as detected by lymphography in the early stages I and II was 25% in 12 cases; the corresponding frequency for the 27 cases of advanced stages III and IV was 59%. Ten patients in advanced clinical stages, but with normal lymphograms were considered cases of secondary peritoneal carcinoma. Lymph node metastases were demonstrated in aortic lymph nodes in 10 cases (Fig. 16) — including the 3 positive findings in stages I and II, in iliac lymph nodes in 4 cases (Fig. 17) and in both lymph node groups in 5 cases of clinical stage IV (Fig. 18). GERTEIS (1967) reports frequencies of lymph node metastases in 57 ovarian tumors of stage I and II of 23% to the iliac region and 16% to the aortic area, with a preference for the aortic region in early stages. FRISCHBIER (1967) found malignant metastases in regional lymph nodes in 7 of 19 patients (41%). Of 21 cases with recurrent malignancy, he detected more extensive findings at lymphographic than at clinical examination in 71%. COLLETTE (1958) was able to detect malignant lymph node metastases in all 5 cases investigated by lymphography. MARKOVITS et al. (1968) report the results of lymphography in 10 cases of seminoma of the ovary. Enlargement of the lymph nodes and filling defects (but without alteration of the lymphatic circulation) were present in cases of malignant metastatic spread to the regional lymph nodes.

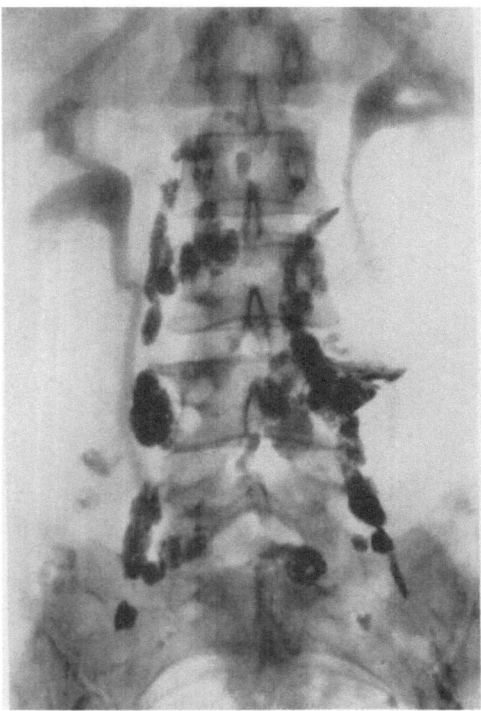

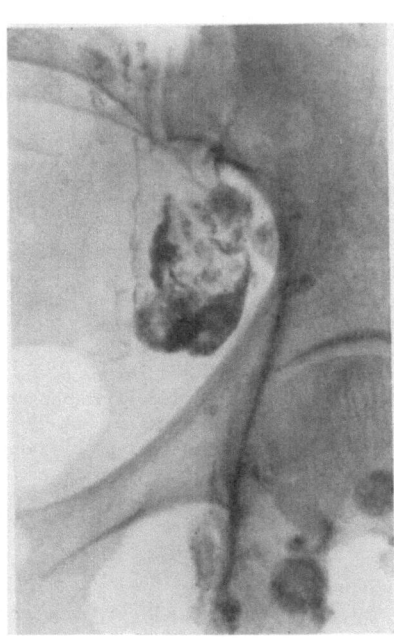

Fig. 17

Fig. 16

Fig. 16. *Carcinoma of the left ovary, stage I*. Metastases in left aortic lymph nodes. Large central filling defects due to malignant growth, displacing to contrast-filled lymphatic tissue. Displacement of the left ureter

Fig. 17. *Carcinoma of the left ovary, stage III*. Metastases in medial external iliac lymph nodes containing large filling defects. Obstruction of the lymphatic circulation

Metastatic spread of malignant ovarian tumors into the regional lymph nodes seems to be more frequent than generally accepted. The aortic node groups are more frequently involved than the iliac nodes, a fact which may be explained anatomically. Cavography is an indispensable aid in evaluating lymphographic results, because the right latero-aortic node groups may not be contrast-filled by lymphography. Metastatic involvement of lymph vessels and lymph nodes occurs predominantly in later stages of the disease, but may be encountered in early cases as well. Consequently, pre-operative lymphography is of great importance as a guide for lymph node excision and irradiation therapy. Negative lymphographs often contrast sharply with clinically massive malignant involvement of the pelvic region. Distant metastases may arise via the peritoneal cavity, through diaphragmatic and retrosternal lymph channels, without involving the retroperitoneal nodes. Displacement of iliac lymph vessels by extensive ovarian tumors has been reported (HAHN et al. 1963), but seems to be rare. Indentation of the urinary bladder and pelvic veins by large tumors is a more frequent occurrence.

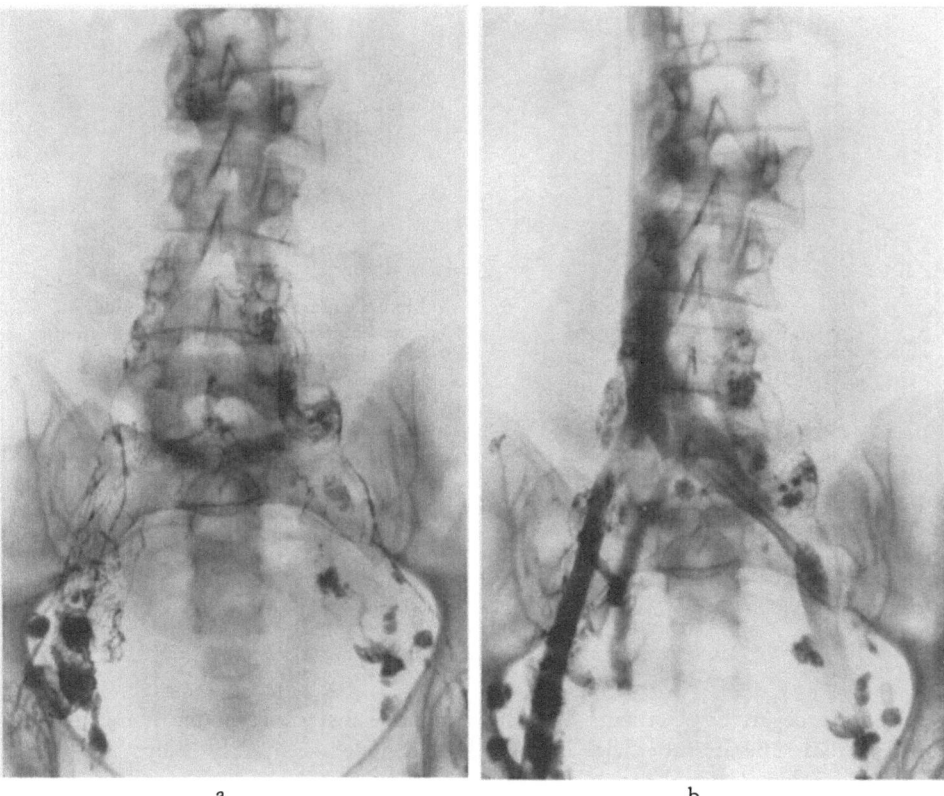

a   b

Fig. 18. *Carcinoma of the ovaries, stage III.* Disseminated metastases in the iliac and aortic lymph nodes. Compression and dislocation of the iliac veins and inferior vena cava

Carcinoma of the Vagina

Anatomy of the Regional Lymph Nodes (Fig. 19)

The lymph vessels of the upper vagina drain into the medial and intermediate external iliac and obturator lymph nodes. The lymphatics of the inferior vagina join the inferior gluteal lymph nodes and to a lesser extent, the obturator lymph node group. Rarely lymph vessels are linked also with medial common and aortic lymph nodes.

In the author's series 9 patients were investigated by lymphography. In 1 case, with the primary tumor reaching the vestibule and clinically normal inguinal lymph nodes, lymphography revealed metastases in deep inguinal lymph nodes, the presence of which was confirmed one month later by extensive malignant infiltration of the parametria (Fig. 20). The 8 remaining lymphograms were normal; 3 proved

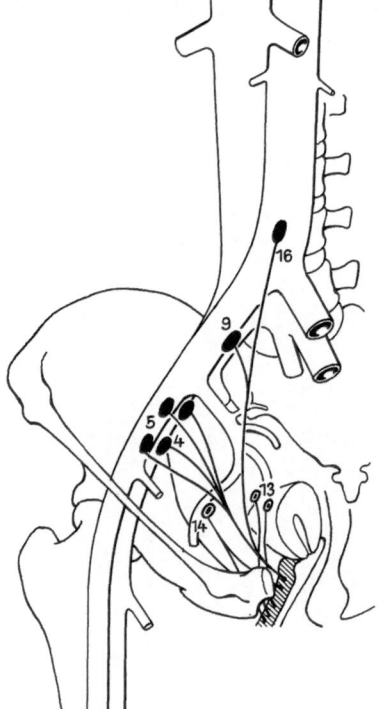

 4 Medial external iliac lymph nodes
 5 Intermediate external iliac lymph nodes
 9 Medial common iliac lymph nodes
13 Inferior gluteal lymph nodes
14 Obturator lymph nodes
16 Pre-retroaortic lymph nodes

● Routinely demonstrated by lymphography.
⊖ Facultatively demonstrated by lymphography.

Fig. 19. *Anatomy of the regional lymph nodes of the vagina*

to be false negative: 2 patients had large palpable metastases in the non-contrast-filled medial superior superficial inguinal lymph nodes verified by biopsy. A third patient developed lymphedema of the leg due to extensive malignant disease 2 months following lymphography.

Carcinoma of the Vulva

Anatomy of the Regional Lymph Nodes (Fig. 21)

The lymphatic drainage of the lower-most part of the vagina below the vestibule, i. e. from the clitoris and labia, is into the medial superior superficial and deep inguinal lymph nodes, which are bilaterally connected. A few deep lymphatics from the clitoris and labia lead to the external iliac lymph nodes. The primary regional lymph nodes of the vagina and vulva are not demonstrated by foot lymphography with the exception of the deep inguinals.

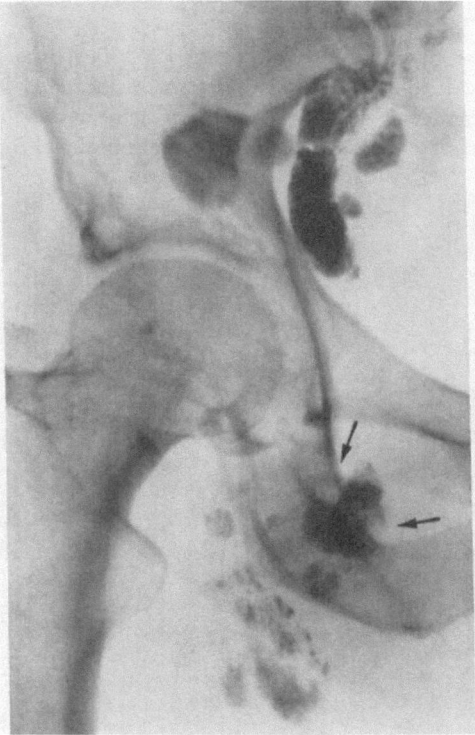

Fig. 20. *Carcinoma of the vagina infiltrating the vestibule.* Metastases in deep inguinal lymph nodes (→). Reactive hyperplasia of the external iliac lymph nodes

2 Deep inguinal lymph nodes
3 Superior superficial inguinal lymph nodes (genital group)
4 Medial external iliac lymph nodes

● Routinely demonstrated by lymphograhy. ⊖ Facultatively demonstrated by lymphography

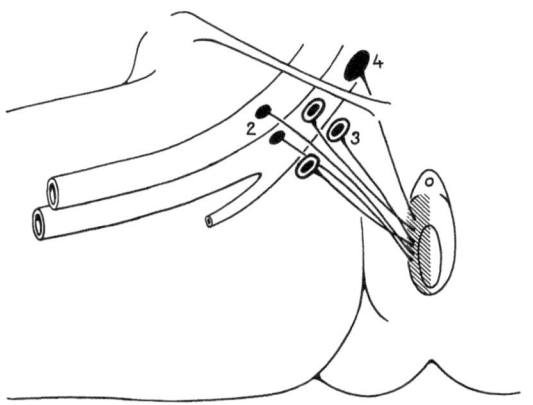

Fig. 21. *Anatomy of the regional lymph nodes of the vulva*

Lymphographic Diagnosis

The author's series of investigations consists of 11 patients, 2 of whom had positive lymphograms. In both cases, metastases were localized in deep inguinal and external iliac lymph nodes (Figs. 22, 23). Of the 9 negative findings, one was incorrect with large metastases present in the superior superficial inguinal lymph nodes.

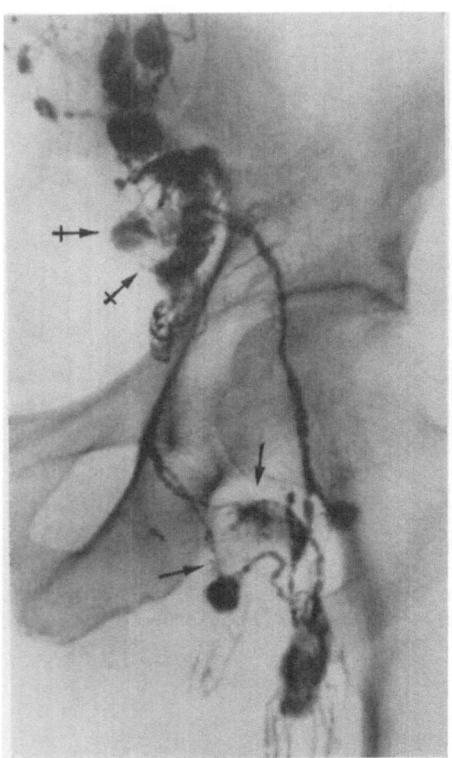 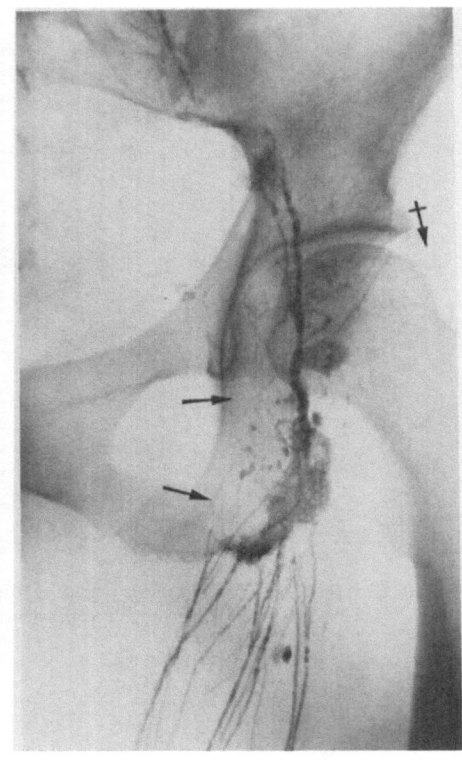

Fig. 22   Fig. 23

Fig. 22. *Carcinoma of the vulva*. Metastases in deep inguinal (→) and medial external iliac lymph nodes (↔)

Fig. 23. *Carcinoma of the vulva*. Metastases in medial inferior superficial and deep inguinal lymph nodes (→). Obstruction of the lymphatic circulation. Collateral lymphatics in the thigh (↔)

FRISCHBIER (1966) investigated 20 patients with carcinoma of the vulva and vagina by lymphography and was able to detect clinically unsuspected malignant metastases in iliac lymph nodes in 3 cases. Five patients with carcinoma of the vulva studied bilaterally by JACKSON (1967) had metastases in the inguinal nodes on 7 sides (i. e. three patients unilaterally and two patients bilaterally) confirmed by histologic examination. On 5 of the affected sides no abnormal findings were observed in lymphography. Pathologic inferior superficial inguinal lymph nodes were excluded from the lymphatic circulation in 1 patient and were not demonstrated by lymphography. On 2 sides medial superficial superior lymph nodes were metastatically involved. Because this node group is not demonstrated by foot lymphography, a false negative radiologic diagnosis was made. Ten patients with vulvar carcinoma were studied by AVERETTE et al. (1964) with lymphography prior to lymphadenectomy. Six patients with definite evidence and 1 patient with suggestive evidence exhibited lymph node involvement. One of the 3 patients with normal lymphograms was found to have metastases in a superior superficial inguinal lymph node. Metastases of the vulva and vagina to regional lymph nodes demonstrated by lymphography have been described in case reports by VIAMONTE et al. (1963), HAHN et al. (1963), PAPILLON et al. (1963), DOLAN (1964) and DANA et al. (1964). Negative lymphographic results are relatively frequent in cases of clinically positive, histologically proven metastases in the medial superior superficial lymph nodes, because this node group is not visualized by lymphography. On the other hand, this node group is readily accessible for clinical palpation. Fibrolipomatous changes within the inguinal lymph nodes lead to considerable difficulties in recognizing metastatic deposits. Definitive diagnosis may be achieved only when extensive marginal filling defects are present in combination with partial obliteration of the lymphatic circulation.

Metastases to the external iliac lymph node groups are detectable only by lymphography. Demonstration of malignant metastatic spread to those nodes inaccessible to clinical investigation is important for the planning of radical vulvectomy and radiation therapy.

Carcinoma of the Breast

Anatomy of the Regional Lymph Nodes (Fig. 24)

Anatomical studies of the regional lymph nodes of the mammary gland have been performed by POIRIER (1898) and ROUVIÈRE (1932) by dissection and by TURNER-WARWICK (1958), who injected vital dyes into patients. Seventy-five percent of the lymph from the breast is drained laterally into the axillary lymph nodes of the corresponding side. The primary regional lymph nodes are those of the pectoral lymph node group, situated at the lateral and inferior margins of the Pectoralis minor muscle. The efferent lymphatics of this lymph node group reach the subscapular and central axillary lymph nodes. From these lymph node groups they continue to the lateral and apical axillary node groups as well as to the supraclavicular lymph nodes. Also, some efferent lymphatics of the mammary gland are connected directly with the apical axillary lymph node group. The remaining 25% of the lymphatic drainage of the breast is directed medially to the parasternal lymph nodes, which are situated along the internal mammary artery between the 5th intercostal space and the supraclavicular region. Lymphography by injecting contrast material into the radial or ulnar subcutaneous lymphatics visualizes lateral and apical axillary lymph nodes as well as supraclavicular nodes (BOBBIO et al. 1962). These groups constitute regional lymph nodes of the breast of the second and third order. The regional node groups of the first order, the pectoral nodes as well as the central axillary and subscapular lymph nodes are not demonstrated by lymphography. Furthermore, the number of apical and lateral axillary lymph nodes and supraclavicular nodes that fills with contrast material is highly variable.

Lymphographic Diagnosis

The diagnostic value of lymphography for detection of malignant metastatic spread into the axillary lymph nodes has been discussed by GOFFRINI et al. (1962), KENDALL et al. (1963), ABBES et al. (1964, 1965, 1968), SHIBATA et al. (1966)

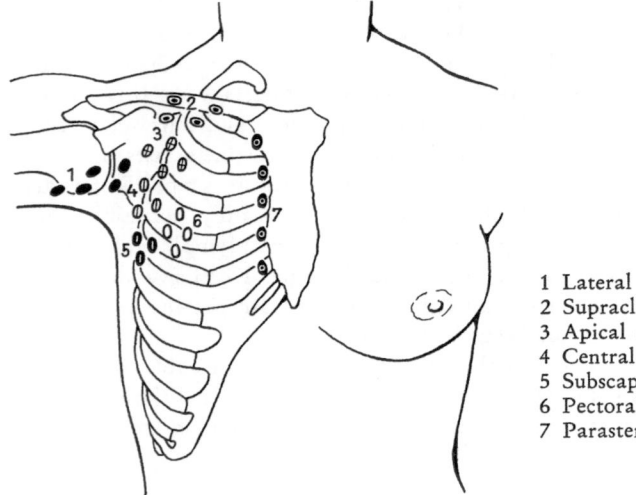

1 Lateral axillary lymph nodes
2 Supraclavicular lymph nodes
3 Apical axillary lymph nodes
4 Central axillary lymph nodes
5 Subscapular lymph nodes
6 Pectoral lymph nodes
7 Parasternal lymph nodes

Fig. 24. *Anatomy of the regional lymph nodes of the breast*

and FUCHS (1967). Because lymphography does not demonstrate all the regional axillary lymph nodes of the mammary gland, the value of this method for preoperative diagnosis of malignant metastatic spread is limited. Moreover, normal lymphographic findings do not rule out the possibility of metastases in the pectoral and subscapular lymph node groups or occasionally in the

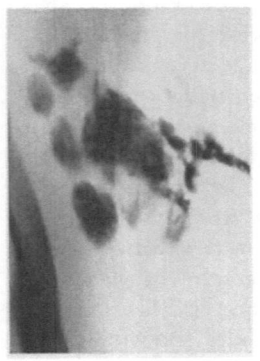

Fig. 25. *Carcinoma of the lateral inferior part of a left mammary lymph node.* Metastases in lateral axillary lymph nodes containing large filling defects. Dislocation of lymphatics by not-contrast-filling metastatic lateral axillary lymph nodes (operative verification)

lateral and apical axillary lymph nodes. LUDVIK and ZAUNBAUER (1966) investigated 22 patients with carcinoma of the breast all verified by lymph node excision. The lymphographic interpretation was positive in 8 cases, negative in 7 cases, false positive in 2 and false negative in 5 cases. SHIBATA et al. (1966) reported

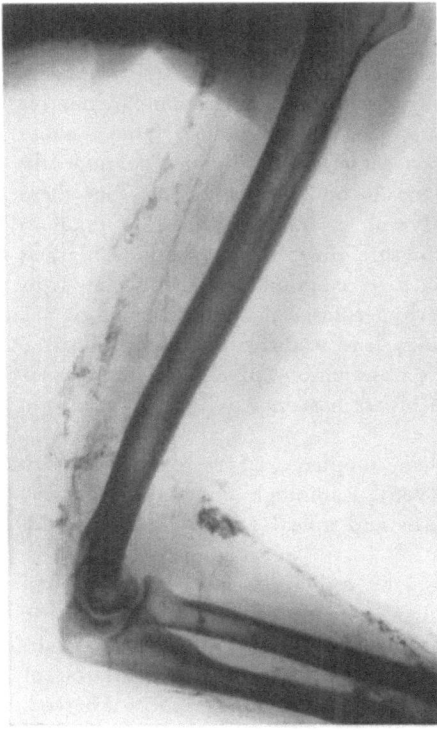

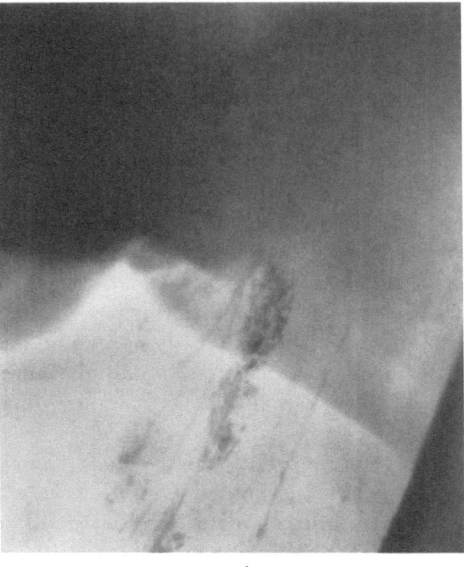

b

Fig. 26. *Recurrent axillary metastases of breast cancer.* a Marked lymphedema, extensive collateral circulation. b Contrast filling of slightly enlarged lateral axillary lymph nodes multiple central containing filling defects

a

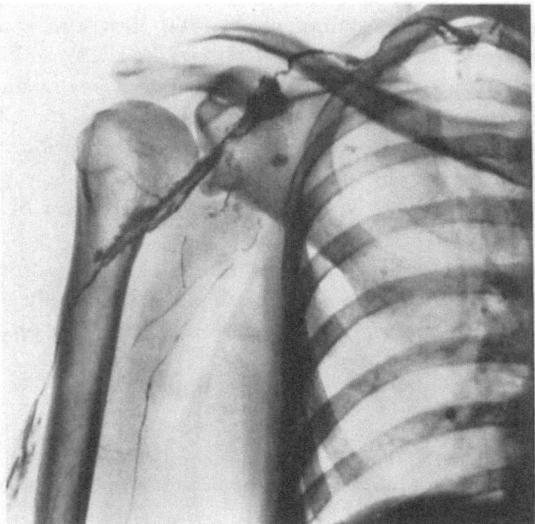

Fig. 27. *Slight secondary lymphedema* of the right arm due to scar formation consequent to surgery and radiation therapy. Normal apical axillary and supraclavicular lymph nodes not removed by operation

the results of 14 cases of axillary lymphography on patients with breast tumors. In 3 cases (2 false negatives and one false positive) the lymphograms did not correlate with the histologic findings. Kendall et al. (1963) investigated 9 patients with breast lesions, 7 of whom had carcinoma. In 4 cases, a detailed comparison was made of the radiologic and histologic findings in all of the 57 lymph nodes removed. Thirty-seven were filled with contrast material; 20 did not contain oily contrast agent. Correct diagnoses were made for 26 of 37 lymph nodes, but there were 10 false negative diagnoses. In the 20 lymph nodes that failed to take up contrast material, 14 manifested malignant growth. Filling defects within enlarged lymph nodes and obstruction of the lymphatic circulation are diagnostic signs indicating cancer metastases (Fig. 25). Reactive hyperplasia and fibrolipomatosis are common within the axillary lymph nodes and may lead to difficulties in diagnosis.

According to these results and the author's observations in a small number of cases, axillary lymphography in cancer of the breast has only a limited diagnostic value.

Preoperative lymphography is of value when complete excision of the axillary lymph nodes is attempted (Kendall et al., 1965). Radiologic controls during the operation insure complete excision of all lateral and apical axillary lymph nodes that filled with contrast agent.

The diagnosis of *malignant recurrency* in the axillary region after surgical excision is very difficult. Considerable impairment and stasis of the lymphatic circulation has occurred, and the contrast material is left within the dilatated subcutaneous and deep collateral lymphatics. Massive paravascular extravasation of the contrast material occurs. Contrast-filling of the axillary region is seldom achieved, even when injecting large doses of contrast material (Fig. 26). The presence of lymphatic obstruction and collaterals is not indicative of malignant infiltration because scar formation, consequent to surgery and radiation therapy often produces identical lymphographic changes (Fuchs et al., 1960; Goffrini et al., 1964; Abbes et al., 1965, 1966, 1968; Cavalot et al., 1965; Mazzeo et al., 1966; Hughes and Patel, 1966; Feldman et al., 1966). Differentiation between malignant infiltration and fibrosis due to scarring by means of lymphography (Figs. 26, 27) is only possible in those rare cases with slight impairment of the lymph circulation.

In the presence of severe obstruction of lymph flow axillary phlebography does not give additional information because complete obstruction of the axillary vein and extensive venous collaterals are encountered.

In summary, lymphography is only of limited usefulness for the diagnosis of malignant metastatic spread in carcinoma of the breast, but only in the preoperative stage. For the diagnosis of postoperative recurrence, it is most often ineffective.

References

Abbes, M.: A proposito di 100 linfografie dell'arto superiore. Minerva Chir. 20, 295 (1965).
—, et G. Juillard: A propos de 250 lymphographies du membre supérieur. Ann. Chir. 22, 1003 (1968).
—, E. Martin, V. Paschetta, A. Pellegrino et P. P. Pratt: La lymphographie en cancérologie. Paris: L'expansion scientifique Française, 1964.
Arvay, N., et J. D. Picard: La lymphographie. Etude radiologique et clinique des voies lymphatiques normales et pathologiques. Paris: Masson & Cie 1963.

AVERETTE, H. E., R. C. HUDSON, and J. H. FERGUSON: Lymphangioadenography. Applications in the study and management of gynecologic cancer (1964).

BACHMANN, F. F.: Die Lymphographie beim Kollum-Karzinom. Med. Welt 20, 1259 (1967).

BENNINGHOFF, D. L., P. G. HERMAN, and J. H. NELSON: Clinicopathologic correlation of lymphography and lymph node metastases in gynecological neoplasms. Cancer 19, 885 (1966).

BOBBIO, P., and F. MANGIONE: The lymphographic method in diagnosis of the grade of axillary metastatic invasion due to breast carcinoma. Ann. ital. Chir. 41, 704 (1965).

—, G. PERRACCHIA e F. PELLEGRINO: Anatomia radiografica del sistema linfatico ascellare e sopraclaveare. Ateneo Parm. 23, 5 (1962).

CHAVANNE, G., D. PELLIER et M. VALATTE: La lymphographie dans les stades I et II du cancer du col utérin. Etude de 150 cas opéres et verifiés histologiquement. J. Radiol. Electrol. 48, 137 (1967).

CAVALOT, F., G. SINISTRERO, E. TETTONI et F. GHILARDI: Aspetti linfografici nelle pazienti mastectomizzati. Minerva Radiol. 10, 76 (1965).

COLLETTE, J. M.: Envahissements ganglionnaires inguino-iliopelviens par lymphographie. Acta radiol. (Stockh.) 49, 154 (1958).

DANA, M., J. P. DESPREZ-CURELY, V. BISMUTH et R. BOURDON: La lymphographie dans les maladies de la peau. Ann. Radiol. 7, 555 (1964).

DARGENT, M., J. L. CHASSARD et D. DARGENT: Valeur prognostique de la lymphographie iléo-pelvienne par voie pédieuse dans le cancer du col utérin. Bull. Cancer 5, 83 (1963).

DOLAN, P. A.: Lymphography. Brit. J. Radiol. 37, 405 (1964).

— Lymphography in genital cancer. Surg. Gyn. Obstet. 118, 1286 (1964).

FELDMAN, M. G., P. KOHAN, S. EDELMAN, and J. H. JACOBSON: Lymphangiographic studies in obstructive lymphedema of the upper extremity. Surgery 59, 935 (1966).

FISCHER, H. W., M. S. LAWRENCE, and J. R. THORNBURY: Lymphography of the normal adult male. Radiology 78, 399 (1962).

—, and J. R. THORNBURY: Lymphangiography in the diagnosis of malignant neoplasms. In: Progress in clinical cancer, p. 213. New York: Grune & Stratton 1965.

FRISCHBIER, H. J.: Experience with lymphography in diagnosis of recurrent female genital carcinoma. Progress in Lymphology. p. 221. Stuttgart: G. Thieme 1967.

— Die Lymphographie, Möglichkeiten und Grenzen der Metastasendiagnostik beim weiblichen Genitalkarzinom. Fortschr. Röntgenstr. 105, 1255 (1966).

FUCHS, W. A.: Lymphographie und Tumordiagnostik. Berlin-Heidelberg-New York: Springer 1965.

— La lymphographie dans le cancer du sein. Méd. et Hyg. (Genève) 25, 483 (1967).

—, and G. BÖÖK-HEDERSTRÖM: Inguinal and pelvic lymphography. Acta radiol. (Stockh.) 56, 340 (1961).

—, M. S. DEL BUONO u. A. RÜTTIMANN: Zur Lymphographie bei chronisch-sekundären Lymphoedemen. Fortschr. Röntgenstr. 92, 608 (1960).

GERTEIS, W.: The frequency of metastases in carcinoma of the cervix and the corpus. Progress in Lymphology. p. 209. Stuttgart: G. Thieme 1967.

— Lymphographic results in recurrence. Progress in Lymphology. p. 222. Stuttgart: G. Thieme 1967.

GOFFRINI, P., P. BOBBIO: Der Lymphkreislauf der oberen Extremität nach Radikaloperation des Mammacarcinoms und seine Beziehung zum Sekundärödem am Arm. Chirurg 35, 145 (1964).

— —, G. PERACCHIA e F. PELLEGRINO: Valore della linfografia e della comparazione anatomico-linfografica nello studio delle metastasi ascellari del cancro della mamella. Ateneo Parm. 23, 33 (1962).

HAHN, G. A., S. WALLACE, L. JACKSON, and G. DODD: Lymphangiography in gynecology. Amer. J. Obstet. Gynec. 85, 754 (1963).

HUGHES, J. H., and A. R. PATEL: Swelling of the arm following radical mastectomy. Brit. J. Surg. 53, 4 (1966).

JANISCH, H., and P. WAGENBICHLER: Lymphographie — diagnostische und therapeutische Hilfsmethoden. Wien. klin. Wschr. 80, 173 (1968).

JACKSON, R. J. A.: Metastatic involvement of the inguinal lymphatics. Progress in Lymphology, p. 207. Stuttgart: G. Thieme 1967.

KENDALL, B. E., J. F. ARTHUR, and D. H. PATEY: Lymphangiography in carcinoma of the breast. Cancer 16, 1233 (1963).

KRITTER, H., N. ARVAY, J. D. PICARD, and G. MANLOT: La lymphographie dans le cancer du col utérin. Ann. Radiol. 5, 55 (1962).

KUNITSCH, G., u. D. R. HOLSTEN: Erfahrungsbericht über 429 Lymphographien bei Geschwulstkranken. Med. Welt 4, 239 (1968).

LUDVIK, W., u. W. ZAUNBAUER: Bedeutung der Lymphographie für die chirurgischen Disziplinen. Fortschr. Röntgenstr. 105, 614 (1966).

MAZZEO, F., e N. SPAMPINATO: La linfografia nel "bracchio grosso" postmastectomia. Minerva Chir. 21, 259 (1966).

MARKOVITS, B., J. GRELLET, CH. GASQUET et D. SARAZIN: La place de la lymphographie dans les séminomes de l'ovaire. Rev. franç. Gynéc. 63, 201 (1968).

MOULINGUET-DOLÉRIS, P., N. ARVAY, J. D. PICARD et G. MANLOT: La lymphographie. Technique, indications et résultats. J. Radiol. Electrol. 42, 281 (1961).

PAPILLON, J., M. DARGENT et J. L. CHASSARD: La lymphographie au lipiodol ultrafluide en cancérologie. J. Radiol. Electrol. 44, 397 (1963).

PICARD, J. D.: La lymphographie en gynécologie. Ann. Chir. 25, 1 (1962).

POIRIER, P.: Traité d'anatomie humaine. Paris: Masson 1898.

REIFFENSTUHL, G.: Der prognostische Wert der Lymphographie beim Kollumkarzinom. Geburtsh. Frauenheilk. 27, 589 (1967).

— The prognostic value of lymphography in carcinoma of the uterine cervix. Progress in Lymphology. Stuttgart: G. Thieme 1967.

— Das Lymphknotenproblem beim Carcinoma colli uteri und die Lymphirradiatio pelvis. München-Berlin-Wien: Urban und Schwarzenberg 1967.

ROUVIÈRE, H.: Anatomie des lymphatiques de l'homme. Paris: Masson & Cie. 1932.

SHIBATA, H. R., P. MCLEAN, J. L. VEZINA, F. G. INGLIS, and E. J. TABAH: Axillary lymphography in carcinoma of the breast. Surgery 60, 329 (1966).

SIEBER, F.: Lymphography in recurrence of carcinoma of the uterine cervix. Progress in Lymphology, p. 218. Stuttgart: G. Thieme 1967.

TURNER-WARWICK, R. T.: The lymphatics of the breast. Brit. J. Surg. 46, 574 (1958).

VIAMONTE, M., D. ALTMAN, R. PARKS, E. BLUM, M. BEVILAQUA, and L. RECHER: Radiographic-pathologic correlation in the interpretation of lymph angioadenograms. Radiology 80, 903 (1963).

VUSKANOVIC, M., M. VIAMONTE, and J. E. MARTIN: The place of lymphadenography in the diagnosis and during the treatment of malignant disease. Amer. J. Roentgenol. 93, 205 (1966).

WOLFF, J. P., P. MARKOVITS, CH. GASQUET, J. GRELLET et H. DABLANC: Valeur de la lymphographie dans les cancers du col utérin au stade I. Rev. franç. Gynéc. 63, 4, 169 (1968).

Male Genital Organs

Malignant Tumors of the Testis

Anatomy of the Regional Lymph Nodes (Fig. 28)

The lymph vessels of each testis — 4—8 channels — drain directly into the aortic lymph nodes situated distal to the renal blood vessels. The lymph vessels of the right testicle drain into the right aortic and preaortic lymph nodes. Those of the left testicle are connected with the left aortic and preaortic lymph nodes. A few lymphatics arising from the medial aspect of the testis and the epidydimis are closely connected with the deferent duct and enter the external iliac lymph nodes (CUNÉO and MARCILLE, 1901). Occasionally, efferent vessels passing to the superficial inguinal lymph nodes are observed (KUBIK, 1967).

Bilateral foot lymphography does not visualize all of the primary regional lymph channels of the testicle. By injection of contrast material directly into the efferent lymphatics of the testis during orchidectomy, one or several lymph nodes are

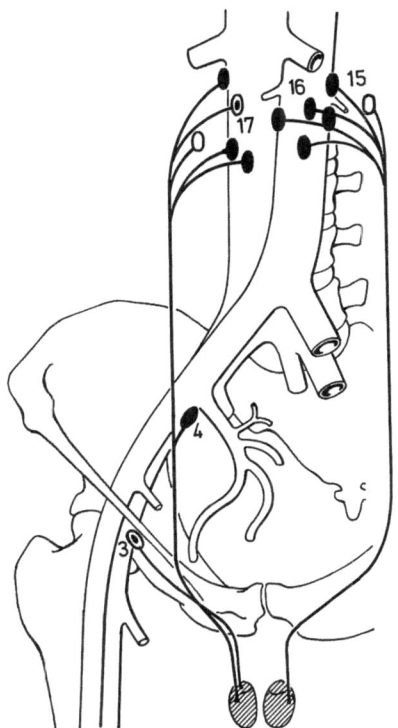

3 Superior superficial inguinal lymph nodes
  (genital group)
4 Medial external iliac lymph nodes
15 Left latero-aortic lymph nodes
16 Pre-retroaortic lymph nodes
17 Right latero-aortic lymph nodes

● Routinely demonstrated by lymphography;
⊖ Facultatively demonstrated by lymphography; ○ Not demonstrated by lymphography

Fig. 28. *Anatomy of the regional lymph nodes of the testes*

filled at the level of L1/2 on the left and at L1/3 on the right side (PELLEGRINI et al., 1957; CHIAPPA et al., 1963; BUSCH and SAYEGH, 1963; SAYEGH et al., 1963; CHAVEZ, 1967). These lymph nodes are situated lateral to the aortic lymph nodes outlined by foot lymphography and are only occasionally demonstrated by the latter method. Consequently, neither foot nor testicular lymphography ensures complete visualization of the regional lymph nodes of the testes. A combined study would give optimal results, but testicular lymphography is tedious for routine use. False negative findings are possible, therefore, in conventional lymphography.

Lymphographic Findings

Seventy-four patients with malignant testicular tumors were investigated, utilizing mainly bilateral foot lymphography after unilateral orchidectomy and prior to radiotherapy. No testicular lymphograms were done. Histologically, 36 cases were seminoma, 16 were embryonal carcinoma, 11 were terato-carcinoma, 4 were teratoma, 2 were chorio-carcinoma and 5 were non-germinal malignant tumors. Thirty-four patients (46%) exhibited pathologic lymphographic findings. Histologic verification was available for only 4 cases, but the clinical course of the disease, cavography, and urography supported the positive lymphographic diagnoses. The frequency of malignant metastatic spread to regional lymph nodes was approximately 50% in embryonal carcinoma, teratoma, terato-carcinoma and chorio-carcinoma, whereas only one-third of the seminoma group exhibited lymph node metastases. Unilateral metastatic involvement of aortic lymph nodes was present in 17 patients (Figs. 29, 30).

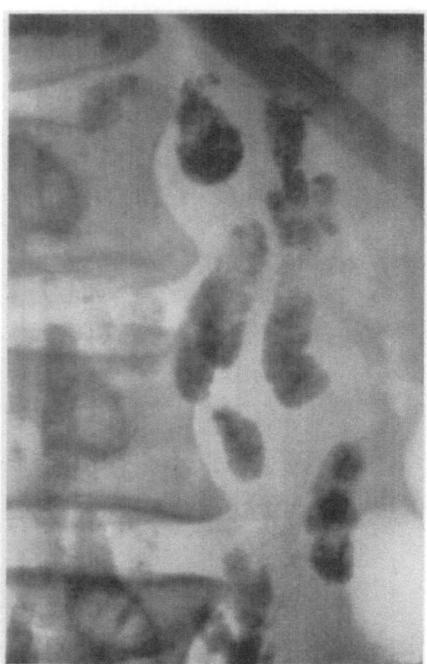

Fig. 29. *Seminoma*. Unilateral metastases in left aortic lymph nodes containing small confluent filling defects

Bilateral metastases in the regional aortic lymph nodes were found in 11 patients (Fig. 31); unilateral metastases to the contralateral side were seen in 2 patients. Additional malignant spread to the iliac node groups was demonstrated in 10 of the above cases of advanced clinical stage with 5 of these showing bilateral involvement (Fig. 32). One patient with malignant infiltration of the scrotum demonstrated evidence of inguinal lymph node metastases (Fig. 33). Inguinal metastases can also be caused by a reflux of tumor cells from the iliac region.

Enlarged lymph nodes with filling defects were present in 31 cases. Dislocation of normal tissue within the lymph nodes with lymph vessel displacement' was observed in 24 cases. Stasis of the lymphatic circulation was observed in 13 patients and non-filling of node groups consequent to malignant infiltration with resultant collateral circulation was observed in 6 cases. Obstruction of the thoracic duct occurred occasionally in cases of very extensive malignant involvement (Figs. 30, 32).

Metastatic involvement of mediastinal lymph nodes developed in 2 cases of seminoma and in one case of embryonal carcinoma at intervals ranging between 10 and 30 months following radiotherapy of the aortic lymph nodes. At the time of lymphography prior to treatment, these mediastinal nodes were contrast-filled and did not reveal pathologic changes, although metastatic spread must have occurred already (Fig. 34). As a consequence, selective prophylactic radiotherapy of the contrast-filled mediastinal lymph nodes must be considered in malignant testicular tumors.

The different histologic types of malignant testicular tumors present identical lymphographic findings. Filling defects in lymph nodes caused by metastatic deposits with tissue dislocation are found in early stages of metastatic spread. Extensive displacement of the remaining lymphatic tissue, complete replacement by malignant tissue, and blockage of the lymphatic circulation indicate advanced stages of malignant disease. Differentiation between the various histologic types of testicular tumors as suggested by CHIAPPA et al. (1963) was not possible in the author's case material. CHIAPPA states that seminoma produces filling defects in lymph nodes more often than the other types of malignant testicular tumors which progress more frequently to blockage of the lymphatic circulation. This difference may arise because patients with seminoma are usually treated in an early stage of the disease, before extensive metastatic spread has occurred.

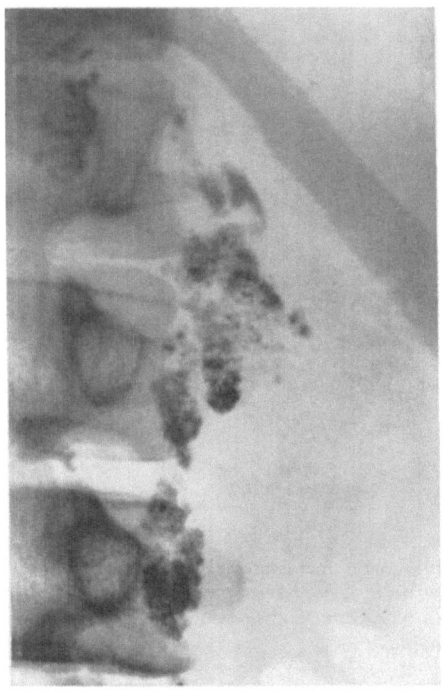 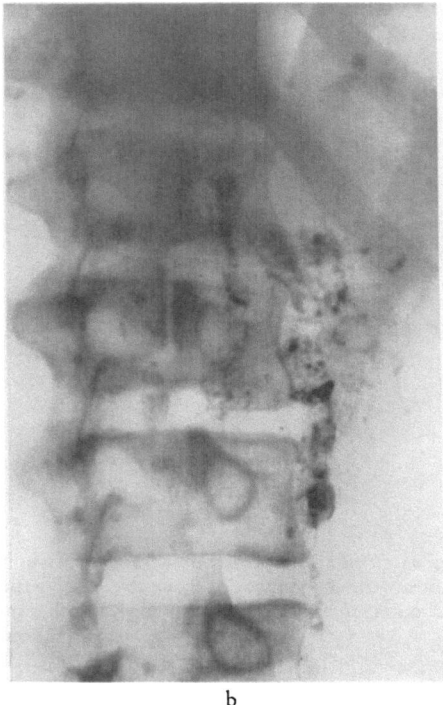

a   b

Fig. 30. *Terato-carcinoma.* a Unilateral metastases in enlarged left aortic lymph nodes. Extensive confluent filling defects. b Recurrency 8 months following radiotherapy with 6000 rad. Bilateral metastases in aortic lymph nodes. Obstruction of the thoracic duct

Diagnosis of metastases in the aortic lymph nodes at the level of the kidneys may be difficult because reactive hyperplasia of this group of nodes is a common finding. Reactive hyperplasia indicates a response of the lymph nodes to tumor cells or to unspecific inflammatory toxic agents, especially after orchidectomy. Follow-up studies and "second-look" lymphograms are necessary to detect metastatic involvement at a later stage. LANGHAMMER (1969) investigated 57 patients with malignant tumors of the testis and stressed the diagnostic difficulties in differentiating fibro-lipomatous reactive and malignant changes in early regional lymph nodes.

Results of lymphographic investigations in testicular tumors have also been reported by other authors. Of 50 patients investigated by PICARD and BABINET (1964), lymphography was positive in 28 cases. COOK et al. (1965) report a series of 26 patients in which lymphography was positive in 10 cases. Sixteen lymphograms were considered to be normal, whereas lymphadenectomy revealed metastatic spread to the regional lymph nodes in 4. The positive lymphographic findings were confirmed by operative exploration in 7 cases.

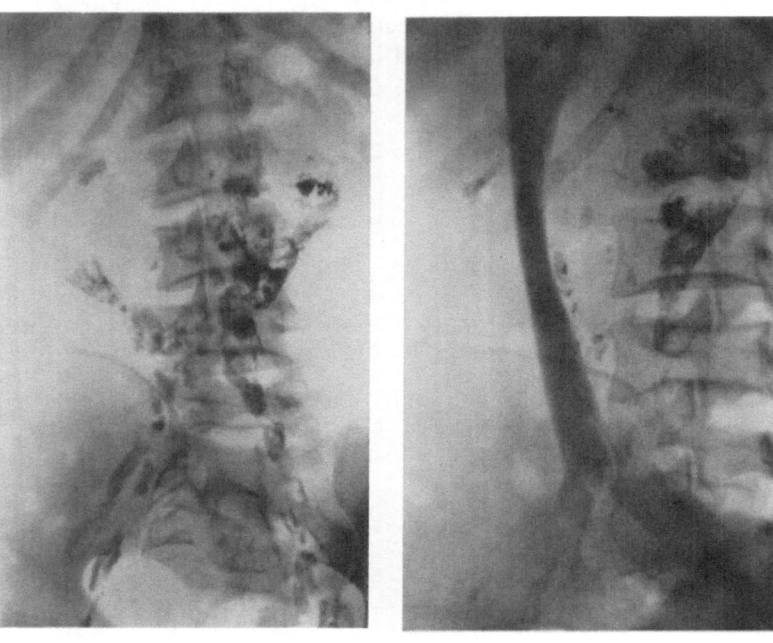

a   b

Fig. 31. *Embryonal carcinoma.* a Extensive bilateral aortic metastases. Dislocation of the contrast-filled lymphatic tissue by malignant growth. b *Lymphographic control:* marked reduction of tumor size following radiotherapy with 5500 rad. Compression and .dislocation of the inferior vena cava

MARKOVITS et al. (1964) report of 35 positive and 13 negative lymphographies in studies on 48 patients. In a series of 71 patients, VON KEISER (1966) reports a high rate of malignant metastatic spread to the regional lymph nodes in cases of malignant teratoma and seminoma. In a series of 17 patients by LUDVIK et al. (1966) 9 lymphograms demonstrated malignant metastatic involvement of the aortic lymph nodes. CHIAPPA et al. (1966) made a study of 36 patients with testicular neoplasm using both testicular and foot lymphography. They conclude, that testicular lymphography is especially indicated to detect early node metastases, whereas foot lymphography is effective to demonstrate widespread lymph node involvement. Similar investigations have been reported by BUSCH et al. (1965).

The great value of lymphography in the detection of malignant metastatic spread is evident from a comparison of the results reported above with the results in 900 cases not investigated by lymphography as published by DIXON and MOORE (1952). The incidences of lymph node metastases diagnosed clinically and with conventional roentgendiagnostic methods in this group were 11% in seminoma, 24% in teratoma and 30% in embryonal carcinoma and terato-carcinoma, whereas lympho-

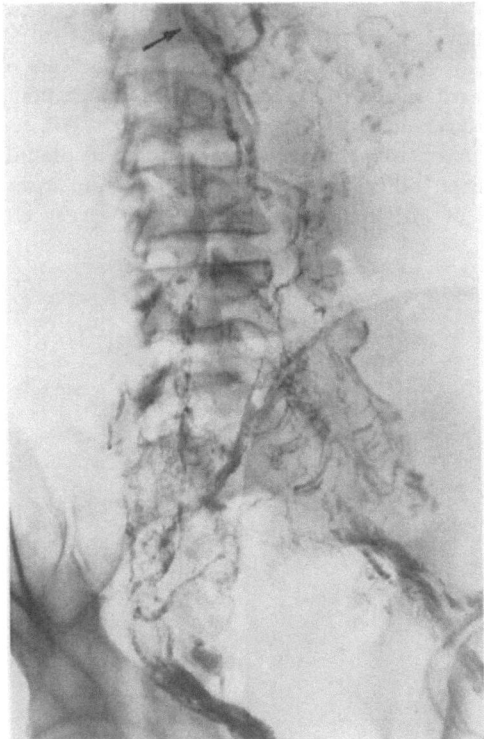

Fig. 32. *Chorio-carcinoma.* Disseminated iliac and aortic metastases. Bilateral obstruction of the thoracic duct (→)

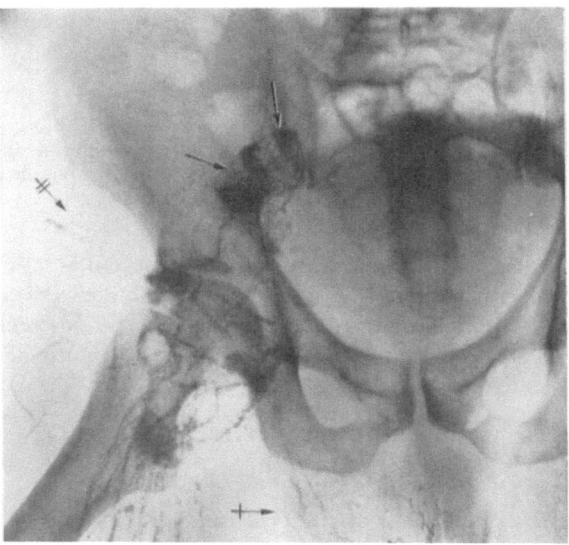

Fig. 33. *Embryonal carcinoma.* Complete obstruction of the lymphatic circulation due to malignant infiltration of the external iliac lymph nodes (→). Extensive collaterals in the edematous scrotum (↔), thigh and abdominal wall (⇢)

graphy demonstrated malignant metastases in 30⁰/o of the case of seminoma, and in 50⁰/o of the cases of each of the following: embryonal carcinoma, teratoma, terato-carcinoma and chorio-carcinoma.

Accurate estimation of the clinical stage and exact planning and control of treatment are the clinical indications for lymphography in cases of seminoma. Pre-operative localization of lymph node metastases is of great importance in terato-

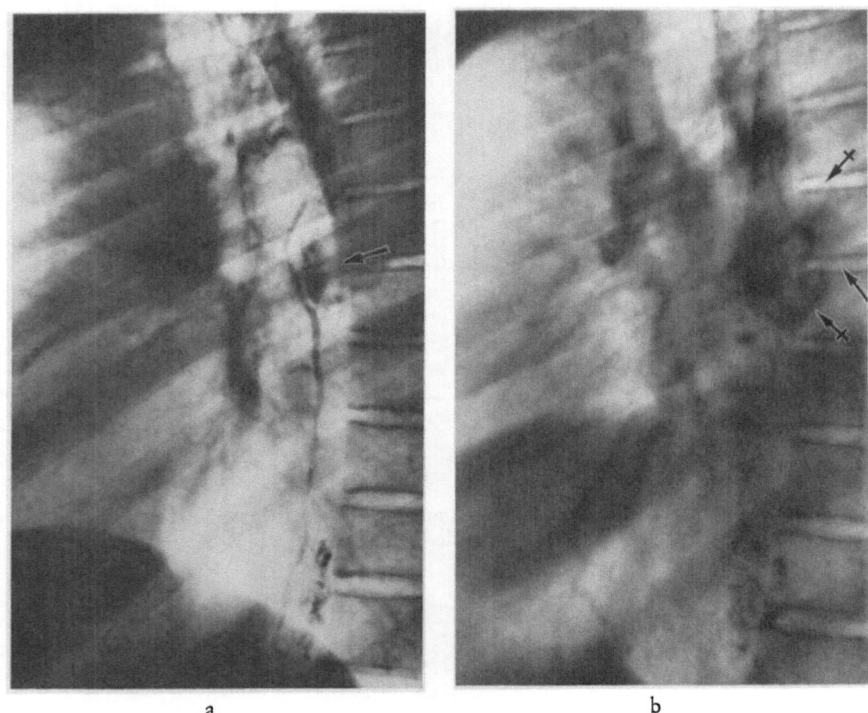

a   b

Fig. 34. *Embryonal carcinoma*. a Contrast filling of normal posterior mediastinal lymph nodes (Th 5/7) (→). b 3 years later metastases at the site of the lymph nodes filled with contrast material at lymphography (↦)

carcinoma because excision of the aortic lymph nodes in unilateral metastases yields good results. Intraoperative radiographic control facilitates the removal of the regional lymph nodes infiltrated by tumor. In cases of chorio-carcinoma, lympho-graphy may yield useful information about prognosis and results of therapy.

Carcinoma of the Penis

Anatomy of the Regional Lymph Nodes (Fig. 35)

The lymph vessels of the skin of the penis and the scrotum lead to the super-ficial inguinal lymph nodes of both the corresponding and the contralateral sides. The efferent vessels of the corpus cavernosum form a plexus below the symphysis, containing one or several small pubic lymph nodes. These vessels continue then to the superficial and deep inguinal lymph nodes of the corresponding and opposite sides. They join the distal medial external iliac lymph nodes and rarely may connect with internal iliac and intermediate external iliac lymph nodes. This topographic arrangement of the regional lymph nodes was confirmed by RIVEROS et al. (1967) in their studies of penis lymphography in 8 normal subjects.

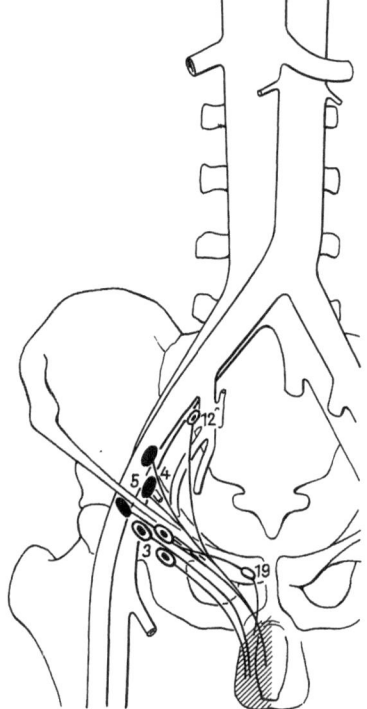

3 Superior superficial inguinal lymph nodes
  (genital group)
4 Medial external iliac lymph nodes
5 Intermediate external iliac lymph nodes
12 Superior gluteal lymph nodes
19 Pubic lymph nodes

● Routinely demonstrated by lymphography;
⊖ Facultatively demonstrated by lymphography; ○ Not demonstrated by lymphography

Fig. 35. *Anatomy of the regional lymph nodes of the penis and scrotum*

Lymphographic Diagnosis

In the author's series of 18 patients with carcinoma of the penis, lymphography was abnormal in 6 cases (33%). Metastatic deposits in external iliac nodes were diagnosed in 3 cases (Fig. 36). Histologic confirmation was not available, but the clinical data were suggestive. One case exhibited histologically proven bilateral metastases in external and common iliac and aortic lymph nodes (Fig. 37). In another patient with malignant involvement of the iliac and aortic nodes, combined with partial obstruction of the lymphatic circulation, the inferior superficial inguinal lymph nodes were contrast-filled showing no abnormalities. Biopsy of clinically enlarged superior superficial inguinal nodes revealed metastatic spread to this node group. Metastases in deep inguinal lymph nodes were correctly diagnosed in the sixth case as confirmed by biopsy (Fig. 38).

Metastases of carcinoma of the penis in regional lymph nodes demonstrated by lymphography have been described in case reports by SCHAFFER et al. (1962), DOLAN

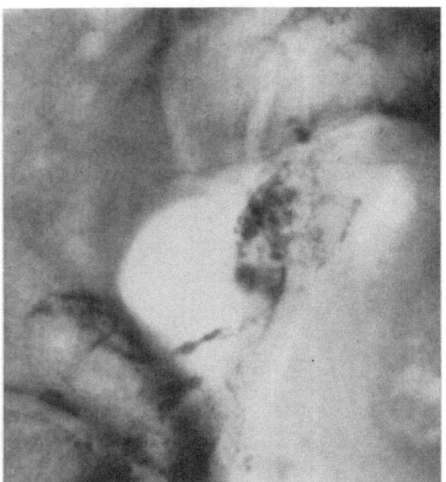

Fig. 36. *Penis carcinoma*. Metastases in medial external iliac lymph nodes containing multiple filling defects (confirmed by lymph node excision)

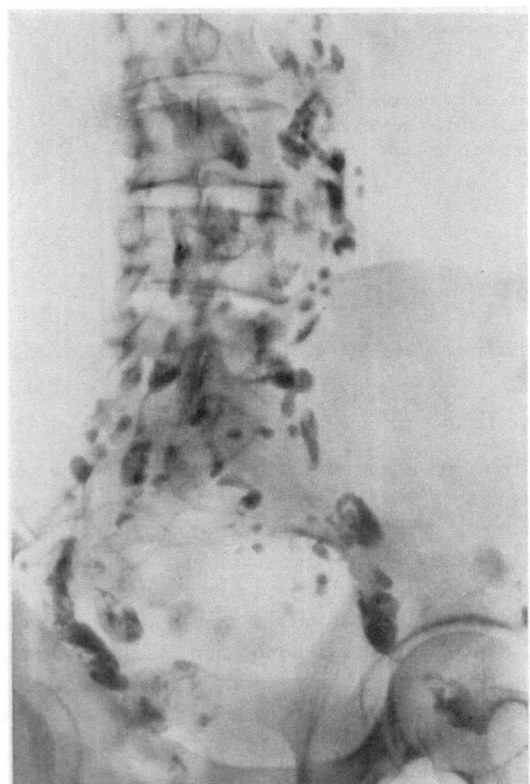

Fig. 37. *Penis carcinoma*. Disseminated metastases in bilateral iliac and aortic lymph nodes (confirmed by lymph node excision)

(1964) and GREGL et al. (1967). RIVEROS et al. (1967) carried out penis lymphography in 4 patients with carcinoma and 2 with inflammatory disease. Among the cases with carcinoma, the positive diagnosis was confirmed by histology in one. In the 2 cases of condyloma accuminatum and syphilitic chancre the regional lymph nodes were enlarged with regular contours and a mottled appearance similar to that of primary lymphoma.

Experience with lymphography in carcinoma of the penis is still limited, but it is evident that the method is of practical value because the planning of surgical and radiation therapy depends chiefly on the extent of the metastatic involvement of regional lymph nodes. Metastatic deposits in the iliac and aortic lymph node groups are detectable only by lymphography. On the contrary clinically enlarged medial superior superficial lymph nodes will not appear on lymphographs as they are not demonstrated by lymphography. Because of the commonly superimposed infection, inflammatory enlargement of the regional lymph nodes is frequent. However, differentiation between metastatic deposits and inflammatory changes is generally possible.

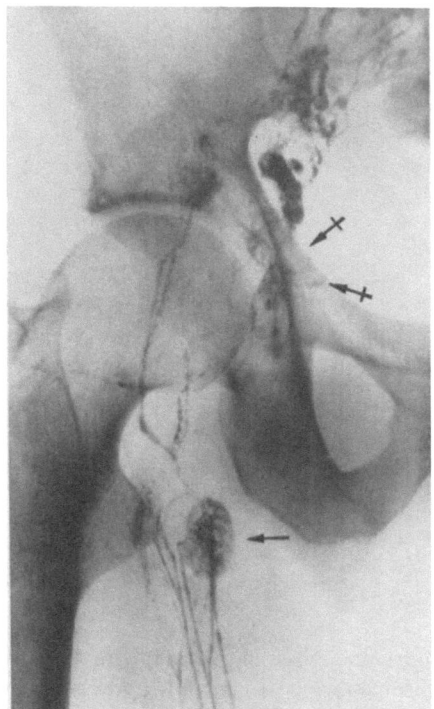

Fig. 38. *Penis carcinoma.* Metastases in superficial inferior inguinal (→) and medial lacunar (↦) lymph nodes. Non-filling of deep inguinal lymph nodes infiltrated by malignant growth. Partial obstruction of the lymph circulation (confirmed by lymph node biopsy)

Carcinoma of the Prostate

Anatomy of the Regional Lymph Nodes (Fig. 39)

Most of the efferent lymph vessels of the prostate leave the organ at its posterior aspect. One group of lymphatics follows the inferior vesical artery and joins the external iliac lymph nodes; the other group, running on the inner aspect of the sacrum, is connected with the lateral sacral and medial common iliac lymph nodes. Paravesical lymph nodes may be interspersed with both groups of lymphatics. A few lymph vessels of the anterior part of the prostate communicate with those of the urinary bladder.

Lymphographic Findings

In the author's series of investigations, 11 cases were examined by lymphography. In 6 clinically advanced cases, metastatic spread to the regional lymph nodes was demonstrated (54%). In only 2 of these patients, metastatic bone involvement was present. Malignant invasion of iliac and latero-aortic lymph nodes occurred in 2 cases (Fig. 40). Bilateral metastatic involvement of external and common iliac

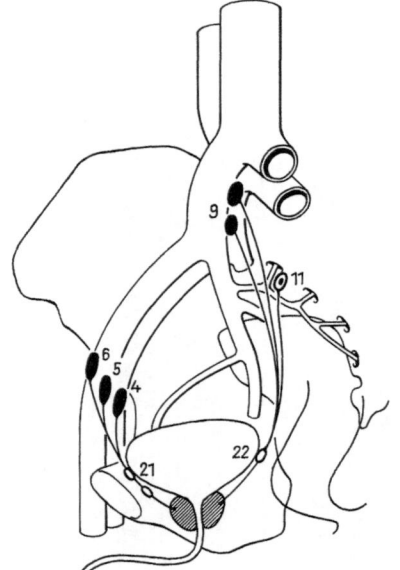

4 Medial external iliac lymph nodes
5 Intermediate external iliac lymph nodes
6 Lateral external iliac lymph nodes
9 Medial common iliac lymph nodes
11 Lateral sacral lymph nodes
   Posterior vesical lymphnodes
21 Lateral vesical lymph nodes

● Routinely demonstrated by lymphography;
⊖ Facultatively demonstrated by lymphography; ○ Not demonstrated by lymphography

Fig. 39. *Anatomy of the regional lymph nodes of the prostate*

nodes was observed in one case (Fig. 41). Metastases to external iliac lymph nodes were confirmed by lymph node excision in another patient. Complete bilateral obstruction of the lymphatic circulation in the iliac nodes and inguinal node metastases were visualized in one case in which collaterals in the thigh and abdominal wall were contrast-filled (Fig. 42). Another patient showed extensive malignant involvement of iliac and aortic lymph nodes with progressive occlusion of the external iliac vein and compression of the inferior vena cava.

Metastases of prostate carcinoma demonstrated by lymphography in regional lymph nodes have been described in case reports by WALLACE et al. (1961, 1962), MAY and BOGASH (1962), VIAMONTE et al. (1963), RÜTTIMANN and DEL BUONO (1964) and ABBES et al. (1964). LUDVIK and ZAUNBAUER (1966) report 14 positive lymphographic findings in 20 patients.

The relative high frequency of malignant metastatic spread to the regional lymph nodes is in direct contrast to the clinical observations of HANSCHKE et al. (1968), who found clinically suspicious inguinal lymph nodes in only 7.7% of 354 cases.

Diagnosis of malignant metastases in regional lymph nodes by lymphography is important to evaluate the operability of the patient. Radical prostatectomy — a treatment with a high rate of cure — is indicated only in cases of early carcinoma strictly limited to the prostate gland (MELLINGER et al., 1967). Therefore, preoperative lymphographic investigations are very important to evaluate exactly the stage of the disease.

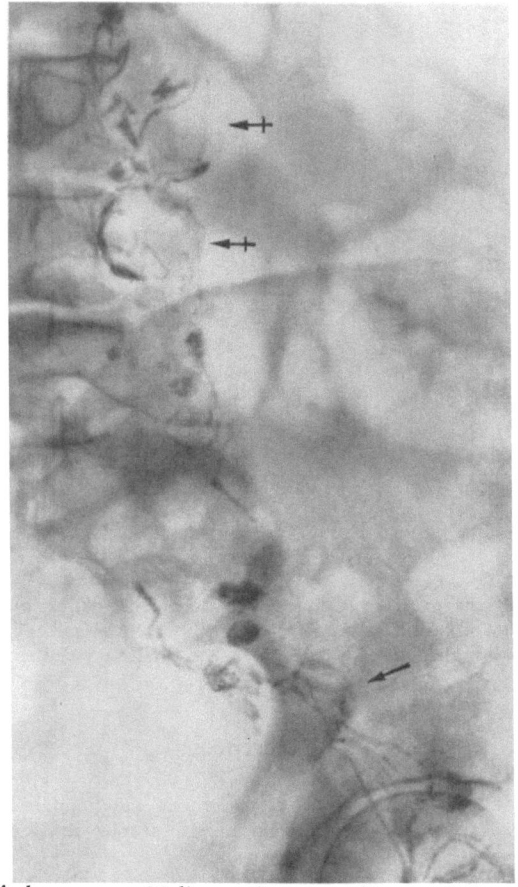

Fig. 40. *Carcinoma of the prostate*. Malignant invasion of external iliac (→) and left aortic (↦) lymph nodes

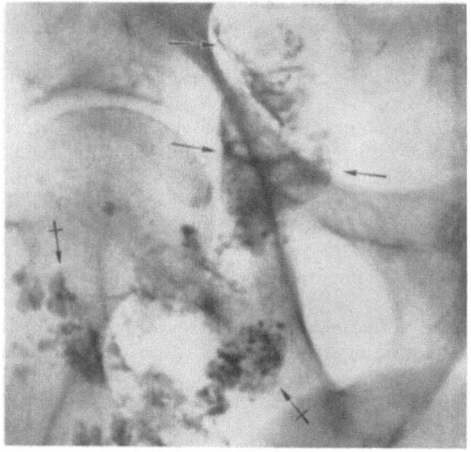

Fig. 41. *Carcinoma of the prostate*. Metastatic involvement of medial external iliac lymph nodes (→). Reactive hyperplasia of the deep inguinal lymph nodes (↦). (Confirmed by lymph node excision)

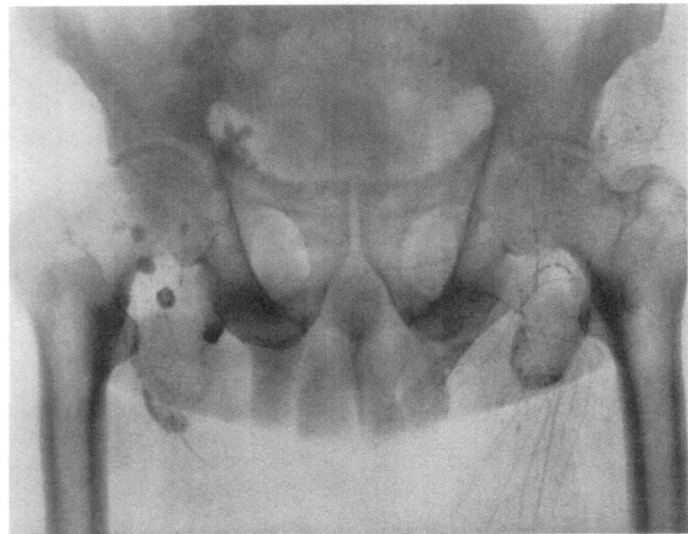

Fig. 42. *Carcinoma of the prostate*. Complete bilateral obstruction of the lymphatic circulation due to malignant invasion of the iliac lymph nodes. Metastases in superficial and deep inguinal lymph nodes. Collaterals in the thigh and abdominal wall

References

ABBES, M., G. JUILLARD et CH. GIRAUD: Les extensions ganglionnaires des cancers urogenitaux de l'homme. Rapport de la lymphographie à propos de 73 cas. J. Urol. Néphrol. 73, 547 (1967).

BURGENER, F. A., und W. A. FUCHS: Die Bedeutung der Lymphographie in der Diagnostik und Therapie maligner Hodentumoren. Schweiz. med. Wschr. 99, 764 (1969).

BUSCH, F. M., u. E. S. SAYEGH: Roentgenographic visualization of human testicular lymphatics; a preliminary report. J. Urol. Néphrol. 89, 106 (1963).

— —, and O. W. CHENAULT: Some uses of lymphography in the management of testicular tumours. J. Urol. Néphrol. 93, 490 (1965).

CHAVEZ, C. M.: Lymphatic drainage of the testicle. Progress in Lymphology. p. 191. Stuttgart: G. Thieme 1967.

CHIAPPA, S., G. GALLI, S. BARBAINI, G. RAVASI et G. BAGLIANI: La lymphographie preoperatoire dans les tumeurs du testicule. J. Radiol. 44, 613 (1963).

—, C. USLENGHI, G. BONADONNA, P. MARANO, and G. RAVASI: Combined testicular and foot lymphography in testicular carcinoma. Surg. Gynec. Obstet. 123, 10 (1966).

COOK JR., F. E., D. D. LAWRENCE, J. R. SMITH, and E. J. GRITLI: Testicular carcinoma and lymphography. Radiology 84, 420 (1965).

CUNÉO, B., and M. MARCILLE: Topographie des ganglions ilio-pelviens. Bull. Soc. anat. Paris 653 (1901).

DIXON, F. J., and R. A. MOORE: Tumors of male sex organs. In: Atlas of tumor pathology. Fasc. 31 B and 32. United States Armed Forces Institute of Pathology, Washington, D. C., 1952.

DOLAN, P. A., and R. R. HUGHES: Lymphography in genital cancer. Surg. Gynec. Obstet. 118, 1286 (1964).

GREGL, A., F. TRUSS, J. KIENLE, F. GRABNER, R. SCHWARTZ u. J. STELZNER: Indikation zur Lymphographie bei den bösartigen Geschwülsten des Urogenitaltraktes. Fortschr. Röntgenstr. 106, 789 (1967).

HANSCHKE, H. J., K. KÖNIG, und W. CASPAR: Spätergebnisse der Behandlung des Prostata-karzinoms. Dtsch. med. Wschr. 47, 2271 (1968).

HOHENFELLNER, R., H. JANISCH, und W. LUDVIK: Die Lymphographie bei malignen Erkrankungen des Urogenitalsystems. Geburtsh. Frauenheilk. 25, 298 (1965).

KUBIK, S.: The efferent vessels and the regional lymph nodes of the kidney, the ureter, the urinary bladder and the male genital organs. Progress in Lymphology. p. 179. Stuttgart: G. Thieme 1967.

LANGHAMMER, H.: Die Lymphographie bei malignen Hodentumoren. Fortschr. Röntgenstr. 110, 191 (1969).

LUDVIK, W., u. W. ZAUNBAUER: Die Bedeutung der Lymphographie für die chirurgischen Disziplinen. Fortschr. Röntgenstr. 105, 614 (1966).

MARKOVITS, P., A. A. ASCARELLI, M. GROSDEMANGE, Y. E. SCHMIERER e J. GRELLET: L'aspetto linfografico della compromissione ghiandulare nei tumori del testiculo. Riv. Radiol. 4, 163 (1964).

MAY, R. E., and M. BOGASH: Lymphangiography as a diagnostic adjunct in urology. J. Urol. 87, 208 (1962).

MELLINGER, G. T., J. C. BAILAR, and L. J. ARDUINO: Treatment and survival of patients with cancer of the prostate. Surg. Gynec. Obstet. 124, 1011 (1967).

PELLEGRINI, P., F. MARGIOTTA, L. ABLEROTANZA e N. DI CAGNO: Tentativi di Visualizzazione Radiologica dei Collettori Linfatici del Testicolo e delle Linfoghiandole Lombo-aortiche. Gazz. int. Med. Chir. 63, 1 (1957).

PICARD, J. D., et J. BABINET: Etude lymphographique de l'extension ganglionnaire dans les tumeurs du testicule. A propos de 50 cas. J. Urol. Néphrol. 70, 595 (1964).

RIVEROS, M., R. GARCIA, and R. CABANAS: Lymphadenography of the dorsal lymphatics of the penis. Cancer 20, 2026 (1967).

RÜTTIMANN, A., u. M. S. DEL BUONO: Die Lymphographie. In: Ergebnisse der medizinischen Strahlenforschung. Neue Folge. Band I. Hrsg. SCHINZ-GLAUNER-RÜTTIMANN. Stuttgart: Thieme 1964.

SAYEGH, E., T. BROOKS, E. SACHSER, and T. BUSCH: Lymphangiography of the retroperitoneal lymph nodes through the inguinal route. J. Urol. 95, 102 (1965).

SCHAFFER, B., S. WALLACE, L. JACKSON, M. JUKER, P. R. LEBERMANN, and T. R. FETTER: Urologic applications of lymphangiography. J. Urol. 87, 91 (1962).

VIAMONTE, M., D. ALTMAN, R. PARKS, E. BLUM, M. BEVILAQUA, and L. RECHER: Radiographic-Pathologic Correlation in the Interpretation of Lymphangioadenograms. Radiology 80, 903 (1963).

VON KEISER, D.: Testicular tumours. Progress in Lymphology. p. 190. Stuttgart: G. Thieme 1967.

Urinary Tract

Malignant Tumors of the Kidney

Anatomy of the Regional Lymph Nodes (Fig. 43)

The efferent vessels of the left kidney drain into the left latero-aortic and pre-aortic lymph nodes; those of the right kidney communicate with the right latero-aortic lymph nodes situated around the inferior vena cava: the latero-caval, pre- and retrocaval and interaortico-caval nodes.

Foot lymphography demonstrates the right aortic lymph nodes at the level of L1/2 in only 30% of the cases, whereas the left aortic lymph node group of this area is visualized in 60%. Non-visualization of the regional lymph nodes of the right kidney by foot lymphography is therefore relatively common. Consequently, cavograph is a supplemental method of great importance for demonstrating regional metastatic spread.

Lymphographic Findings

Twenty-one patients with carcinoma of the kidney were investigated by lymphography. Eight lymphograms demonstrated malignant metastatic spread to the regional aortic lymph nodes, which was confirmed in 5 cases by lymph node excision

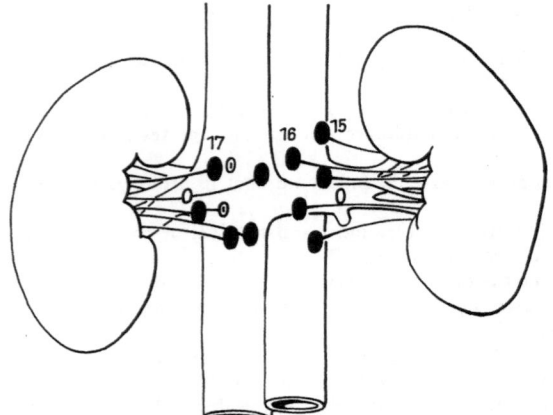

15 Left aortic lymph nodes
16 Pre-retro aortic lymph nodes
17 Right aortic lymph nodes

● Routinely demonstrated by lymphography; ⊖ Facultatively demonstrated by lymphography; ○ Not demonstrated by lymphography

Fig. 43. *Anatomy of the regional lymph nodes of the kidney*

(Figs. 44, 45). In one patient the positive lymphographic finding was supported by compression of the inferior vena cava in cavography. A questionable positive lymphographic diagnosis in 1 patient was not confirmed histologically. Lymphography in a 2-year old boy with a nephroblastoma of the left kidney (Wilm's tumor) demonstrated obstruction of the left aortic lymph vessels and metastatic deposits within pre-aortic lymph nodes at the level of L2, a finding confirmed by lymph node excision (Fig. 46).

VON KEISER (1966) studied 16 patients with malignant kidney tumors by lymphography and found 8 lymphograms to be abnormal. In all cases the lymph nodes in the hilar region of the kidney were involved. In 5 cases metastatic deposits in lymph nodes situated at the bifurcation of the aorta and iliac area were observed. In one case of recurrent hemangioendothelioma of the right kidney, obstruction and collateral circulation were present.

ELKE and RUTISHAUSER (1967) investigated 6 cases of renal tumors. Four lymphograms were considered to be indicative of tumor metastases to the regional lymph nodes, findings which were confirmed by lymph node excision in 2 cases. An interesting feature was the storage of contrast material within the tumor cells of metastases in 3 patients (ELKE, 1965). Case reports on the diagnostic value of lymphography in tumors of the kidney have been published by RÜTTIMANN and DEL BUONO (1964), ALTMAN et al. (1962), VIAMONTE et al. (1963), PUJOL and LAMARQUE (1964) and GREGL et al. (1967).

McDONALD (1966) considered lymphography to be valuable in patients with renal carcinoma, because in 50% of his cases metastatic involvement of the regional lymph nodes was demonstrated by this method.

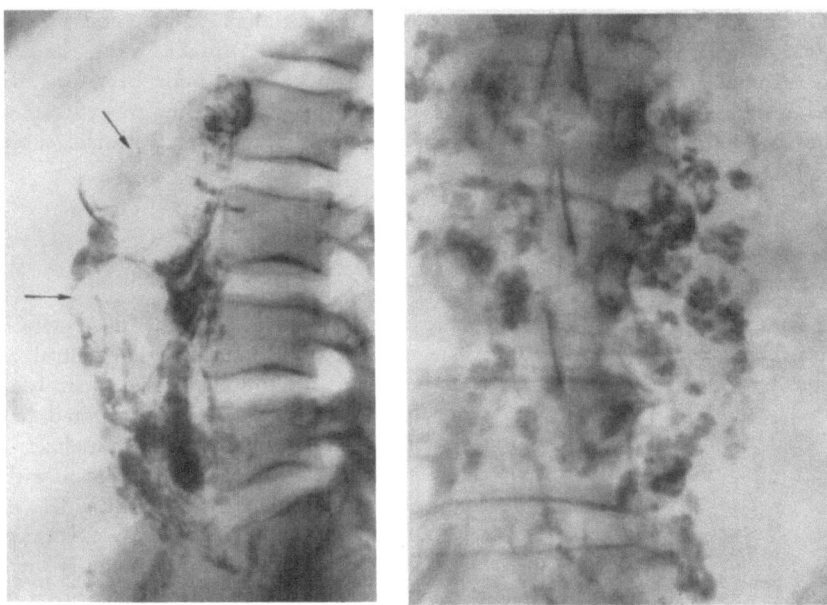

Fig. 44   Fig. 45

Fig. 44. *Carcinoma of the left kidney.* Extensive filling defects in enlarged aortic lymph nodes caused by malignant metastases (→) (confirmed by lymph node excision)

Fig. 45. *Carcinoma of the left kidney.* Multiple small filling defects in slightly enlarged metastatic aortic lymph nodes (confirmed by lymph node excision)

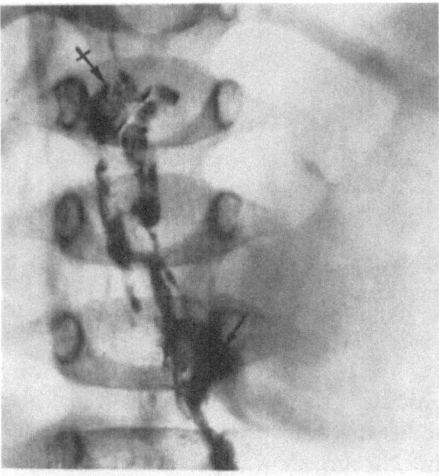

Fig. 46. *Nephroblastoma of the left kidney.* Obstruction of the left aortic lymphatics (→). Metastatic deposits within pre-retro aortic lymph nodes (↦) (confirmed by lymph node excision)

According to Staehler (1959) metastases to the regional lymph nodes in renal carcinoma are observed in 25%, according to Robson (1963) in 22.5% of the cases. Because regional lymph node metastases are indicative of a poor prognosis with local recurrencies usually fatal within a short time, it is important to evaluate the condition of the regional lymph nodes by lymphography prior to radical surgery (Zingg, 1966).

Malignant Tumors of the Adrenal Gland

Anatomy of the Regional Lymph Nodes

The lymphatics of the suprarenal gland form a superficial and a deep network which are connected by anastomoses. The efferent lymphatics of the ventral and dorsal border enter the primary regional lymph nodes which are the aortic lymph nodes of the corresponding side, situated at the level of L1/2. Lymphography visualizes the right aortic lymph nodes at this level with a frequency of only 30% and of the left side with a frequency of 60%. Therefore cavography is of great importance supplementally in localizing metastatic spread arising from the right suprarenal gland.

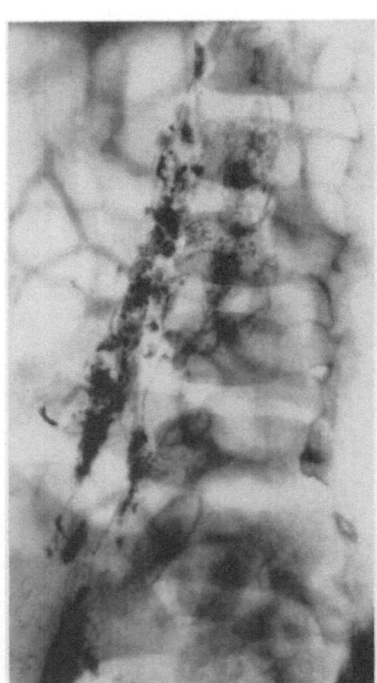

Fig. 47. *Sympaticoblastoma.* Enlarged aortic lymph nodes containing multiple large filling defects indicative of metastatic deposits

Lymphographic Findings

Malignant tumors of the suprarenal gland are carcinoma, neuroblastoma (sympaticogonioma, sympaticoblastoma) and pheochromoblastoma. Lymphographic investigations in cases of sympaticoblastoma have been reported by Gasquet et al. (1967), who studied 24 children with the disease. In each of the cases, pathologic changes within the aortic lymph vessels and nodes were observed. Dislocations of the lymph vessels by malignant growth and partial and complete obstructions of the lymphatic circulation within the aortic and iliac regions were common findings. The lymph nodes were enlarged and contained multiple large filling defects indicative of metastatic deposits. The lymphographic findings were seen by the author in the cases of a 2-year old girl and a 4-year old girl with large tumors of the left adrenal glands, verified by angiography (Fig. 47). Radiotherapy was prescribed because of the massive malignant lymph node involvement. No surgery was performed. The systematic lymphographic investigations by the group of Gasquet (1967) demonstrate clearly the high frequency of lymph node metastases in sympaticoblastoma. The great extent of lymphatic involvement explains the inoperability of most of these cases. Radiotherapy and chemotherapy are essential and may reduce the malignant growth to a size which may be surgically removed.

There are no published reports of lymphographic investigations in cases of carcinoma and pheochromocytoma of the adrenal gland. In the author's series of investigations a 16-year old girl with a tumor of the left adrenal gland was studied by lymphography. No malignant involvement of the regional lymph nodes was detectable.

Carcinoma of the Urinary Bladder

Anatomy of the Regional Lymph Nodes (Fig. 48)

The lymphatics of the anterior bladder wall drain into the anterior and lateral vesical lymph nodes which are connected with the external iliac lymph nodes. The lymphatics of the posterior bladder wall drain to the posterior and lateral vesical

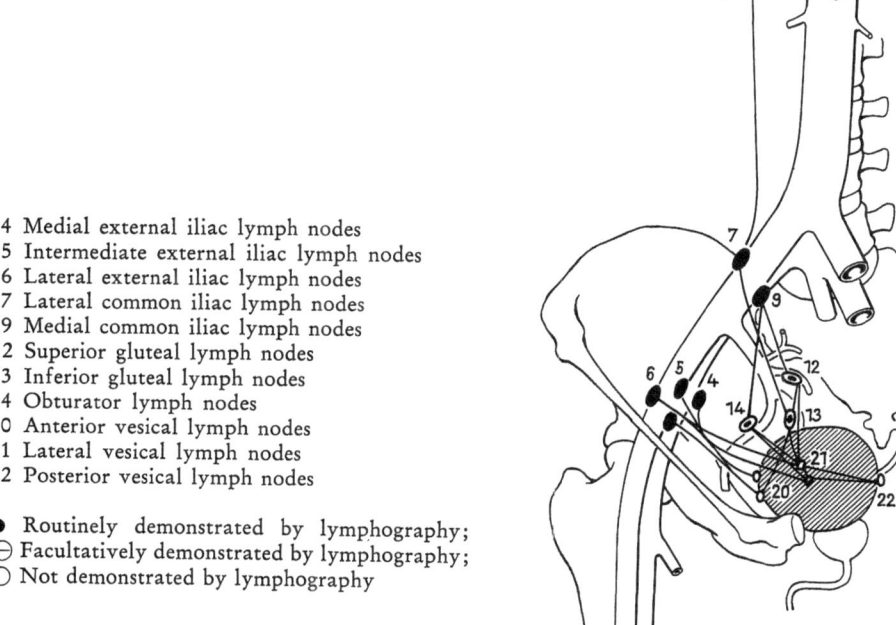

 4 Medial external iliac lymph nodes
 5 Intermediate external iliac lymph nodes
 6 Lateral external iliac lymph nodes
 7 Lateral common iliac lymph nodes
 9 Medial common iliac lymph nodes
12 Superior gluteal lymph nodes
13 Inferior gluteal lymph nodes
14 Obturator lymph nodes
20 Anterior vesical lymph nodes
21 Lateral vesical lymph nodes
22 Posterior vesical lymph nodes

● Routinely demonstrated by lymphography;
⊖ Facultatively demonstrated by lymphography;
○ Not demonstrated by lymphography

Fig. 48. *Anatomy of the regional lymph nodes of the urinary bladder*

lymph nodes and also join the external iliac node group. Some efferent lymph vessels of the urinary bladder are directly connected with the superior and inferior gluteal and obturator lymph nodes. The efferent lymphatics of the gluteal node group communicate with the common iliac lymph nodes. The major primary regional lymph node groups of the urinary bladder, the anterior, lateral and posterior vesical lymph nodes, situated in the perivesical tissue, are not demonstrated by foot lymphography. The remaining primary regional lymph nodes, the inferior and superior gluteal and obturator lymph nodes, are very inconstantly contrast-filled. Malignant metastatic deposits within these lymph nodes are rarely observed. Consequently foot lymphography demonstrates only regional lymph nodes of the second and third order, namely the common and external iliac node groups.

Lymphographic Findings

One hundred-and-nine patients with malignant tumors of the urinary bladder of varying size and histology were investigated, most often employing bilateral lymphography. The clinical investigation, usually under general anaesthesia, included cytoscopy and bimanual palpation. Electrocoagulation of the tumor, partial bladder

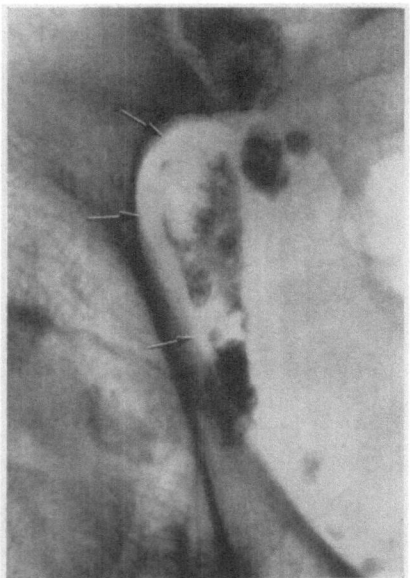

Fig. 49

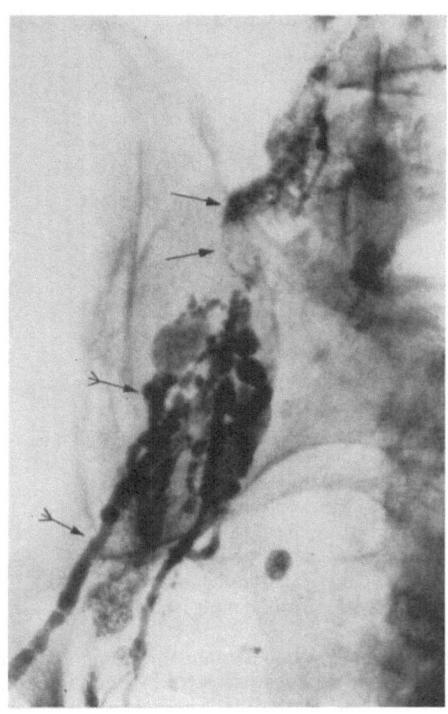

Fig. 50

Fig. 49. *Carcinoma of the urinary bladder*. Metastases in medial external iliac lymph nodes containing large marginal filling defects (→) caused by metastatic foci

Fig. 50. *Carcinoma of the urinary bladder*. Metastases in lateral common iliac lymph nodes (→). Partial obstruction of the lymphatic circulation, dilatation of the afferent lymphatics (↔)

resection, and in rare cases total cystectomy were performed. Most patients were treated by radiotherapy with high speed electrons and high voltage.

In 85 cases lymphography did not reveal pathologic changes. Twenty-four patients (22%) had positive lymphographic findings in regional lymph nodes of the second and third order. Of the 24 positives, 17 exhibited malignant metastatic spread exclusively within the external iliac lymph nodes of one side (Fig. 49) and in one case bilateral involvement of the external iliac nodes was demonstrated. In 2 cases tumor metastases were present in a single common iliac lymph node (Fig. 50).

There was also a single case of unilateral involvement of the external iliac and deep inguinal lymph nodes, a single case of bilateral involvement of dissimilar groups — a lateral common iliac node on the left and a medial external iliac on the right (Fig. 51), and a single case of iliac-aortic node involvement.

In 2 cases with localization of the primary tumor within the dorsal part of the left half of the urinary bladder, bilateral metastatic spread within the common and external iliac lymph nodes with partial blockage of the lymphatic circulation was found (Fig. 52). The presence of collateral vessels in the para-vertebral region

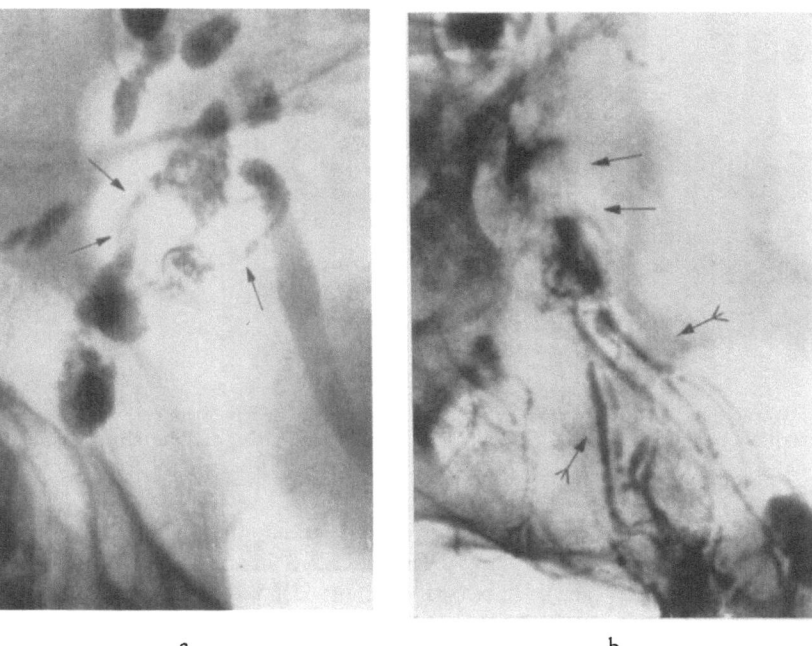

a   b

Fig. 51. *Carcinoma of the urinary bladder.* a Metastases in two right medial external iliac lymph nodes. Well demarcated large central filling defects (→). Dilatation but no dislocation of the right ureter. b Malignant metastatic spread to a left lateral common iliac lymph node. Marginal and central filling defects (→). Slight stasis of the afferent lymphatics (↔)

indicated additional malignant infiltration within the left lateral aortic lymph nodes. All lymph nodes infiltrated by malignant tissue were enlarged and showed marginal and central filling defects of various size. Eleven cases with obstruction of the lymph circulation were counted.

Seventy-six of the 108 patients were studied by angiography of the urinary bladder prior to lymphography. In 16 of the 47 patients (34%) with malignant infiltration of the perivesical region, as seen on the angiogram, lymphography revealed metastatic deposits within the regional lymph nodes.

Cavography as a complimentary method to lymphography was performed in 47 of the series of 108 patients. Thirty-eight cavograms with normal lymphograms did not show pathologic findings including 20 cases with perivesical tumor infiltration in the angiogram. Five patients with positive lymphographic findings had compression of the iliac veins because of tumor growth.

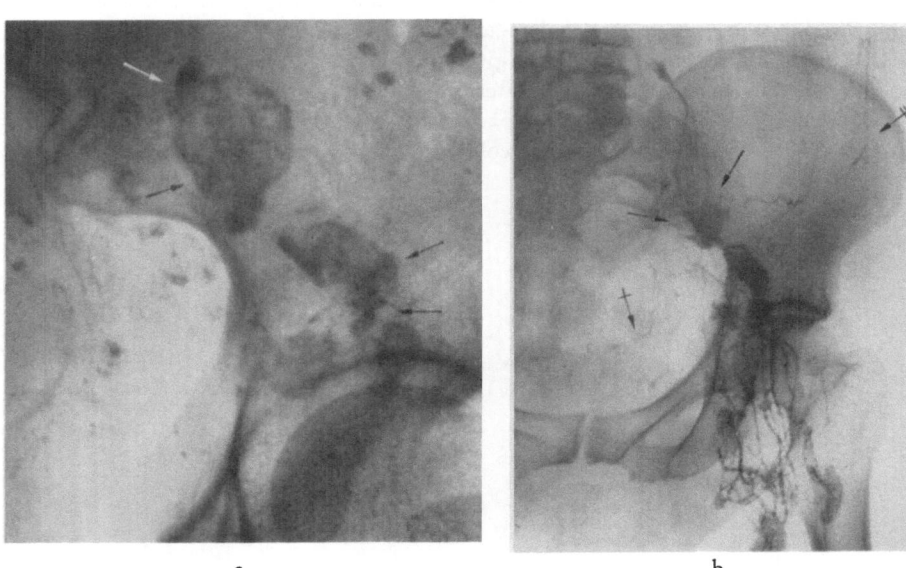

a   b

Fig. 52. *Carcinoma of the urinary bladder.* a Metastatic involvement of the external and common iliac lymph nodes (→). b Collateral lymphatics in the paravertebral, lumbar (↔) and pelvic region (–‖→)

Metastases of carcinoma of the urinary bladder in regional lymph nodes demonstrated by lymphography have been described in case reports by COLLETTE (1958), SCHAFFER et al. (1962), VIAMONTE et al. (1963), VAUGHAN and VAREY (1964), DE ROO (1964), BELTZ and THURN (1965), ELKE and RUTISHAUSER (1967) and GREGL et al. (1967). WILJASALO (1965) investigated 31 patients with bladder cancer without discussing the specific diagnostic problems in detail.

McDONALD and WALLACE (1965) reported the lymphographic findings in 31 patients with malignant bladder tumors. Lymphographic diagnoses were checked against histologic control in 12 cases: 10 diagnoses were correct and 2 were false negatives. Four patients had metastases in the external and common iliac lymph nodes. LUDWIK and HOHENFELLER (1966) reported tumor metastases within the iliac lymph nodes in one third of 46 patients examined by lymphography.

MAJOR et al. (1963), and RÜTTIMANN (1964, 1966) stress the importance of combined angiographic and lymphographic investigation of patients with malignant tumors of the urinary bladder. The primary regional lymph nodes of the urinary bladder, the anterior, posterior and lateral vesical lymph nodes, are situated within the perivesical tissue and are not demonstrated by lymphography. Bladder angiography may indicate penetration of the bladder wall by a malignant tumor and infiltration of the perivesical tissue (BOIJSEN and NILSSON 1963, MARANTA et al. 1964, LANG et al. 1966, NILSSON 1967). Perivesical tumor infiltration implies direct invasion of the regional lymph nodes situated in the perivesical tissue, and the presence of metastases within these lymph nodes cannot be assumed if the malignant tumor is not penetrating the bladder wall.

The other primary regional lymph nodes of the urinary bladder, the superior and inferior gluteal and the obturator lymph nodes are only occasionally demonstrated by lymphography. Malignant metastatic spread to these lymph node groups cannot be diagnosed by lymphography, because these lymph nodes are not contrast-filled when infiltrated by malignant tumor cells.

In conclusion, angiography should be performed in all cases of urinary bladder malignancy. Lymphography is indicated in those cases exhibiting perivesical tumor infiltration because experience has shown that one-third of these cases have positive lymphograms.

References

ALTMAN, D., W. SHAVER, and M. VIAMONTE: Lymphangiography in children. Amer. J. Dis. Child 104, 335 (1962).

BELTZ, L., u. P. THURN: Das Lymphogramm beim tumorösen retroperitonealen Lymphblock. Fortschr. Röntgenstr. 102, 278 (1965).

BOIJSEN, E., and J. NILSSON: Angiography in diagnosis of tumors of the urinary bladder. Acta radiol. (Stockh.) 57, 241 (1962).

COLLETTE, J. M.: Envahissements ganglionnaires inguino-iliopelviens par lymphographie. Acta radiol. (Stockh.) 49, 154 (1958).

DE ROO, T.: Lymphografie. Van Gorcum's Med. Bibl. Nr. 182 (1964).

ELKE, M.: Speicherung von öligem Kontrastmittel in Lungenmetastasen eines hypernephroiden Karzinoms nach Lymphographie. Fortschr. Röntgenstr. 103, 625 (1965).

—, u. G. RUTISHAUSER: Die Lymphographie als Zusatzuntersuchung bei urologischen Tumoren. Fortschr. Röntgenstr. 107, 224 (1967).

FUCHS, W. A.: Die Lymphographie bei Harnblasentumoren. Radiologe 8, 180 (1968).

GASQUET, C., P. MARKOVITS, M. GROSDEMANGE et O. SCHWEISSGUTH: La lymphographie dans les sympathomes de l'enfant. Ann. Radiol. (Paris) 10, 501 (1967).

GREGL, A., F. TRUSS, J. KIENLE, F. GRABNER, T. SCHWARTZ u. J. STELZNER: Indikation zur Lymphographie bei den bösartigen Geschwülsten des Urogenitaltraktes. Fortschr. Röntgenstr. 106, 789 (1967).

LANG, E. K., M. H. NOURSE, W. N. WISHARD, JR., and J. H. O. MERTZ: The accuracy of preoperative staging of bladder tumors by arteriography. A 5 year study. J. Urol. 95, 363 (1966).

LUDVIK, W., u. R. HOHENFELLNER: Die Lymphographie beim Blasencarcinom. Urol 4, 77 (1966).

MARANTA, E., F. CAMPONOVO u. M. S. DEL BUONO: Die Beckenangiographie. Fortschr. Röntgenstr. 101, 229 (1964).

MAYOR, G., F. CAMPONOVO, F. PUPATO, E. ZINGG, J. WELLAUER, A. RÜTTIMANN, M. DEL BUONO u. A. SCHNAUDER: Spezielle röntgendiagnostische Untersuchungen bei Malignomen des Urogenitaltraktes. Urologe 2, 76 (1968).

McDONALD, J. S.: Discussion note. Diseases of the kidneys and ureters. Progress in Lymphology. p. 183. Stuttgart: G. Thieme 1967.

—, and E. N. K. WALLACE: Lymphangiography in tumours of the kidney, bladder and testicle. Brit. J. Radiol. 38, 93 (1965).

Nilsson, J.: Angiography in tumors of the urinary bladder. Acta radiol. (Stockh.) suppl. 263 (1967).

Pujol, H., et J. L. Lamarque: Ilio-cavographie et lymphographie dans la recherche des adenopaties retroperitoneales. Paris: Masson & Cie 1964.

Robson, C. J.: J. Urol. **89**, 37 (1963).

Rüttimann, A.: Erkrankungen des retroperitonealen Lymphsystems. Lehrbuch der Röntgendiagnostik, Vol. 5. Stuttgart: G. Thieme 1965.

— u. M. S. Del Buono: Die Lymphographie. In: Ergebnisse der medizinischen Strahlenforschung. Neue Folge. Band I. Hrsg. Schinz-Glauner-Rüttimann. Stuttgart: Thieme 1964.

Schaffer, B., S. Wallace, L. Jackson, M. Juker, P. R. Lebermann, and T. R. Fetter: Urologic applications of lymphangiography. J. Urol. **87**, 91 (1962).

Staehler, W.: Klinik und Praxis der Urologie. Stuttgart: G. Thieme 1959.

Vaughan, B. F., and J. F. Varey: The lymphographic appearances of malignant pelvic lymph node involvement. Chir. Radiol. **15**, 329 (1964).

Viamonte, M., D. Altman, R. Parks, E. Blum, M. Bevilaqua, and L. Recher: Radiographic-pathologic correlation in the interpretation of lymphangioadenograms. Radiology **80**, 903 (1963).

von Keiser, D.: Renal tumors. Progress in Lymphology. p. 182. Stuttgart: G. Thieme 1967.

Wiljasalo, M.: Lymphographic differential diagnosis of neoplastic diseases. Acta radiol. (Stockh.) suppl. 247 (1965).

Zingg, E.: About the question of therapy in the kidneys with hypernephroma. Progress in Lymphology. p. 183. Stuttgart: G. Thieme 1967.

Gastrointestinal Tract

Carcinoma of the Anus

Anatomy of the Regional Lymph Nodes (Fig. 53)

The lymph vessels arising from the external anal region form a network within the subcutaneous tissue and drain via the medial aspect of the thigh into the medial superior superficial lymph nodes. The lymphatic drainage of the internal anal region is directed towards the anorectal lymph nodes which are connected with internal and common iliac lymph nodes.

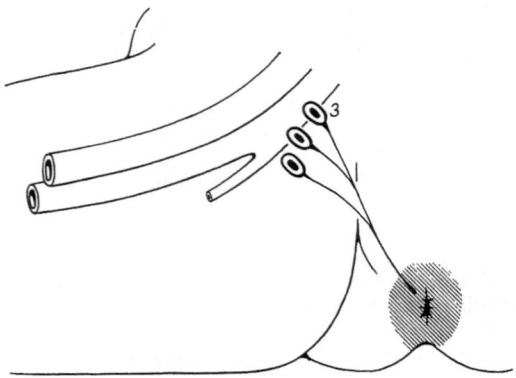

⊖ Facultatively demonstrated by lymphography

Fig. 53. *Anatomy of the regional lymph nodes of the anus.* 3 Superior superficial inguinal lymph nodes (perineal group)

Lymphographic Findings

In the author's series of investigations 7 patients with anal carcinoma were studied by lymphography. Metastatic deposits in regional lymph nodes were identified in 5 cases. In one patient, tumor metastases were demonstrated in right medial external iliac lymph nodes and, in a later stage, in right latero-aortic nodes. Two patients in clinically early tumor stages demonstrated metastases in external iliac lymph nodes, findings which were confirmed by lymph node excision (Figs. 54, 55).

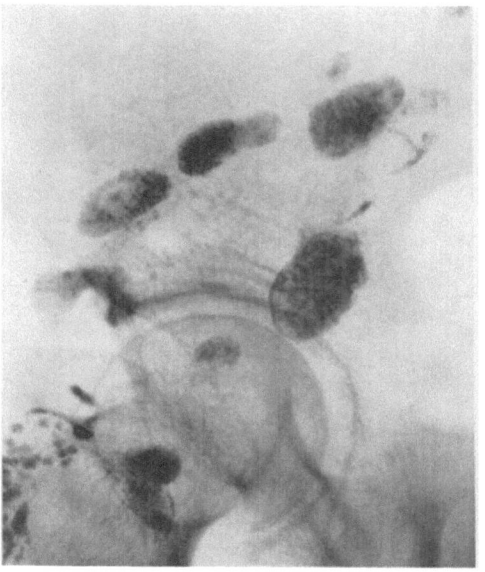

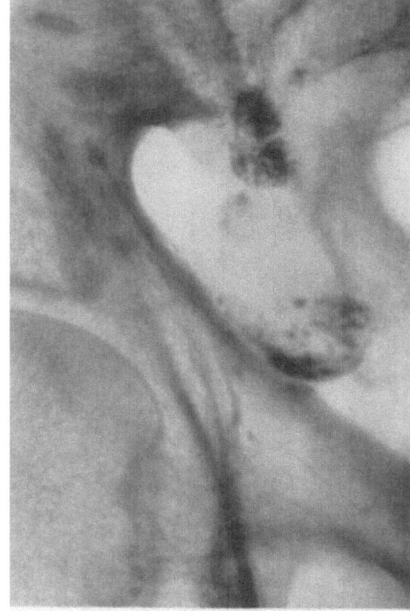

Fig. 54

Fig. 55

Fig. 54. *Anal carcinoma.* Metastases in lateral and medial external iliac lymph nodes containing multiple small central and marginal filling defects (confirmed by lymph node excision)

Fig. 55. *Anal carcinoma.* Metastases in enlarged medial external iliac lymph nodes. Large central filling defects (confirmed by lymph node excision)

Clinically suspicious metastases to inguinal and medial external iliac lymph nodes were demonstrated by lymphography in one patient, and later confirmed by biopsy (Fig. 56). In the remaining patient with extensive malignant invasion causing edema of the leg and scrotum, lymphography visualized tumor infiltration of the inguinal iliac and aortic lymph nodes. Partial obstruction of the lymphatic circulation was demonstrated (Fig. 57).

The high frequency of malignant involvement of regional lymph nodes, in particular the external iliac nodes, indicates clearly the diagnostic value of lymphography in carcinoma of the anus. However, it must be remembered that the primary regional lymph nodes of the anal region are not contrast-filled by foot lymphography. Prior to abdomino-peritoneal resection of the rectum and anus with lymph node excision, preoperative radiation therapy is performed on the basis of lymphographic findings. Prophylactic curative or palliative radiation therapy is indicated according to the extent of malignant metastatic involvement of the regional lymph nodes.

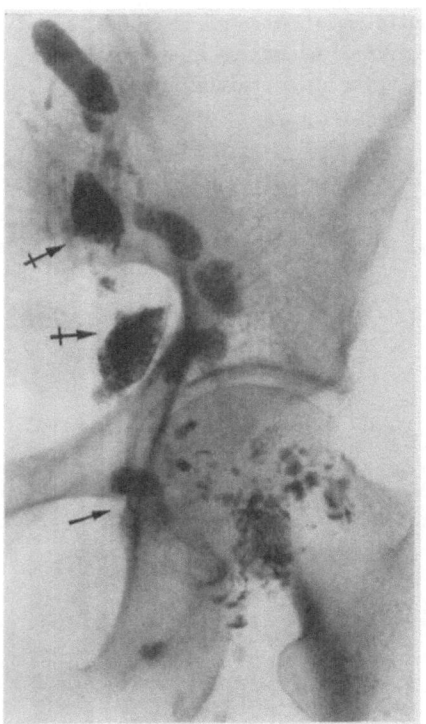

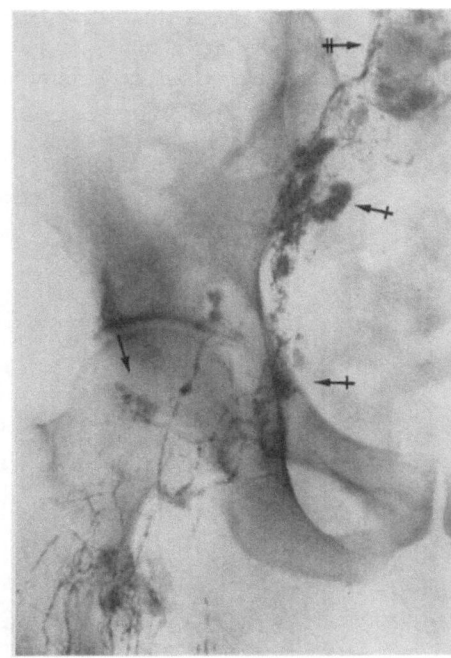

Fig. 57

Fig. 56

Fig. 56. *Anal carcinoma.* Metastases to the deep inguinal (→) and medial external iliac lymph nodes (↔). Slight obstruction of the lymphatic circulation (confirmed by lymph node excision)

Fig. 57. *Anal carcinoma.* Extensive malignant invasion of the inguinal (→) iliac (↔) and aortic (⊣→) lymph nodes. Partial obstruction of the lymphatic circulation, leading to lymphedema of the leg and scrotum

Carcinoma of the Rectum

Anatomy of the Regional Lymph Nodes (Fig. 58)

The primary regional lymph nodes of the rectum are the para-rectal and superior hemorrhoidal lymph nodes. The efferent lymphatics of these nodes are connected with inferior and superior gluteal lymph nodes which are inconstantly visualized by lymphography. Their efferent lymph vessels enter the medial common iliac lymph nodes, which are normally contrast-filled by lymphography.

Lymphographic Findings

In the author's series of investigations, 30 patients with carcinoma of the rectum were investigated by lymphography. In 23 cases, the malignant lesion was limited to the rectum; 7 tumors were situated in the recto-sigmoidal area. In 5 of the 25 patients with clinically advanced tumor propagation or recurrencies, lympho-

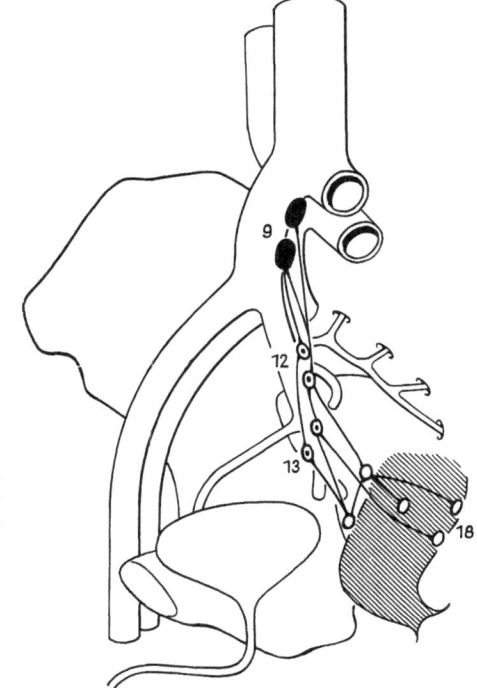

9 Medial common iliac lymph nodes
12 Superior gluteal lymph nodes
13 Inferior gluteal lymph nodes
18 Superior rectal lymph nodes

● Routinely demonstrated by lymphography; ⊖ Facultatively demonstrated by lymphography; ○ Not demonstrated by lymphography

Fig. 58. *Anatomy of the regional lymph nodes of the rectum*

graphy demonstrated malignant involvement of the regional lymph nodes. Positive lymphographic findings were observed in one of 6 cases, in which clinical investigations considered the malignant tumor to be strictly limited to the rectum. Malignant metastases were demonstrated in right common iliac lymph nodes in 3 cases (Fig. 59), in the external iliac nodes in 1 case (Fig. 60), in both the iliac and aortic lymph nodes in 2 cases (Fig. 61).

Cavography was positive in 2 cases, and 7 patients were found to have hydronephrosis, predominantly of the left kidney — caused by tumor infiltration of the pelvic region. PALANTIA et al. (1965) carried out preoperative lymphographic studies in 28 cases with malignant neoplasm of the rectosigmoid, 5 of which also presented involvement of the anal region. According to their results, the authors stress the frequency of metastases to the epicolic and paracolic lymph nodes not demonstrated by lymphography in contrast to the negative lymphographic and histologic findings of the inguinal and iliac lymph nodes. Similar observations have been made by

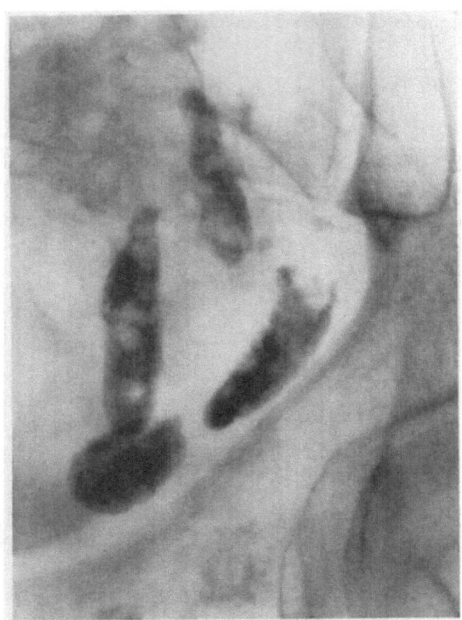

Fig. 59. *Rectal carcinoma.* Metastases in enlarged right external and common iliac lymph nodes containing large marginal and central filling defects (confirmed by lymph node excision)

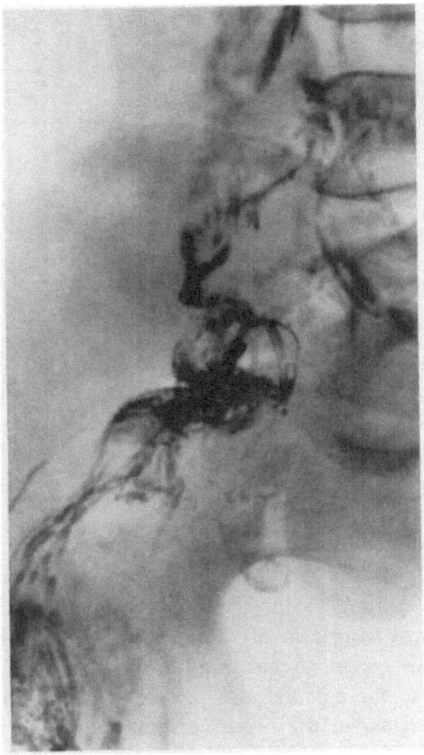

Fig. 60. *Carcinoma of the recto-sigmoidal area.* Metastases in external and common iliac lymph nodes containing numerous small marginal and central filling defects

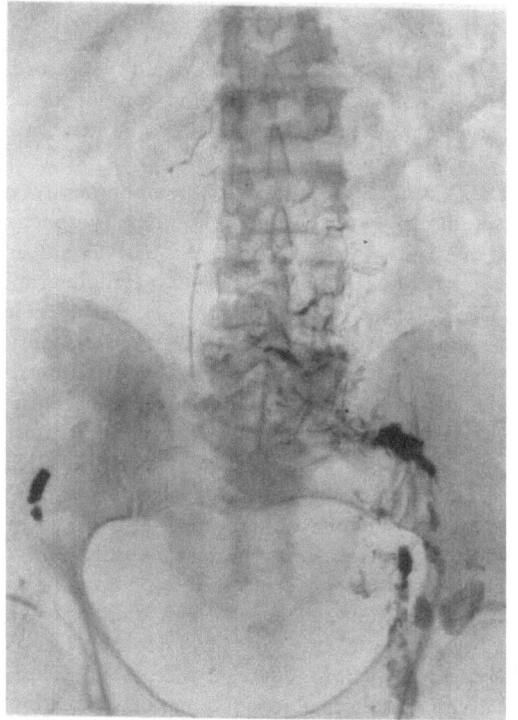

a

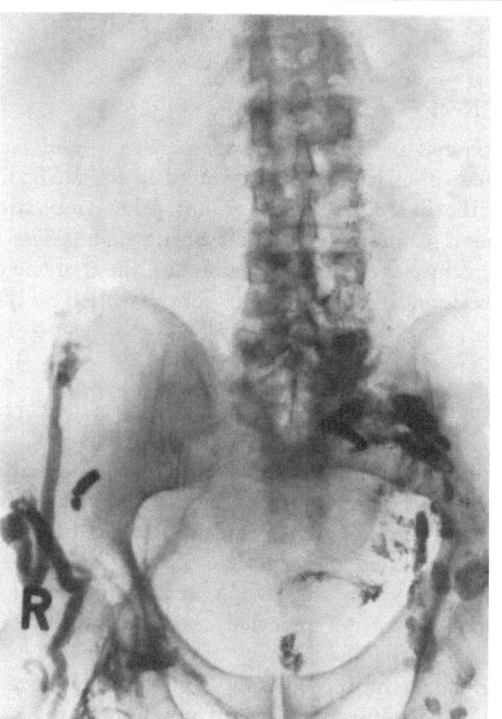

b

Fig. 61. *Rectal carcinoma*. Extensive bilateral metastatic spread into the iliac and aortic lymph nodes. Complete obstruction of the lymphatic circulation and occlusion of the pelvic veins on the right side. Contrast material in the appendix and large bowel

Sinistrero et al. (1965). Ludvik and Zaunbauer (1966) studied 9 patients with carcinoma of the rectosigmoid by lymphography, four of which were also verified by lymph node excision. Five lymphographies were positive, 3 negative and 1 false positive.

Gregl et al. (1967) report the results of lymphography in 30 patients with carcinoma of the rectum. In 6 of 17 operable cases, lymphography demonstrated malignant metastases of regional lymph nodes. Nine of 13 inoperable tumor patients exhibited metastases to regional lymph nodes by lymphography. Chiappa et al. (1967) investigated 36 patients, 13 of whom were recurrencies, showing clinical signs of malignant metastatic spread. Lymphography was positive in all 13 cases of advanced tumor stage. In 9 of the 23 patients with clinically operable tumors, positive lymphographic diagnoses were made. Four lymphograms were only suggestive of metastatic deposits in lymph nodes, and 10 lymphograms were normal. The positive lymphographic diagnoses were verified in 3 of the 9 cases by lymph node excision. In 2 cases with positive lymphograms no metastases were found at operation. Lymphographic control studies were able to demonstrate metastatic involvement after a normal appearance at the first investigation.

The relative high percentage of positive lymphographic findings in cases of operable carcinoma of the rectum reflects the high diagnostic value of preoperative lymphography. Therapy planning and prognosis depend largely on the presence of metastases within the regional lymph nodes. Furthermore, extensive metastatic spread suspected by clinical investigations is objectively demonstrated by lymphography.

Carcinoma of the Colon

Anatomy of the Regional Lymph Nodes (Fig. 62)

The efferent lymphatics of the descending, transverse and ascending colon drain into the para- and mesocolic lymph nodes situated in the mesocolon. The lymphatics of the coecum enter the ileo-coecal node groups. The lymphatic circulation of the left half of the colon is connected with left aortic nodes. The lymph of the right half of the colon drains into the intestinal trunk and the thoracic duct. Consequently, none of the primary regional lymph nodes are contrast-filled by lymphography.

Lymphographic Findings

In the author's small series of investigations, 7 cases of carcinoma of the colon were investigated by lymphography. The lymphograms in 2 cases of malignant tumor of the sigmoid were negative although the carcinomatous infiltration had reached the pelvic wall. In 1 patient with a large carcinoma of the left colic flexure, lymphedema of the leg, and malignant infiltration of the external iliac and inguinal region, lymphography confirmed the complete obstruction of the lymphatic circulation (Fig. 63). Lymphography was negative in 1 case with a malignant lesion situated in the ascending colon. Operation revealed metastatic deposits in regional lymph nodes which were not contrast-filled.

In 3 cases of carcinoma of the coecum, lymphography was normal. However, one of these patients had extensive malignant invasion of the peritoneal cavity and the ovaries.

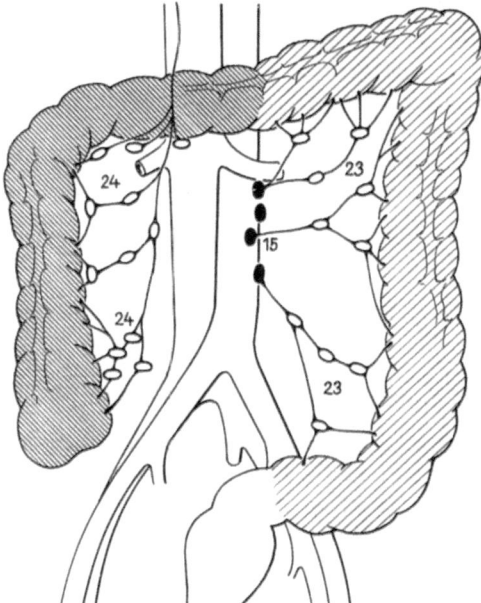

15 Left aortic lymph nodes
23 Para- and mesocolic lymph nodes
   of the left colon
24 Para- and mesocolic lymph nodes
   of the right colon

● Routinely demonstrated by lymphography; ○ Not demonstrated by
lymphography

Fig. 62. *Anatomy of the regional lymph nodes of the colon*

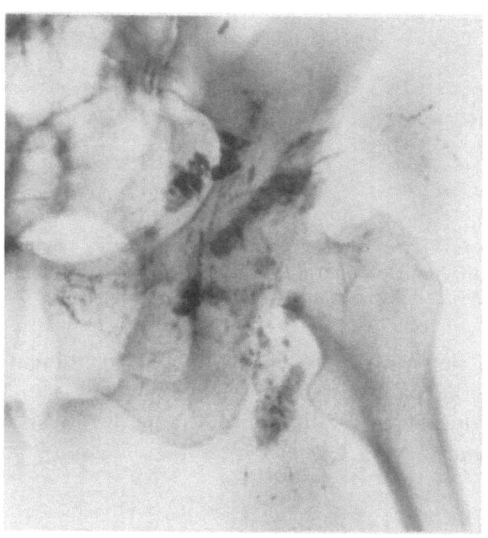

Fig. 63. *Carcinoma of the left colic flexure.* Malignant infiltration of the iliac region. Complete obstruction of the lymphatic circulation. Numerous collateral lymphatics in the thigh
and abdominal wall

The disappointing diagnostic results of lymphography are explained by the fact that foot lymphography demonstrates only secondary and tertiary regional lymph node groups. Similar negative results of lymphography in cancer of the large intestine have been reported by Viamonte et al. (1963) and Rüttimann and Del Buono (1964).

Clinical indication for lymphography in cases of malignant tumors of the large intestine without involvement of the anus and rectum is therefore very limited. However, if extensive metastatic spread is suspected by clinical investigations, positive lymphographic findings may objectively demonstrate the extent of the disease.

Carcinoma of the Upper Gastrointestinal Tract

Anatomy of the Regional Lymph Nodes

The regional lymph nodes of the stomach are the gastric, spleno-pancreatic and superior aortic node groups. The lymphatics of the duodenum drain into the superior pancreatic and pancreatico-duodenal nodes. The lymphatics of the jejunum and ileum enter the mesenteric lymph nodes. All these node groups including the regional lymph nodes of the pancreas and liver are connected with the intestinal lymph

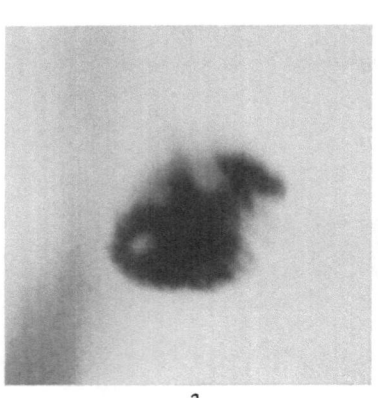 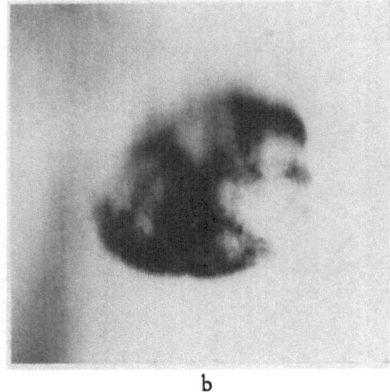

a   b

Fig. 64. *Scirrhous carcinoma of the stomach.* a Tumor metastasis in an enlarged supraclavicular lymph node containing multiple marginal filling defects. b Rapid tumor growth within 17 days. Increase of lymph node size and metastatic foci

trunks. Therefore, they are not contrast-filled by foot lymphography. Only a few efferent lymphatics of the pancreas enter the aortic nodes situated distal to the renal hilus. Consequently the possibility of detecting metastases in cancer of the upper gastrointestinal tract is very limited.

Lymphographic Findings

In the author's small series 8 patients with carcinoma of the stomach were studied by lymphography, which did not reveal metastatic foci within the aortic lymph nodes demonstrated. An enlarged supraclavicular lymph node was contrast-filled in a patient with a scirrhous type of gastric carcinoma. Well demarcated marginal filling defects due to metastatic foci were present (Fig. 64 a). A rapid growth rate of the metastatic node was observed during a period of 17 days, indicating the high malignancy of the carcinoma (Fig. 64 b).

Similar negative results of foot lymphography in cancer of the upper gastrointestinal tract were reported by Viamonte et al. (1963) in carcinoma of the stomach, and by Arvay and Picard (1963) in cancer of the pancreas. Displacement and complete obstruction of the thoracic duct in advanced cases of esophageal carcinoma has been observed by Leger et al. (1962) and Arvay and Picard (1963).

In conclusion, foot lymphography is very rarely indicated in cancer of the esophagus, stomach, duodenum, small intestine or pancreas, because diagnosis of malignant metastatic spread of these tumors is beyond the range of foot lymphography, consequent wholly to anatomic relations.

References

Arvay, N., et J. D. Picard: La lymphographie. Etude radiologique et clinique des voies lymphatiques normales et pathologiques. Paris: Masson & Cie. 1963.

Chiappa, S., G. Bonnadonna, C. Uslenghi, and U. Veronesi: Lymphangiography in the diagnosis of retroperitoneal node metastasis in rectal cancer. Brit. J. Radiol. 40, 584 (1967).

Gregl, A., J. Kienle, H. Uebel u. H. G. Weber: Lymphangiographie beim Rektumkarzinom. Fortschr. Röntgenstr. 106, 351 (1967).

Léger, L., M. Prémont et G. Hugon: Lymphographie du canal thoracique dans les cancers oesophagiens. Gaz. méd. Fr. 69, 2801 (1962).

Ludvik, W., u. W. Zaunbauer: Die Bedeutung der Lymphographie für die chirurgischen Disziplinen. Fortschr. Röntgenstr. 105, 614 (1966).

Palantia, A., A. Martelli, G. Gozetti u. M. Villa: Die Lymphographie im Stadium der lymphatischen von bösartigen Tumoren im Mastdarmsigma. Langenbecks Arch. Klin. Chir. 310, 83 (1965).

Rüttimann, A., u. M. S. Del Buono: Die Lymphographie. In: Ergebnisse der medizinischen Strahlenforschung. Neue Folge. Band I. Hrsg. Schinz-Glauner-Rüttimann. Stuttgart: Thieme 1964.

Sinistrero, G., G. Toscano, P. F. Carrazone e G. Da Rosa: Quadri linfografici nel carcinoma del retto. Minerva radiol. fisioter. radiobiol. (Torino) 10, 51 (1965).

Viamonte, M., D. Altman, R. Parks, E. Blum, M. Bevilaqua, and L. Recher: Radiographic-pathologic correlation in the interpretation of lymphangioadenograms. Radiology 80, 903 (1963).

Malignant Tumors of the Head and Neck

The diagnostic value of cervical lymphography in the diagnosis of malignant metastatic spread to the regional lymph nodes has been extensively investigated by Fisch (1966, 1968). In his monograph, he describes in detail the lymphographic findings in 128 patients with carcinoma of the head and neck. The primary tumors were situated mainly in the larynx (50 cases), hypopharynx (19 cases), tongue (18 cases), maxillary region (9 cases), and tonsils (9 cases). In 31 patients the lymph nodes were removed by radical neck dissection and investigated histologically.

Malignant metastatic deposits in cervical lymph nodes may be identified by lymphography by the presence of marginal filling defects and partial or complete obstruction of the lymphatic circulation (Fig. 65). Blockage of the oily contrast material is not characteristic for carcinoma in the cervical area; it may also be due to *reticular or follicular hyperplasia* of the lymph nodes. This important limitation must be considered when evaluating cervical lymphography for the detection of metastases in the cervical lymph nodes. Furthermore, only the deep lateral lymphatic system of the neck is visualized in a normal cervical lymphogram. The contrast material will not fill all the nodes which drain a given area of the cervical lymphatic

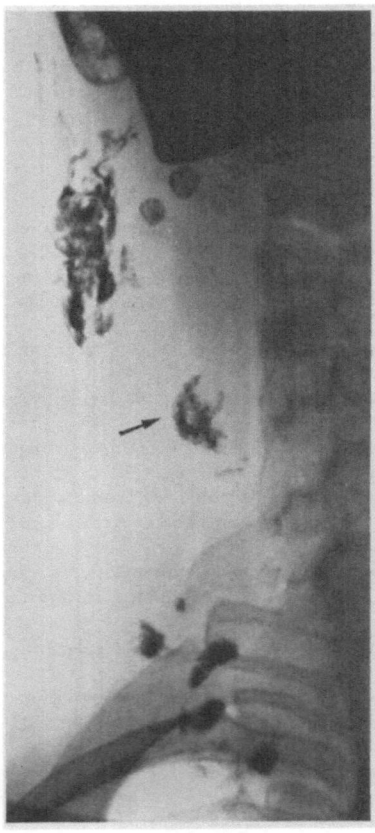

Fig. 65. *Branchiogenic carcinoma of the right neck.* Extensive lymphatic obstruction in the jugular and spinal lymph nodes by malignant and unspecific inflammatory lesions. Contrast filling of a single jugular lymph node (→) containing 3 marginal filling defects, the upper-most caused by malignant metastatic foci, the intermediate by the hilum of the node, and the lower-most by unspecific inflammatory reaction (confirmed by lymph node excision). (By Courtesy of U. Fisch, M. D., Zurich)

system and of course, cancer metastases to these nodes will not be demonstrated on the lymphogram. Moreover, the clinical use of lymphography in the cervical region is significantly limited by its technical difficulties. The rate of successful investigations reported by Fisch (1966, 1968) is only 50%.

Cervical lymphography is of great value in evaluating the extent of an abnormal reaction, demonstrating its presence in the deep lateral lymphatic system of the neck. The drainage area of a primary carcinoma may be correctly determined and, following complete neck dissection, thoroughly examined histologically. Cervical lymphography is at the present time not a true clinical, but an investigative method which has contributed to a very detailed analysis of clinical and histologic evaluation of the lymphatic system of the neck.

References

Fisch, U.: Lymphographische Untersuchungen über das zervikale Lymphsystem. Fortschr. Hals-Nas.-Ohrenheilk. Vol. 14. Basel-New York: Karger 1966.
— Lymphography of the cervical lymphatic system. Philadelphia-London-Toronto: Saunders 1968.

Malignant Melanoma

in lymph node metastases of undifferentiated squamous cell carcinoma of the skin. 48 patients with malignant melanoma. Positive lymphographic findings were present in 21 cases (45%). Control lymphograms and "second-look" lymphography were

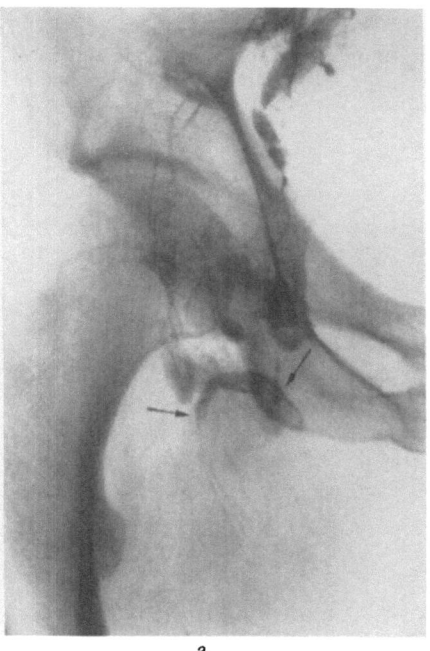
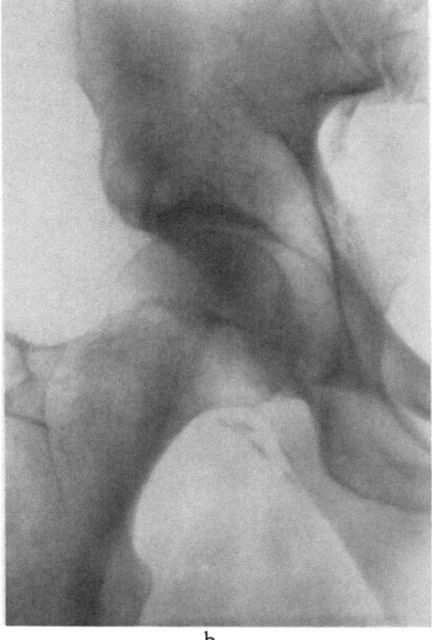

a   b

Fig. 66. *Malignant melanoma of the thigh.* a Enlarged inferior superficial inguinal lymph nodes with extensive central filling defects due to malignant tissue. Preserved contrast-filled lymphatic tissue in the peripheral area (→). b Complete surgical removal of the metastatic node

positive in 3 cases following normal primary lymphograms, and in 1 case cavography demonstrated lymph node metastases at a later stage. Pathologic lymphograms showed enlarged lymph nodes with extensive central filling defects and displacement of the remaining lymphatic tissue towards the periphery of the nodes.

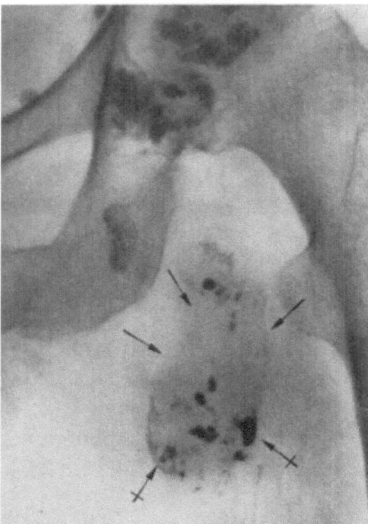

Fig. 67. *Malignant melanoma of the big toe.* Enlarged inferior superficial inguinal lymph nodes containing large central and marginal filling defects (→). Drop-like deposition of contrast material (↔)

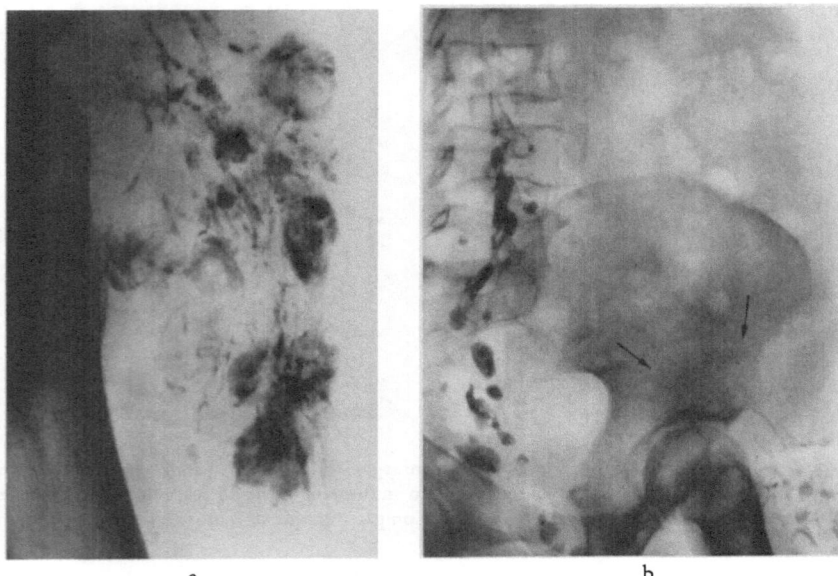

a   b

Fig. 68. *Malignant melanoma of the lower abdominal wall.* a Metastatic superior superficial inguinal lymph nodes containing large central filling defects. b Obstruction of the lymphatic circulation in the iliac region. Collateral lymphatics. Metastases in medial external iliac lymph nodes

Multiple, irregular confluent filling defects caused by malignant tumors in lymph nodes were present in the positive lymphograms of 10 patients. Partial or complete obstruction of the lymphatic circulation secondary to metastases was seen in 5 of the 21 positive cases. Large, coalescent, central filling defects with peripheral semi-ulnar areas of contrast-filled lymphatic tissue are frequent but not pathognomonic findings in lymph node metastases of malignant melanoma. The malignant tumors were localized in the *skin of the lower extremities* in 32 patients. In 17 of these,

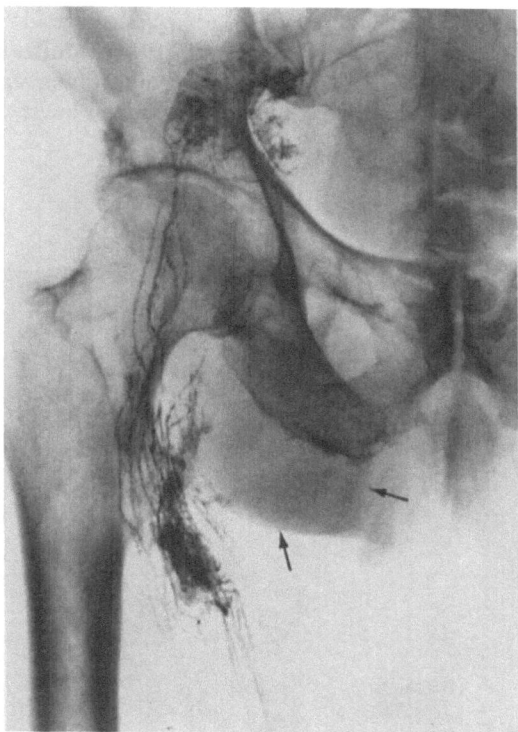

Fig. 69. *Malignant melanoma of the anal region.* Complete obstruction of the medial inguinal lymphatics by metastases in superior superficial inguinal lymph nodes (→). Metastatic involvement of the external iliac lymph nodes (confirmed by lymph node excision)

lymphography demonstrated malignant involvement of the inguinal lymph nodes (Fig. 66). In 7 of these cases malignancy had spread to the external iliac lymph node groups (Fig. 67). Eight of these positive lymphographic findings were verified by lymph node excision. Three of the 4 patients with malignant melanoma of the *skin of the lower abdominal wall* showed a negative lymphographic study, but malignant metastases within the medial superior superficial inguinal lymph nodes were proven histologically. One patient had extensive metastases in superior superficial inguinal lymph nodes and complete obstruction of the lymphatic circulation in the iliac region (Fig. 68). In 2 of 4 patients with the melanoma localized within the *anal region,* lymphography revealed malignant metastases to inguinal and lateral iliac nodes, leading to lymphatic obstruction. (Fig. 69). In one patient, the diagnosis was negative, but lymphographic control 3 months later showed evidence of malignant invasion of the inguinal nodes.

Eight patients with the primary tumor situated in the drainage area of the axillary lymph nodes *(shoulder, scapular area and upper arm)* were studied by arm lymphography. Two cases exhibited malignant involvement of contrast-filled axillary nodes as proven by subsequent histology (Fig. 70). Three lymphograms were negative. In one patient lymphography did not visualize any enlarged malignant axillary lymph nodes, a finding verified by lymph node excision.

Fischer et al. (1962), Wallace et al. (1962), Viamonte et al. (1963), Arvay and Picard (1963), Dolan (1964), Dana et al. (1964), McPeak (1966), de Roo and Thomas (1967) described similar pathologic lymphograms exhibiting predominantly central filling defects. However, similar lymphographic findings are observed

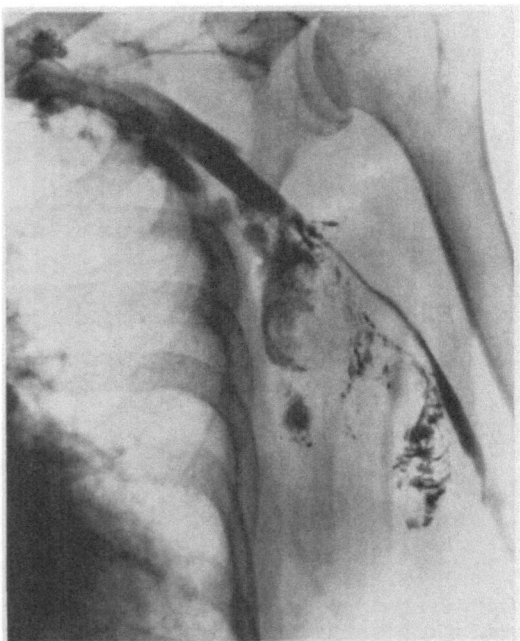

Fig. 70. *Malignant melanoma of the scapular area.* Large metastatic lateral axillary lymph nodes with extensive central filling defects and displacement of the remaining lymphatic tissue. Stasis of the lymphatic circulation. Compression of the axillary vein

in lymph node metastases of undifferentiated squamous cell carcinoma of the skin. On the other hand, filling defects in the marginal sinus because of tumor tissue are present in lymph nodes with metastases of both carcinoma and malignant melanoma. Both histologic types of malignant tumors have a tendency to obstruct the lymphatic circulation. Therefore, the lymphographic appearance of lymph nodes with metastases is similar in both carcinoma and malignant melanoma, however, malignant melanoma shows a tendency to produce large central filling defects.

The *diagnostic value* of lymphography in malignant melanoma has been carefully investigated by Cox et al. (1966) correlating histologic and lymphographic findings in 17 melanoma patients. Of 228 lymph nodes of the inguinal and axillary region examined histologically, 63 had filling defects. Nine nodes were diagnosed as containing tumor and 5 were questionably positive. Only 6 of the 9 diagnosed as containing tumor and none of the 5 questionable nodes were shown by histology

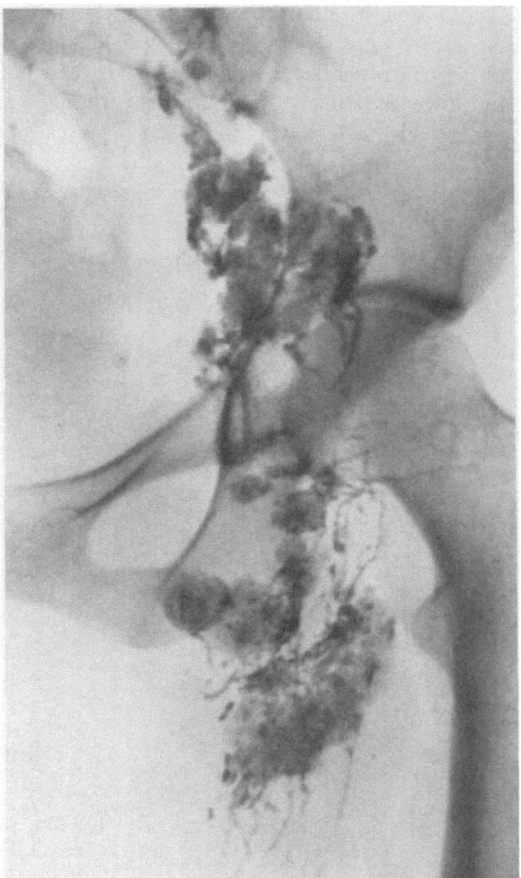

Fig. 71. *Squamous cell carcinoma of the big toe.* Enlarged inguinal and external iliac lymph nodes. Confluent central filling defects due to metastatic foci (verified by lymph node excision)

to exhibit tumor involvement. Four nodes were interpreted as false negative. Small deposists of tumor, less than 3 mm in size, were found in 4 other nodes without discernable radiographic filling defects. In another study by McPeak (1966) correlations between clinical lymphography and histologic findings were studied in 21 patients with melanoma. The lymphographic diagnosis was correct for 12 patients (60%), 8 of whom were correctly positive and 4 of whom were correctly negative. In 6 patients the lymphographic findings were inconclusive and in 2 other patients the lymphogram was interpreted incorrectly: one was a false positive, the other a false negative diagnosis.

The relatively high frequency of inconclusive or incorrect diagnoses reported
in these studies concurs with the author's experience and may by explained by the
difficulty of distinguishing filling defects caused by malignant invasion from the
filling defects caused by chronic inflammatory reaction and fatty involution, which
are so common to the axillary and inguinal nodes.

Secondary invasion of lymph nodes in malignant melanoma is demonstrated by
foot and arm lymphography only if the regional lymph nodes are situated within
the drainage area of the contrast-filled lymph vessels. In cases of malignant melanoma of the upper and lower extremities, the particular drainage area of the affected
skin region must be filled with a contrast agent (e. g. In a case of malignant mela-

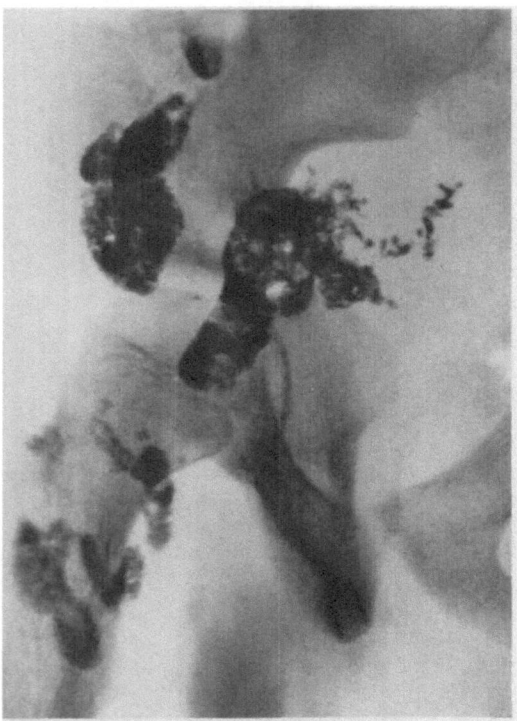

Fig. 72. *Round cell sarcoma of the gluteal region.* Metastatic enlargement of the external iliac
lymph nodes with loosening of the storage pattern and confluent filling defects

noma of the calf, the lymphatics of the lesser saphenous vein group must be contrast-
filled). Regional metastases of the skin of the trunk are demonstrated only if the
drainage area is situated close to the inguinal or axillary region.

Carcinoma of the Skin

In the author's series of investigations, 4 patients with carcinoma of the skin of
the lower extremities were investigated by lymphography. In 2 cases with squamous
cell carcinoma of the skin of the calf, lymphography was negative. One patient with
squamous cell carcinoma of the big toe showed enlarged inguinal and external

iliac lymph nodes with extensive central filling defects and displacement of the remaining lymphatic tissue towards the periphery of the nodes. The changes were similar to those observed in malignant melanoma (Fig. 71). In a case of cancroid of the skin in the popliteal area, lymphographic findings were observed suggestive of malignant metastatic spread to the inguinal region.

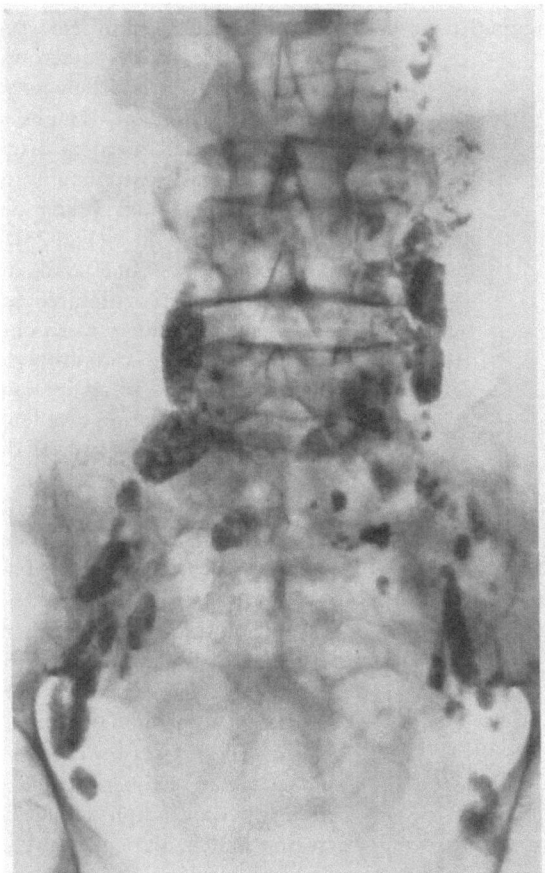

Fig. 73. *Polymorph cell sarcoma of the abdominal wall.* Confluent rounded filling defects in enlarged aortic lymph nodes

As in melanoma, lymph node metastases of skin carcinoma are demonstrated by foot and arm lymphography only if the regional lymph nodes are situated within the drainage area of the contrast-filled lymph vessels. Because the regional lymph nodes of the skin are frequently affected by inflammatory and degenerative changes, lymphographic diagnosis is difficult and not infrequently inconclusive.

Localized Sarcoma

Malignant metastatic spread to lymph nodes in sarcoma not originating from the lymphatic system is relatively rare. In the author's series, 23 patients with different histologic sarcoma types not arising from the lymphatic system were examined by lymphography. Three of 16 patients with sarcoma (polymorph cell, round cell, spindle cell, leiomyomyxo- and fibrosarcoma, synovioma) originating in the lower extremity and lower trunk areas, had metastases in regional inguinal lymph nodes that were demonstrated by lymphography. One patient with round cell sarcoma of the gluteal region had metastases in the medial external iliac lymph nodes (Fig. 72). Another case of polymorph cell sarcoma of the gluteal region with clinically apparent bilateral inguinal metastases, exhibited considerably enlarged iliac and aortic lymph nodes with numerous, regularly distributed, round filling defects similar to those of primary malignant lymphoma. In a case of polymorph cell sarcoma originating in the abdominal wall, lymphography revealed large, confluent, irregular filling defects of enlarged aortic lymph nodes (Fig. 73).

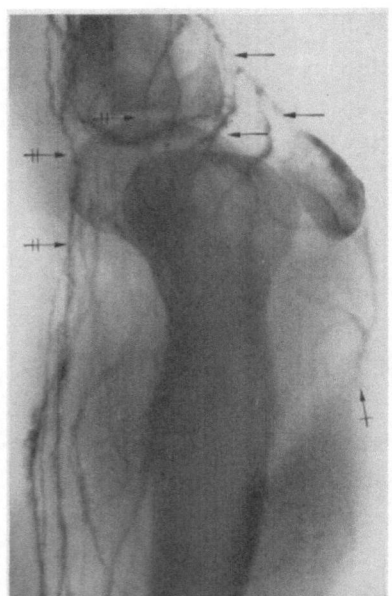

Fig. 74. *Chondromyxosarcoma of the femur.* Obstruction of the lymphatics on the ventral and medial side of the tumor (↔). Slight dilatation of peripheral lymphatics (→). Collateral circulation via medial and dorsal lymphatics (⊣⊢→)

In 5 cases of bone sarcoma (chondrosarcoma, osteosarcoma, reticulosarcoma), 3 positive lymphographic findings were observed. An extensive, infiltrating chondromyxosarcoma of the lower femur led to complete obstruction of the lymphatic circulation on the ventral and medial aspects of the tumor and of the collateral circulation (Fig. 74). In a case of osteochondrosarcoma of the femur, control lymphography revealed metastatic spread to iliac and aortic lymph nodes confirmed by biopsy 6 weeks after amputation (Fig. 75).

In another patient with recurrent reticulosarcoma of the humerus, lymphography demonstrated extensive filling defects of enlarged axillary lymph nodes caused by malignant invasion (Fig. 76). In a case of *infiltrating neurinoma* of the retroperitoneum, complete obstruction of the lymph circulation in the aortic region and in the collateral lumbar lymphatics was demonstrated by lymphography and later verified during operation (Fig. 77). Extensive *retroperitoneal neuroblastoma* in a child did not directly involve the lymphatic system. Radiation fibrosis of the retroperitoneal lymph vessels and lymph nodes, but not obstruction and infiltration, was demonstrated by lymphography (Fig. 78). During operation prior to radiotherapy, large retroperitoneal tumor masses were found.

Negative lymphographic findings in soft tissue sarcoma and osteosarcoma have been reported by Viamonte et al. (1963) and Boyd and Altmaier (1963). Large lymph node metastases having the characteristic of primary malignant lymphoma may be found lymphographically in Ewing's sarcoma (Rüttimann and Del Buono, 1964).

Sarcoma not originating from the lymphatic system rarely involves the lymphatic system secondarily. The lymphographic appearance is that of metastases of primary carcinoma or primary malignant lymphoma. As a consequence the rare

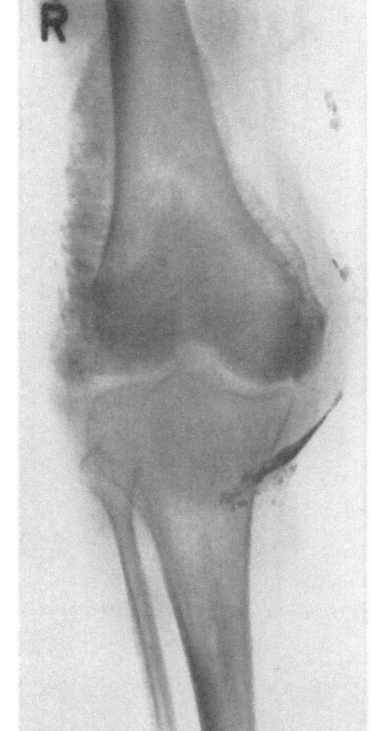

Fig. 75 a–c. *Osteochondrosarcoma of the femur.*
a Dislocation and obstruction of the anterior
medial group of lymphatics by the malignant
tumor. b Reactive hyperplasia of the external
iliac lymph nodes. c Lymphographic control
4 months later demonstrating metastases in the
external and common iliac lymph nodes

a

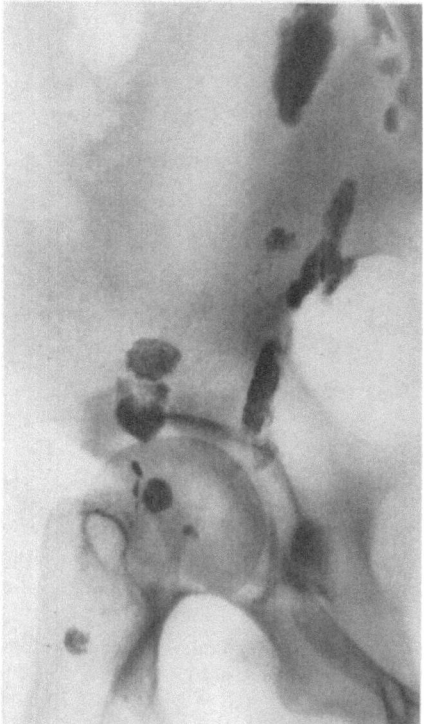

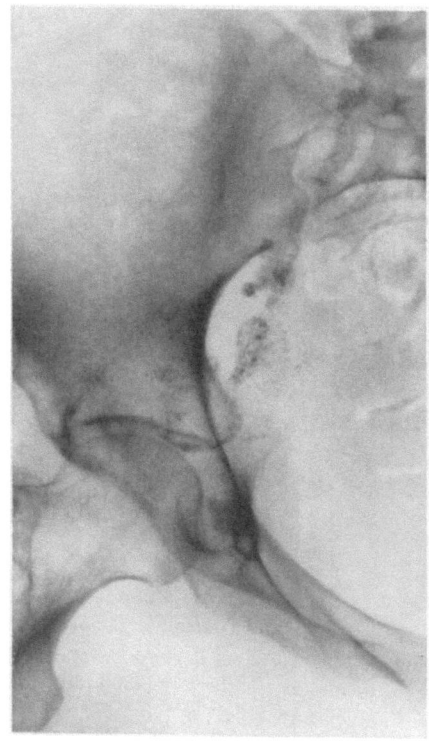

b   c

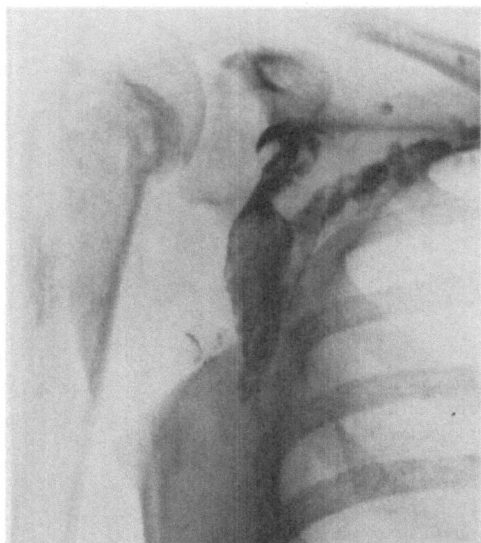

Fig. 76. *Reticulosarcoma of the humerus.* Metastases in enlarged lateral axillary lymph nodes. Large central filling defects

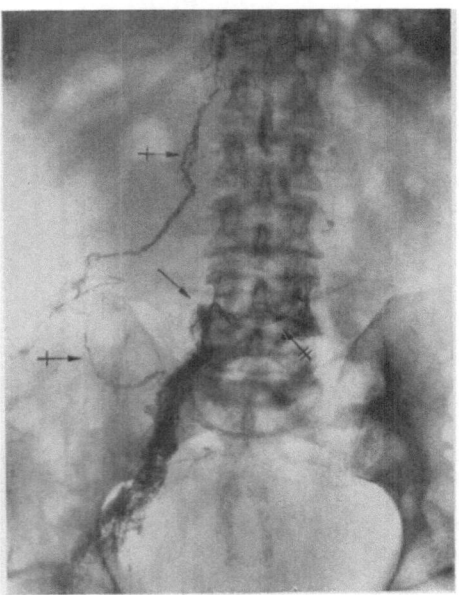

Fig. 77

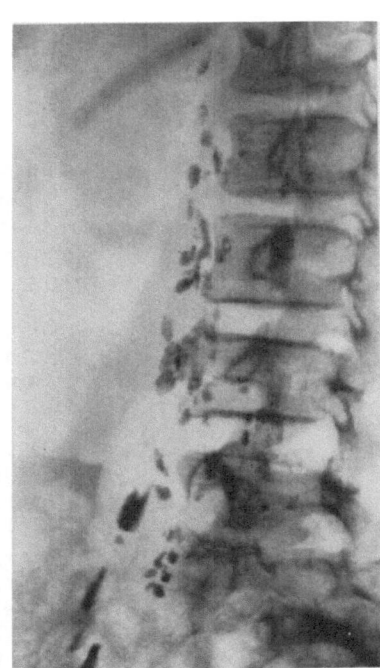

Fig. 78

Fig. 77. *Infiltrating neurinoma.* Complete obstruction of the lymphatic circulation at the level of the left common iliac lymph nodes (→) Collateral lymphatics in the lumbar fossa (↔) and contralateral aortic lymph vessels (⊣→) (verified by operation)

Fig. 78. *Retroperitoneal neuroblastoma.* Fibrosis of the aortic lymph nodes following radiotherapy (2500 rad.) (confirmed by lymph node excision)

lymphatic propagation of sarcoma not originating from the lymphatic system has various characteristic lymphographic manifestations, and extensive sarcomatous infiltration may not touch the lymphatic system at all.

References

ARVAY, N., et J. D. PICARD: La lymphographie. Etude radiologique et clinique des voies lymphatiques normales et pathologiques. Paris: Masson & Cie. 1963.

BOYD, A. D., and W. A. ALTMEIER: Lymphography in management of malignant neoplasms of lower extremities. Arch. Surg. 85, 911 (1963).

COX, K. R., W. S. C. HARE, and P. T. BRUCE: Lymphography in melanoma. Correlation of radiology with pathology. Cancer 19, 637 (1966).

DANA, M., J. P. DESPREZ-CURELY, V. BISMUTH et R. BOURDON: La lymphographie dans les maladies de la peau. Ann. Radiol. 7, 555 (1964).

DE ROO, T., and P. THOMAS: Lymphography with supplementary tomographic examination in the preoperative analysis of melanosarcoma. Chir. Radiol. 18, 83 (1967).

DOLAN, P. A.: Lymphography. Brit. J. Radiol. 37, 405 (1964).

FISCHER, H. W., M. S. LAWRENCE, and J. R. THORNBURY: Lymphography of the normal adult male. Radiology 78, 399 (1962).

McPEAK, C. L.: Lymphography in melanoma. In: Progress in lymphology, p. 155. Stuttgart: G. Thieme 1967.

RÜTTIMANN, A., u. M. S. DEL BUONO: Die Lymphographie. In: Ergebnisse der medizinischen Strahlenforschung. Neue Folge. Band I. Hrsg. Schinz-Glauner-Rüttimann. Stuttgart: Thieme 1964.

VIAMONTE, M., D. ALTMAN, R. PARKS, E. BLUM, M. BEVILAQUA, and L. RECHER: Radiographic-pathologic correlation in the interpretation of lymphangioadenograms. Radiology 80, 903 (1963).

WALLACE, S., and R. R. GREENING: Clinical applications of lymphography. Amer. J. Roentgenol. 88, 97 (1962).

Chapter 8

Malignant Lymphoma

James W. Davidson

With 35 Figures

Thesis

Lower extremity lymphography has added new dimensions to the understanding of malignant lymphomas in two ways. First, by demonstration of abnormalities in lymph nodes which are not readily accessible to clinical examination, and second, by the display of alteration in normal lymph node architecture.

In Hodgkin's disease, preliminary observations suggest that there are two distinct patterns which correlate well with the histological classification (Lukes). With lymphocyte predominance, abnormal lymph nodes have been found principally in superficial and retroperitoneal groups. The nodular sclerosing type has involved the mediastinum and its contiguous lymph nodes in the lower neck and upper abdomen Lymphographic appearances indicate varying stages of evolution of the pathological process within lymph nodes of different regions, and presentations with mixed cellularity may accompany either of the basic distributions.

In lymphosarcoma and reticulum cell sarcoma, similar studies have been commenced.

Introduction

Long term survival [15] and cure [5, 6] are now practical considerations in management of patients with malignant lymphomas. Although the pathogenesis and mode of progression of primary malignant neoplasms of lympho-reticular structures are poorly understood, it has been noted that the most important single factor influencing the progress and ultimate survival of patients with Hodgkin's disease is the extent of involvement on institution of treatment [17]. Similar considerations may apply to lymphosarcoma and to reticulum cell sarcoma. In new patients presenting with localized adenopathy due to malignant lymphoma, bilateral lower extremity lymphography is part of routine pre-management assessment in many centres. Similar investigation may be used to reassess the extent of lympho-reticular disease when recurrence of malignant lymphoma is suspected.

Radiographic patterns of contrast medium in lymph nodes in each of the lymphomas have been frequently described [3, 7, 27, 28]. However, recent clarification of the histological subtypes of the malignant lymphomas and further experience with lymphography allows more practical interpretation of lymphographic findings. This account is based on results of such investigation at The Ontario Cancer Institute of patients suffering from histologically proven lymphomas (Table 1). For purposes of analysis, lymphograms have been considered in terms of radiographic appearances and their significance with regard to clinical staging and the natural history of each of the malignant lymphomas. Such studies may be classed as initial lymphograms when performed in new patients, and as reassessment lymphograms when used in reappraisal of those in whom clinical breakdown has occurred at an interval following a course of therapy.

Table 1. *Lymphography in lymphomas*

	No. of patients	No. of lymphograms	Initial	Reassessment	Repeat	Abnormal	Normal	Equivocal
Hodgkin's disease	278	302	160	118	24	167	106	29
Lymphosarcoma	107	110	62	45	3	71	34	5
Reticulum cell sarcoma	77	78	61	16	1	43	28	7
Other lymphomas	4	4	3	1		4		
Total	466	494	286	180	28	285	168	41

Lymphographic findings have been assessed in each individual patient with prior knowledge of the clinical presentation, site of biopsy, and histological diagnosis. Factors affecting the size and morphology of lymph nodes, such as previous radiotherapy, chemotherapy including steroid administration, regional sepsis, skin changes, and the age and sex of the patient must be considered. Similar storage patterns to those of malignant lymphomas have been described in a variety of conditions including metastatic malignancy, sarcoidosis, tuberculosis, histoplasmosis, infectious mononucleosis, and reactive hyperplasia secondary to infections, collagen diseases, and antigens of all kinds. Nevertheless, in each of the malignant lymphomas, architectural changes within lymph nodes demonstrated by lymphography have proven an useful in vivo reflection of the underlying cellular abnormality, and provide valuable evidence on their natural history.

Introductory Pathology

The term "malignant lymphoma" includes all primary malignant neoplasms of lympho-reticular tissues. Classification of each subtype is based on analysis of the cellular composition and pattern [19] of a lymph node following biopsy (Table 2). Those consisting mainly of primitive reticular cells or their histiocytic derivatives cover a spectrum of histological patterns encompassed by the older term "reticulum cell sarcoma", including the stem cell type and those with mixed lymphocytic-histiocytic types. Those derived from lymphocytes or their precursors fall into two groups, differentiated and undifferentiated, giving the lymphocytic and lymphoblastic tumours. For diagnosis of Hodgkin's disease, characteristic Reed-Sternberg cells must be identified. In each of the above cellular subtypes, a nodular or diffuse pattern may occur. Such neoplasms often initially affect only one lymph node group or extra-nodal site, and may be usefully considered under the three main pathological groups, reticulum cell sarcoma, lymphosarcoma, and Hodgkin's disease. A further lymphoma described in African children but believed to have a more widespread geographical distribution, is the Burkitt tumour [4], in which characteristic, but non-specific, large histiocytes giving a "starry-sky" appearance, are found.

Table 2. *Classification of malignant lymphoma*

Table 3. *Classification of Hodgkin's disease*

By courtesy of Dr. ROBERT J. LUKES

Using the subtypes of Hodgkin's disease proposed by LUKES, BUTLER and HICKS [13], and later modification (Table 3) [12], histological features may be related to clinical stages and survival. Abnormalities of lymph nodes displayed by lymphography may also be considered in terms of such alterations of cellularity. It is suggested that the numerous histological expressions found in Hodgkin's disease represent manifestations of differences in the host response. The lymphocytic and histiocytic types describe diffuse cellularity throughout each individual lymph node, with few Reed-Sternberg cells. These are commonly associated with Stage I disease and prolonged median survival. Uniformity of cellular proliferation gives compression, but rarely obliteration, of intranodal sinusoids. Nodular sclerosis, identified by the occurrence of birefringent collagen bands with a tendency to nodule formation and the presence of distinctive large cytoplasmic Reed-Sternberg cells, is thought to be a regional manifestation of disease arising in the mediastinum. It is of uncertain evolution but shows a natural tendency to undergo sclerosis. Diffuse fibrosis and reticular subtypes are associated with lymphocyte depletion, widely disseminated disease, higher clinical stages, and a poor prognosis. Mixed Hodgkin's disease is thought to be an intermediate form reflecting changing cellularity, and shows histiocytes, mature neutrophils, plasma cells, and lymphocytes in varying proportions, usually with a slight to moderate degree of disorderly fibrosis. Focal necrosis may be present. Such a process of variable degree may frequently extend throughout the entire node, and is associated with obliteration of sinusoids and follicles. The role of the lymphocyte in host response is expressed in the most recently adopted classification.

The Place of Lymphography

For more meaningful analysis of lymphographic appearances of individual lymph nodes, architectural abnormality depicted by distortion and obliteration of sinusoids filled with radiopaque contrast material, should be considered in terms of altered cellularity. The great variability in the histological features of the malignant lymphomas gives similar diversity of radiographic patterns. Fairly characteristic lymphographic findings have been described in lymphosarcoma, reticulum cell sarcoma, and Hodgkin's disease [26]. It is evident, however, that as diagnosis is based on cellular characteristics identified by microscopy, specific patterns of contrast material in sinusoids corresponding to each subtype of the malignant lymphomas cannot be accurately identified. Nevertheless, correlation of such radiographic findings with lymph node histology at biopsy or autopsy, shows that lymphography is a highly accurate method of detecting involvement by malignant lymphomas. Despite limitations, the radiologist has the advantage of examining in vivo a large area of the lympho-reticular system. Thus, lymphographic findings interpreted with prior knowledge of the site of biopsy and histological features, allow assessment of the extent of disease, and evolution of the pathological process may be elicited from individual lymph node architecture.

Clinical Considerations

In the widely adopted system of clinical staging of patients with Hodgkin's disease, the diaphragm is an important practical anatomical line of division [20]. Patients in clinical stages I and II are those with involvement of lympho-reticular structures on one side of the diaphragm, and should disease be detected on the opposite side, the stage is advanced to III. If in addition, extra-nodal tissues are affected, the patient is placed in Stage IV. Similar concepts have been applied to appraisal of patients with lymphosarcomas and reticulum cell sarcomas. By displaying lymph node groups in clinically occult pelvic and retroperitoneal regions, bilateral lower extremity lymphography has proven the most valuable procedure in this respect. Inferior vena cavography by outlining soft tissue abnormalities above the aortic lymph nodes but still below the diaphragm is a useful supplement to lymphographic study [2]. Chest radiography, including tomographs of the mediastinum and whole lung, accurately delineates disease within the thorax.

The first recognized sites of involvement in a series of patients seen at The Ontario Cancer Institute [16] are documented in Table 4. Enlargement of cervical lymph

Table 4. *Lymphomas—1957 to 1965. First recognized site of involvement*

	R.C.S. (%)	L.S. (%)	H.D. (%)
Peripheral nodes	30	50	82
Mediastinum	2	3	5
Para-aortic nodes or spleen	7	7	4
Alimentary tract and/or Mesentery	37	22	4
Skin or skeletal	15	7	1
Other extranodal	9	11	4
	100%	100%	100%

By courtesy of Dr. VERA PETERS

nodes has been the most frequent presentation in Hodgkin's disease, and has been less common in the other lymphomas. Involvement of the alimentary tract and mesentery, often first discovered at laparotomy, was relatively more common in reticulum cell sarcoma and lymphosarcoma. In the majority of such new patients with apparently localized lymphoma, bilateral lower extremity lymphography has been performed to examine femoral, iliac, and aortic nodes. As mediastinal and periclavicular nodes may frequently be opacified, information useful in clinical staging can be obtained if mediastinal tomography is performed subsequent to lymphography. Interpretation of vascular procedures, such as inferior vena cavography, is also aided by prior opacification of the lymph nodes. Thus, plain film of chest, bilateral lower extremity lymphography, mediastinal tomography, and supplementary vascular procedures is considered the optimal sequence of investigation.

Hodgkin's Disease

"Hodgkin's disease appears clinically to be a disturbance ... of cellular immunity associated with progressive neoplasia. The pattern varies from one which is benign, localized, lymphocytic predominant, and eminently curable, to one which is malignant, rapidly disseminated, shows lymphoid depletion, and is fatal. A few patients may die of immunological failure and overwhelming infection with little, if any, tumour detectable post-mortem. Definition is not so much our need as a clearer understanding of the whole process involved" [23]. Architectural alterations within individual lymph nodes infiltrated by Hodgkin's disease may be usefully displayed in clinically occult regions by lymphography. The results of such studies (Table 5) are documented according to the histological interpretation of lymph node biopsy. These lymphographic findings are further considered in terms of radiographic appearances, influence on clinical management, and the natural history of Hodgkin's disease.

Table 5. *Lymphography in Hodgkin's disease*

Pathology		No. of patients	No. of lympho- grams	Ab- normal	Normal	Equivocal
JACKSON and PARKER		65	68	42	19	7
	Lymphocytic and histiocytic	54	60	34	19	7
	Nodular sclerosis	46	52	27	20	5
LUKES	Mixed	72	78	36	34	8
	Diffuse fibrosis	3	3	3		
	Reticular	10	11	9	2	
Unclassified		28	30	16	12	2
Total		278	302	167	106	29

Radiographic Appearances
Lymphocyte Predominance

Case 1: At the age of 11 years, a male patient received local radiotherapy to the right side of the neck for Hodgkin's disease. The biopsy diagnosis was Hodgkin's paragranuloma, and on review was reclassified as the lymphocytic and histiocytic type. After more than 20 years of good health, he was investigated in hospital for vague pain in the lumbar region, sweating, and weakness, of short duration. Lymphography (Fig. 1 a) demonstrates moderately enlarged lymph nodes in the left common iliac region. Fine sinusoids and areas of diffuse granular contrast pattern are seen within and adjacent to confluent translucent areas outlined by the opacified marginal sinus. Apart from a few small scattered filling defects, even distribution of contrast material is seen within the remaining nodes of normal size. Biopsy (Fig. 1 b) at laparotomy showed that the lymphographic changes corresponded to diffuse lymphocytic and histiocytic infiltration of the node with displacement of fine sinusoids filled with oily contrast medium. Reed-Sternberg cells confirmed the diagnosis of Hodgkin's disease with lymphocyte predominance.

Comment: Preservation of sinusoidal patency within enlarged lymph nodes is demonstrated both by lymphography and histology in a patient who remained in apparent good health for more than 20 years following low-dose radiotherapy to the neck. Areas of homogeneous storage pattern and enlarged nodes are seen in addition to lymphographically normal nodes.

Case 2: A middle-aged woman complained of a small lump in the right axilla. Biopsy revealed a lymph node infiltrated with Hodgkin's disease of mixed type. Lymphography (Fig. 2 a) showed granular superimposed nodes of variable size in the aortic chains. Several nodes of similar pattern were projected above the medial end of the left clavicle (Fig. 2 b). Radiography of the largest node following its removal (Fig. 2 c) showed diffusely distributed contrast medium within the parenchyma. Confluent areas and fine radiopaque sinusoids are noted with good architectural perservation. Histology (Fig. 2 d) shows Reed-Sternberg cells with diffuse proliferation of lymphocytes and histiocytes adjacent to well preserved sinusoids containing clear globules of oily contrast medium.

Comment: Excellent preservation of sinusoidal architecture is present within diffuse cellular proliferation due to Hodgkin's disease with lymphocyte predominance. This corresponds to a granular homogeneous storage pattern of lymphographic contrast medium. Variability in the histological picture between the presenting site and further disease revealed by lymphography is illustrated.

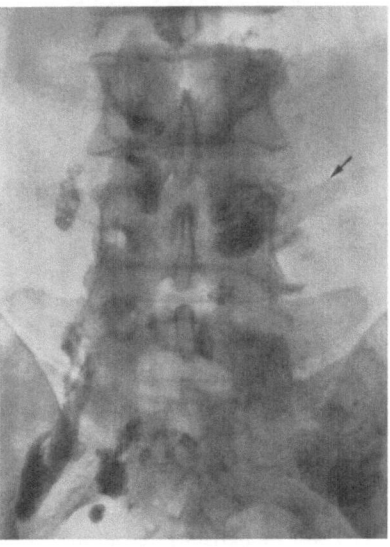

a

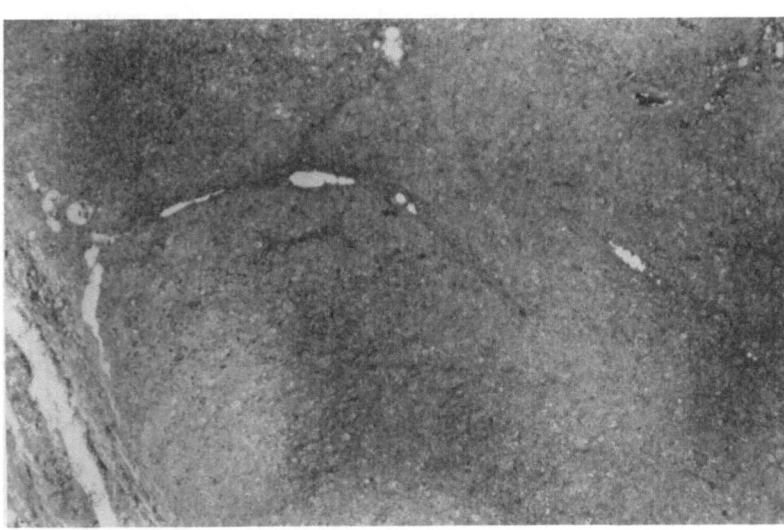

b

Fig. 1. Hodgkin's disease—Lymphocytic and histiocytic type. a Lymphadenogram—Fine contrast filled sinusoids within radiolucent filling defects and homogeneous contrast filled areas in enlarged left common iliac and lower aortic lymph glands. b Biopsy (arrow)—Lobular oily contrast material in fine sinusoids adjacent to patent marginal sinus

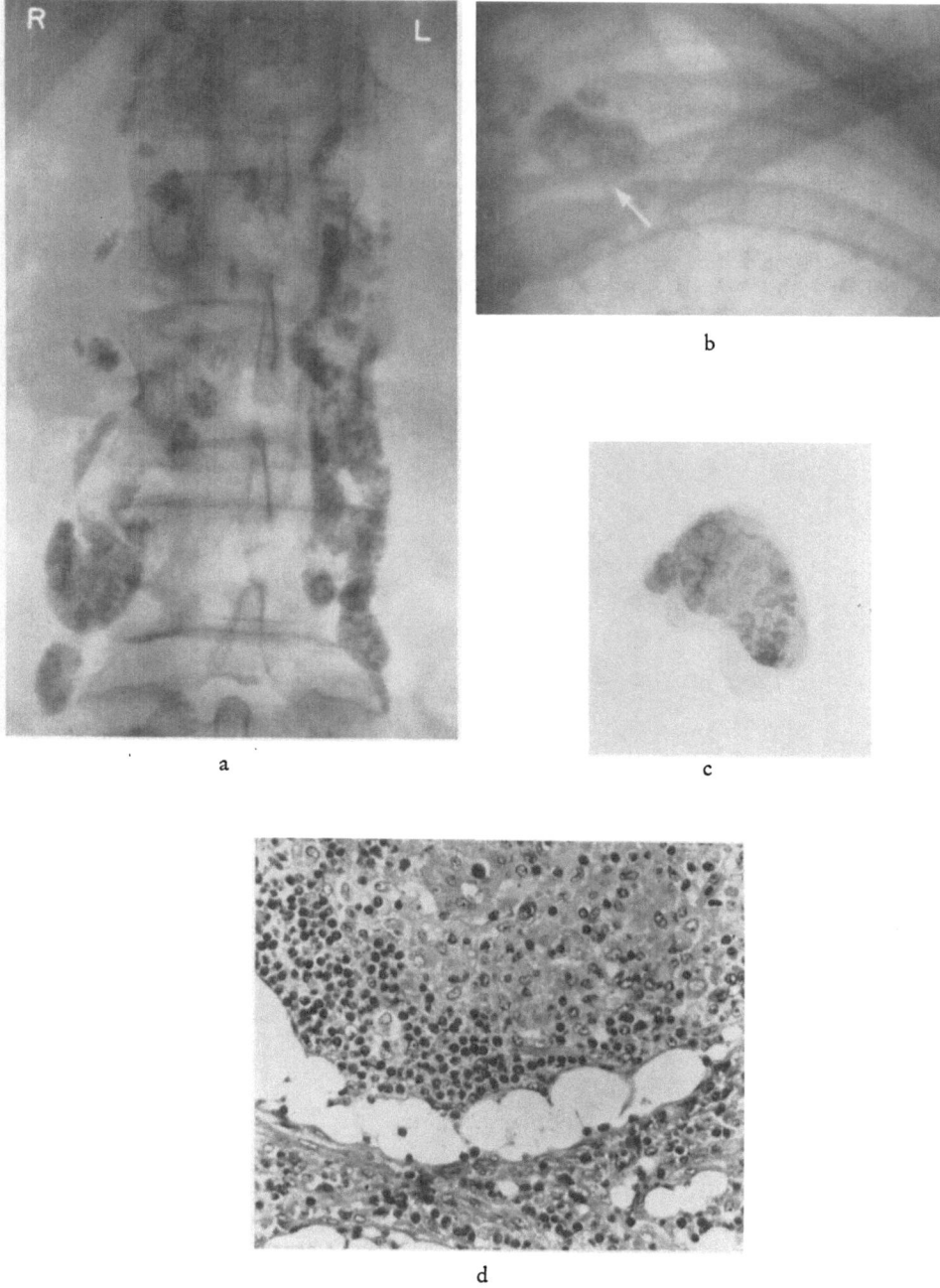

Fig. 2. Hodgkin's disease—Lymphocyte predominance. a Granular aortic nodes. b "Scalene" node with diffuse granular contrast pattern. c Radiograph of biopsy specimen. Note fine radiopaque sinusoids. d Histology of biopsy specimen. Globular oily contrast material within patent sinusoids—adjacent lymphocytic and histiocytic infiltration with Reed-Sternberg cells

Case 3: A 23-year-old female was found to have an enlarged lymph node in the left axilla. No further clinical evidence of abnormality was elicited. Biopsy revealed diffuse lymphocytic and histiocytic Hodgkin's disease. Lymphography (Fig. 3 a) shows irregularly filled lymph nodes in the upper aortic region projected on both sides of the spine and consistent with a marked architectural abnormality. A homogeneously opacified, slightly enlarged lymph node, and several smaller nodes projected above the left clavicle were visualized on tomography (Fig. 3 b). Radiographic appearances suggest variations in architectural abnormality in different lymph node groups, and are consistent with a more advanced type of disease in the extreme upper aortic nodes.

Comment: Hodgkin's disease with lymphocyte predominance presenting in Stage I has been altered to Stage III following lymphography.

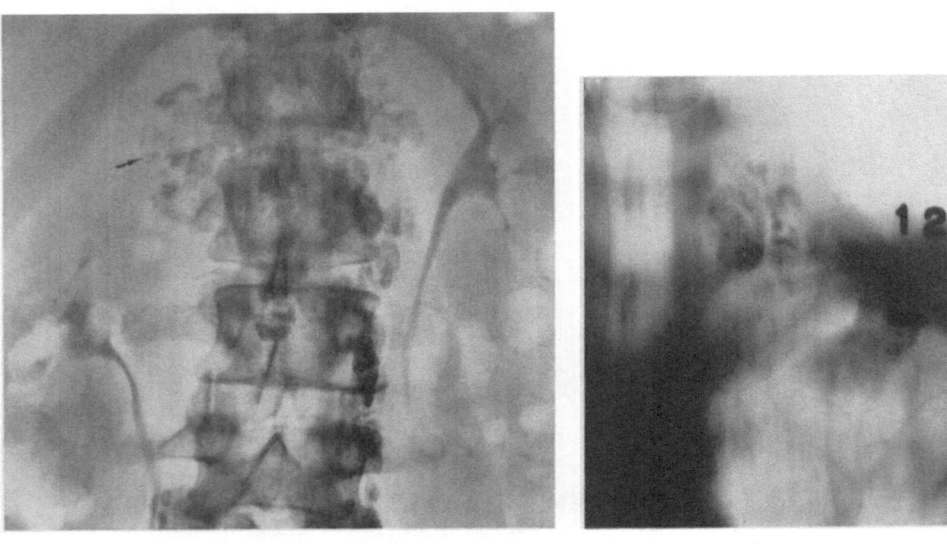

a   b

Fig. 3. Lymphocytic and histiocytic Hodgkin's disease. a Enlarged irregularly filled upper aortic node. b Scalene node with granular pattern and adjacent small nodes extending towards the left axilla

Nodular Sclerosis

Case 1: A male, aged 26 years, who complained of intermittent fatigue and night sweats during the previous year, was found to have a palpable node in the right anterior triangle of the neck. Biopsy disclosed Hodgkin's disease of nodular sclerosing type. Chest radiography showed broadening of the mediastinal shadow, confirmed by tomography (Fig. 4 a) to be due to enlarged lymph nodes in paratracheal, right hilar and subcarinal regions. Lymphography (Fig. 4 b and c) displayed numerous irregular lymph nodes in the aortic and right iliac groups. Moderately enlarged nodes with extensive confluent radiolucent defects in the storage pattern are most evident on the right side. Nodes of homogeneous texture and normal size or slight enlargement are seen at a lower level in close proximity. Numerous small dense nodes and lymphoid aggregates are demonstrated in the right paravertebral region at thoraco-abdominal level.

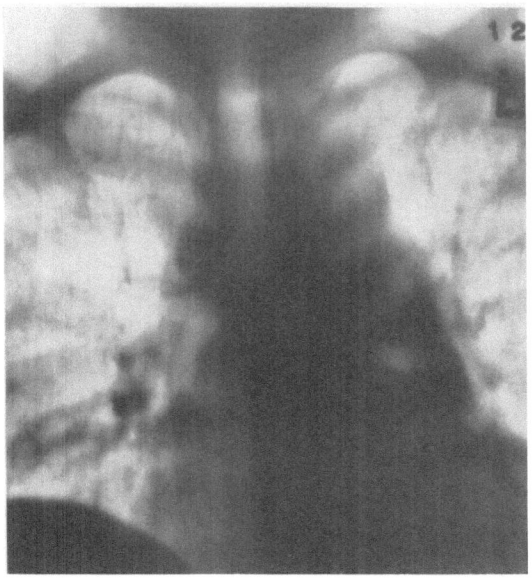

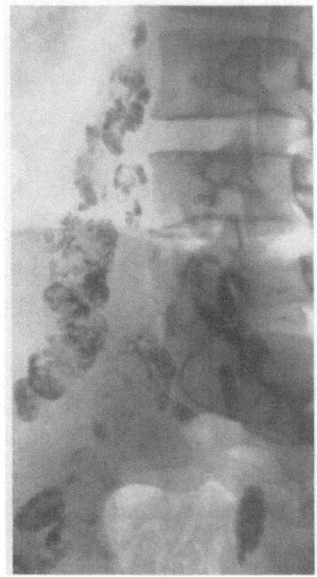

Fig. 4. Hodgkin's disease—Nodular Sclerosis. a Tomograph—paratracheal, subcarinal and hilar adenopathy. b and c Lymphogram—irregular filling in enlarged aortic and right common iliac nodes

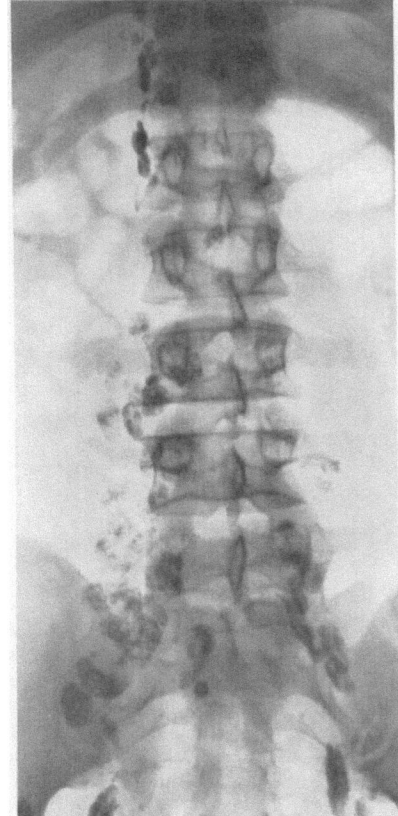

Comment: Presentation in the neck is accompanied by extensive mediastinal involvement and widespread distribution of abnormality in the retroperitoneal nodes. Filling defects in the storage pattern are consistent with infiltration of an advanced type. The clinical stage has been advanced to III following lymphography.

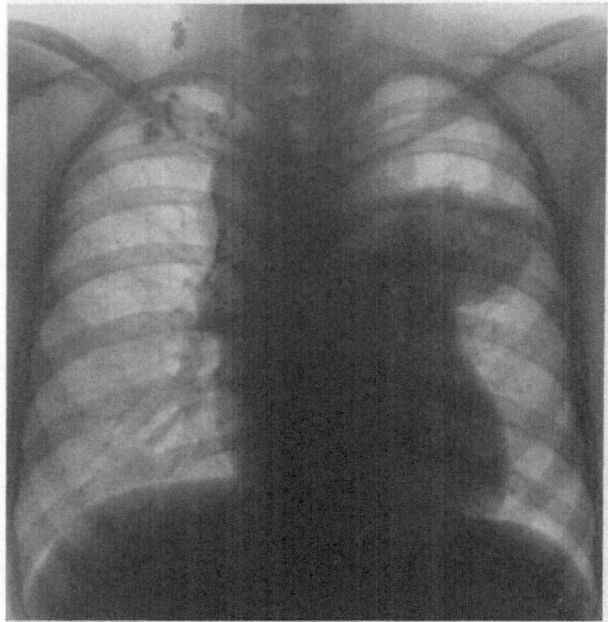

a

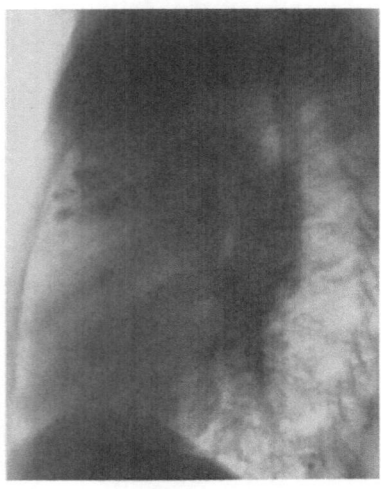

b   c

Fig. 5. Hodgkin's disease—Nodular Sclerosis. a Chest film showing gross widening of the mediastinum and a large soft tissue mass projected over the left lung field. Opaque nodes are best seen in the right periclavicular region. b Left lateral chest film showing opacified anterior mediastinal lymph node adjacent to an extensive soft tissues mass. c Spot radiograph showing irregular confluent filling defects in several nodes within the thorax. d Lymphadenogram— Slight regional hyperplasia left upper aortic region. e A.P. tomograph—Minor irregularities and small radiolucent filling defects in several. f Oblique film of simple magnification showing normal granularity in upper aortic nodes

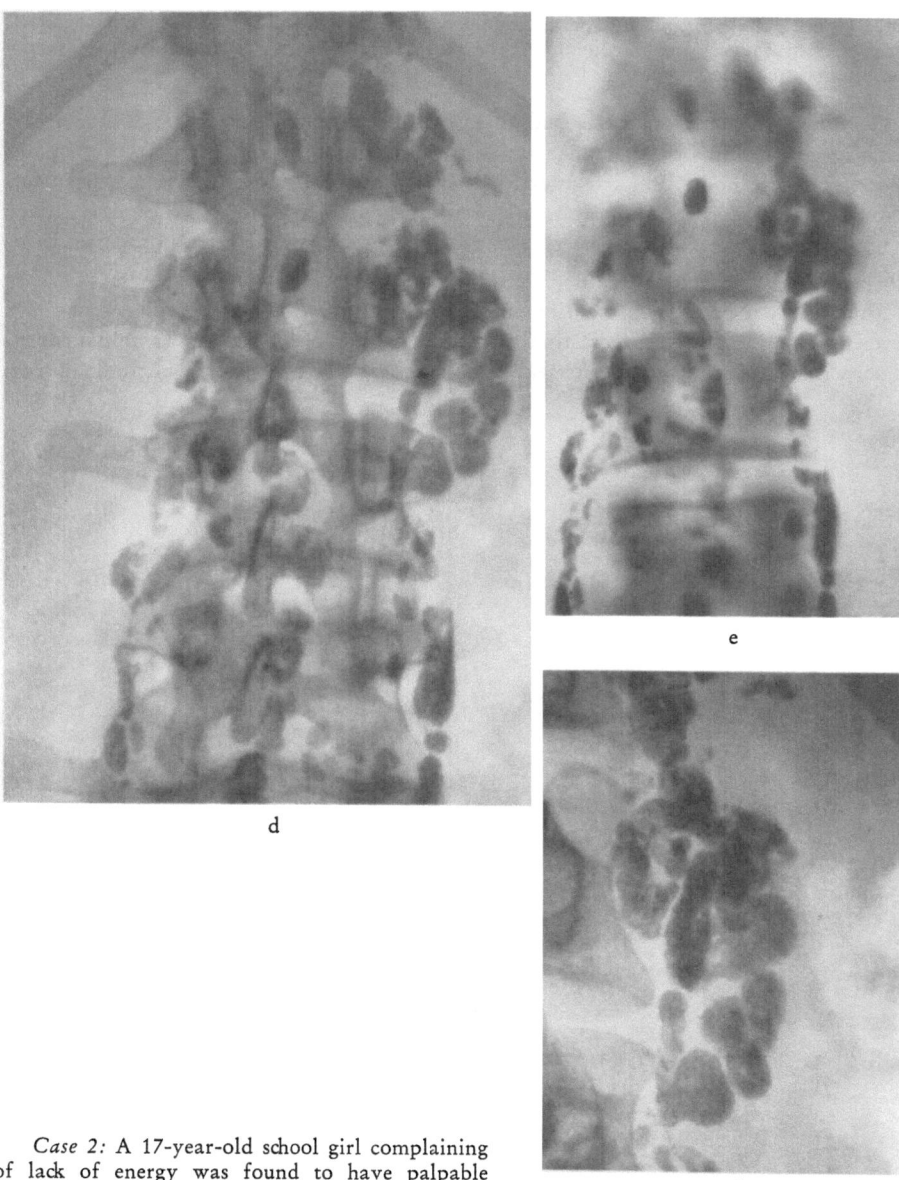

d

e

f

Case 2: A 17-year-old school girl complaining of lack of energy was found to have palpable discrete 1 cm nodes at the base of the neck on both sides. Biopsy reveal a lymph node infiltrated with Hodgkin's disease of nodular sclerosing type. Chest radiographs (Fig. 5 a and b) showed an extensive mediastinal soft tissue mass with posterior bowing of the trachea. A large extrapleural mass contiguous with the mediastinum was projected over the left lung field. Radiopaque lymph nodes were noted in the anterior and mid mediastinum. Spot film (Fig. 5 c) of a mediastinal node showed gross irregularity in contrast distribution consistent with abnormal architecture, and several smaller partly filled adjacent lymph nodes are noted. Lymphography (Fig. 5 d) showed multiple small lymph nodes in the aortic groups. Tomography (Fig. 5 e) showed irregularity of the margins and small translucencies in several glands. Oblique spot film with simple magnification (Fig. 5 f) showed homogeneous distribution of the contrast medium with normal granularity in the parenchyma of many superimposed small nodes.

Comment: Extensive mediastinal disease is present, and gross architectural abnormality is seen in opacified mediastinal nodes. Slight regional hyperplasia in the upper left aortic nodes and irregularity of small adjacent nodes indicates a need for surveillance by repeat radiographs at intervals to detect progressive disease at the earliest possible time. However, in the presence of advanced intrathoracic disease, there is no evidence of extensive aortic lymph node architectural abnormality.

Thus, in two patients presenting in the neck with Hodgkin's disease of nodular sclerosing type, extensive mediastinal abnormality has been present. Lymphography has shown widespread retroperitoneal lymph node disease in Case 1, but only minor

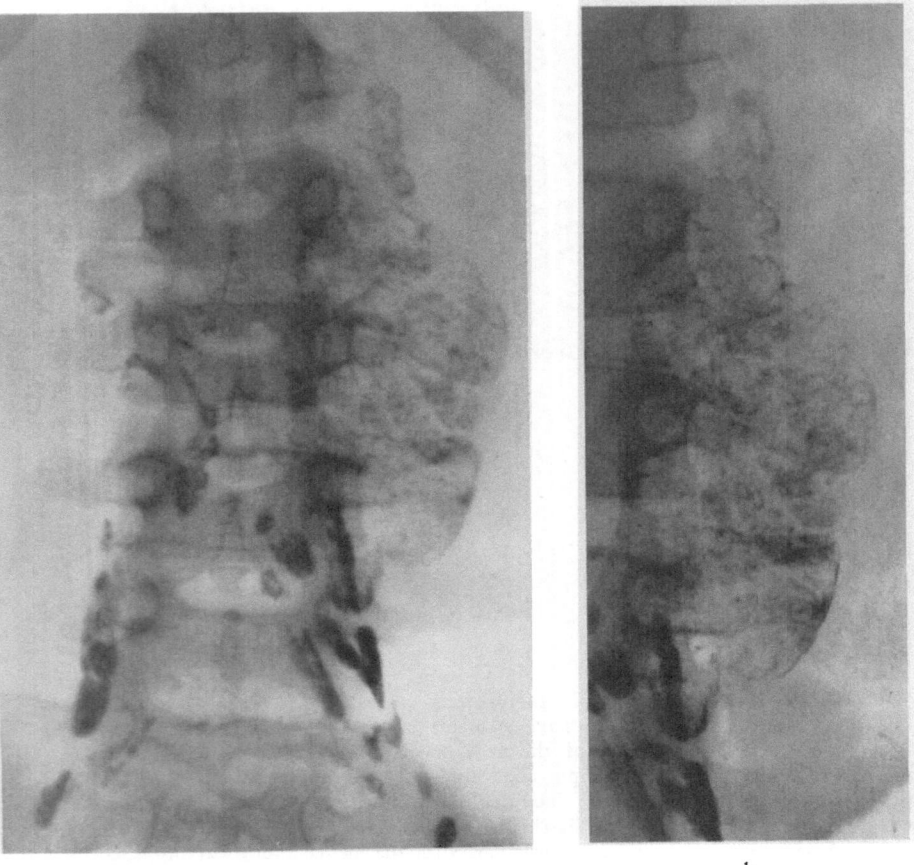

a   b

Fig. 6. Hodgkin's disease—Mixed cellularity type. a A.P. b Left posterior oblique radiograph. Extensive aortic node enlargement with confluent filling defects is noted. Marginal preservation is seen in several nodes

changes in the aortic nodes in the second patient insufficient for definite diagnosis of change associated with lymphoma, although the mediastinal involvement appears of more advanced type.

Mixed Hodgkin's Disease

Case 1: A boy, aged nine years, had a palpable swelling in the right side of the neck of ten days' duration. For four months, intermittent malaise, fever, and cough had been noted. Biopsy from the neck revealed a lymph node infiltrated with Hodgkin's disease of mixed cellularity type. Chest radiography showed a moderate increase in the upper mediastinal shadow, and enlarged paratracheal nodes were confirmed by tomography. Lymphography (Fig. 6 a and b) shows enlargement of aortic nodes with irregular filling defects up to several millimetres in diameter. No normal storage patterns were demonstrated above the external iliac region. Following radical irradiation to the neck, mediastinum, axillae, and abdomen, this patient continued to deteriorate and died four months from the date of the lymphogram.

Comment: Gross architectural abnormality consistent with massive replacement in retroperitoneal nodes is seen. The radiographic abnormality indicates a more advanced pathological stage in widely distributed, generalized Hodgkin's disease in a patient with a poor response to therapy.

Case 2: A 24-year-old man consulted his doctor because of a lump in the left groin which had been present for two years. On biopsy, this was found to be a lymph node infiltrated with Hodgkin's disease of mixed nodulare type (Fig. 7 b). Lymphography (Fig. 7 a) demonstrates enlarged lymph nodes in the left iliac groups with widely distributed somewhat floccular contrast material. Scattered irregular radiolucent areas of variable size and most marked in the submarginal regions can be seen (Fig. 7 d). In the right aortic region (Fig. 7 c), slightly enlarged nodes of normal granularity are noted. In the left aortic region (Fig. 7 e), smaller granular of varying shape are revealed.

Comment: Variability in the size and storage pattern of lymph node groups in different regions is seen. Confluent filling defects (Fig. 7 d) in a coarse "cotton-wool" contrast pattern reflect a mixed nodular type of lymphoma. These variable radiographic appearances display the evolution of the pathological process in different areas.

Case 3: A young woman who had noticed a swelling in the right lower neck for several weeks was found on biopsy to be suffering from Hodgkin's disease of mixed cellularity type. Chest X-rays showed an extensive soft tissue mass in the upper and mid mediastinum consistent with gross adenopathy. Lymphography (Fig. 8 a) showed lymph nodes of normal size in both aortic regions. Sharply demarcated, rounded and irregular punched-out filling defects were present in several of the nodes. Despite radical irradiation of the neck, axillae, and mediastinum, the patient succumbed three months after lymphography. At autopsy, histological examination of aortic nodes (Fig. 8 b) showed marked lymphocyte depletion with almost total node replacement by Hodgkin's disease of reticular type.

Comment: Following presentation in the neck with Hodgkin's disease showing mixed cellularity, this patient succumbed to progressive intrathoracic disease. Small abnormal aortic nodes on the lymphogram correspond to lymphocyte depleted reticular Hodgkin's disease.

Two of these patients presenting in the neck have been found to show gross architectural abnormality in aortic nodes consistent with partial replacement. Cases 1 and 3 presenting in the neck, both show filling defects in large and small aortic nodes

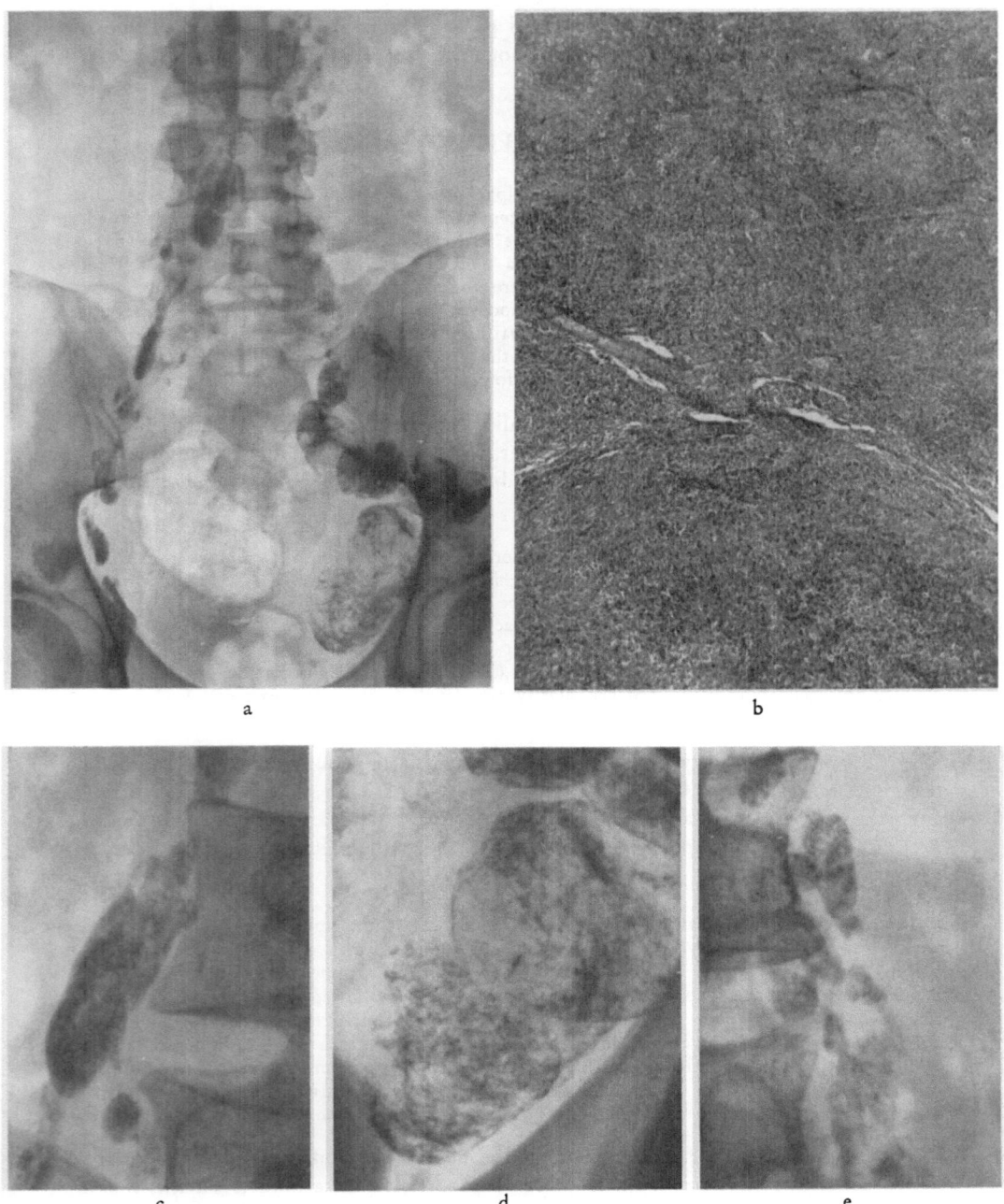

Fig. 7. Hodgkin's disease—Mixed nodular type. a Lymphogram—Variations in the size and contrast patterns in different regions. b Histological section from left groin node—patent sinusoids in a mixed nodular background. c Irregular opacification in right aortic nodes. d Iliac nodes simple magnification—floccular contrast material with confluent filling defects. e Granular left aortic node

respectively suggesting an advanced type of disease and a rapid downhill course ensued. In case 2, the most advanced abnormality in larger nodes is present in the groin and iliac nodes with preservation of architecture in the aortic region. Thus, distinctive patterns of involvement may be seen in these patients with a similar presenting histological picture.

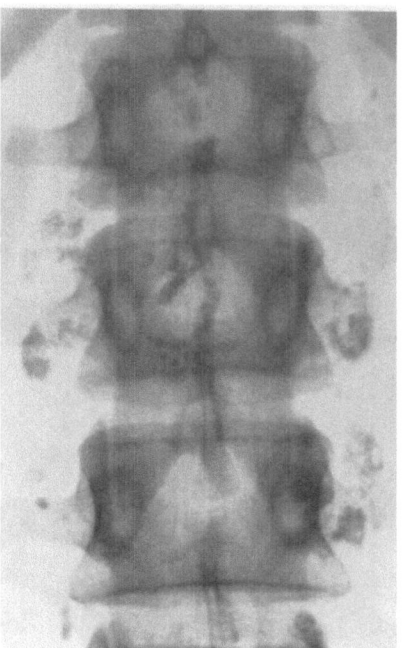

a

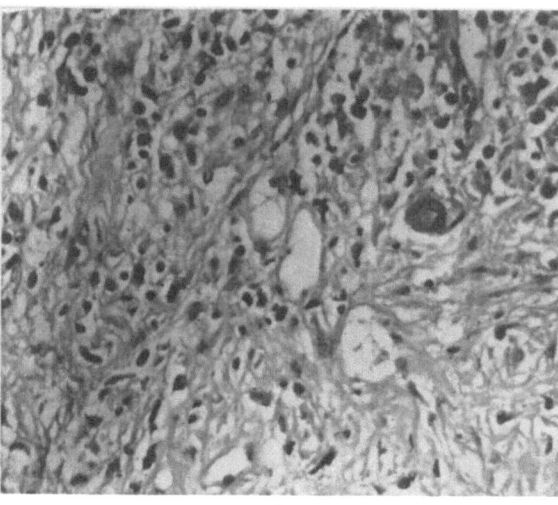

b

Fig. 8. Hodgkin's disease—Mixed cellularity type from neck node. a Irregular filling defects in small nodes. b Histology—Aortic node showing reticular Hodgkin's disease

Diffuse Fibrosis

A male, aged 40 years, complained of cough and weight loss for several months. A 1 cm lymph node was palpated at the base of the neck on the left side. Chest radiograph (Fig. 9 a) revealed gross broading of the mediastinal shadow. Biopsy from the left side of the neck disclosed a lymph node infiltrated with a diffuse sclerosing form of Hodgkin's disease with lymphocyte depletion. Lymphography (Fig. 9 b and c) opacified lymph nodes of normal size in the aortic chains. Apart from a few small filling defects in the contrast pattern in the upper left aortic nodes, the appearances are normal.

Comment: With radiographic evidence of extensive mediastinal disease and lymph node involvement at the base of the neck by a pathologically advanced form of Hodgkin's disease, minimal changes are present in aortic lymph nodes. The further course of this patient has been slowly progressive disease with no significant response to irradiation or chemotherapy.

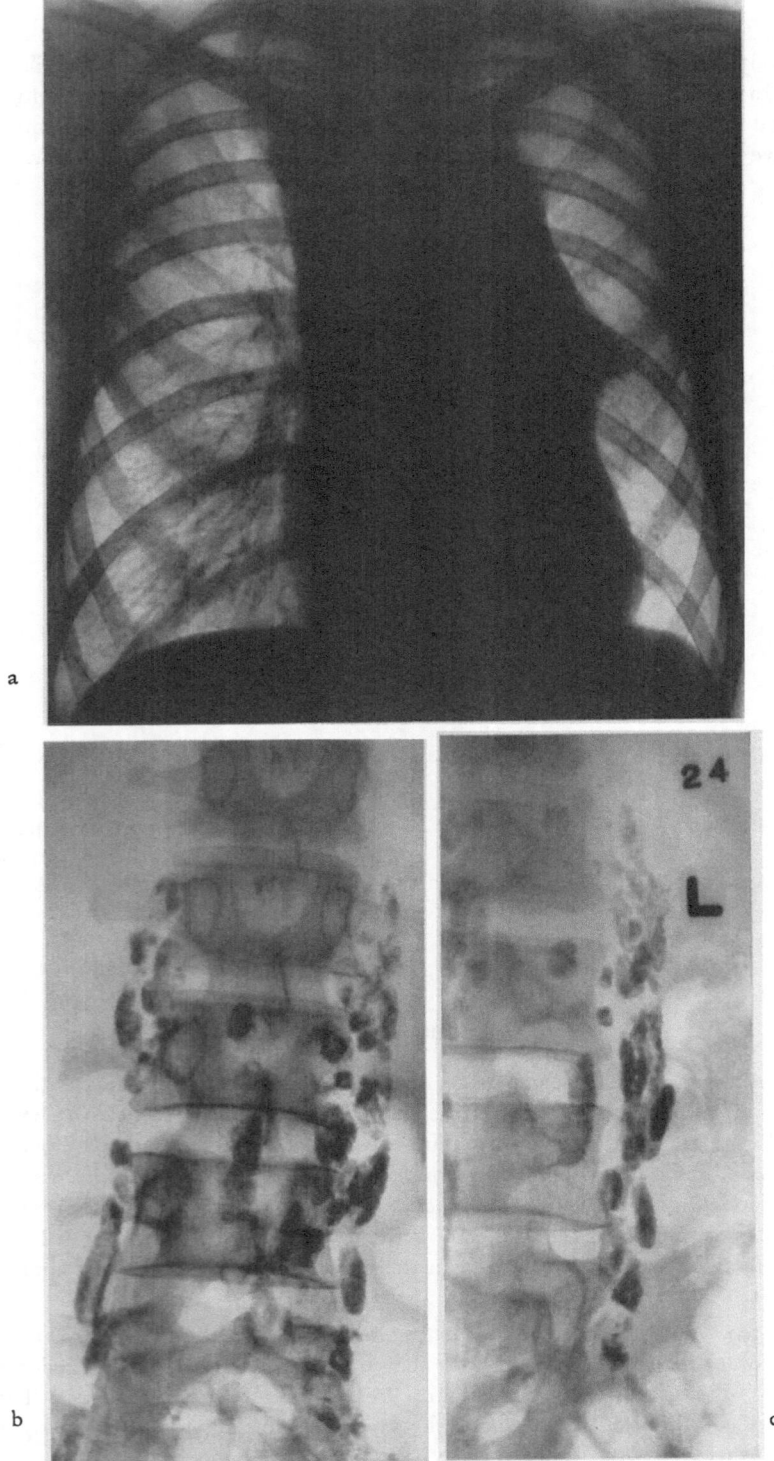

Fig. 9. Hodgkin's disease—Diffuse fibrosis. a Extensive mediastinal soft tissue mass. b Lympho-gram showing small nodes without definite abnormality. c Left posterior oblique showing multiple translucent defects in upper aortic nodes of normal size

Reticular Hodgkin's Disease

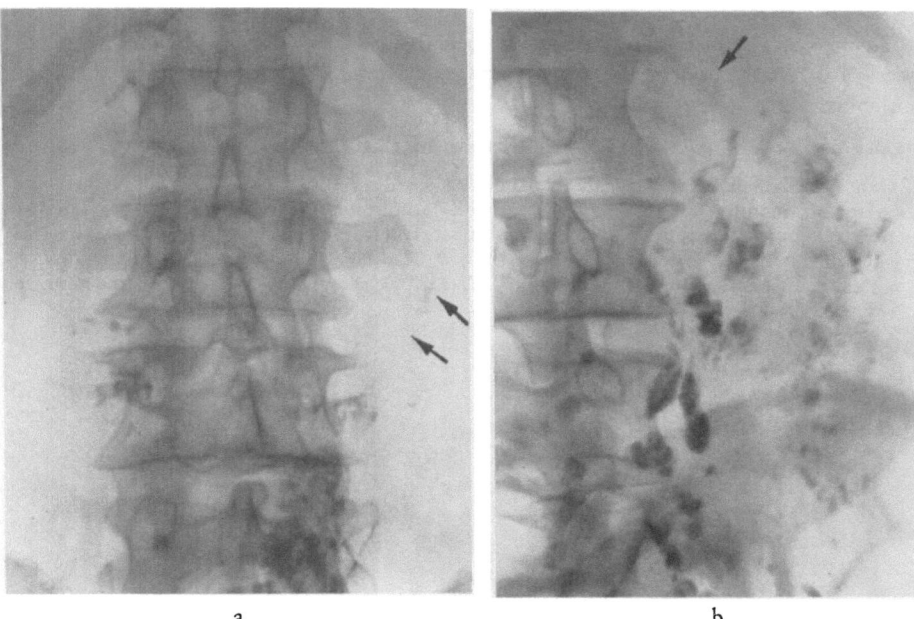

a   b

Fig. 10. Hodgkin's disease—Reticular type. a Displacement of aortic lymph vessels (→).
b Irregular poorly filled nodes and faintly opacified nodes (→)

Case 1: A male, aged 67 years, had suffered from vague
abdominal discomfort for eight months. Because of clinical
suspicion of a deep-seated abdominal mass, laparotomy was
performed. Biopsy of retroperitoneal lymph nodes revealed
Hodgkin's disease of reticular type with lymphocyte depletion.
Lymphography shows several displaced marginal vessels in the
aortic regions (Fig. 10 a). The lymphadenogram (Fig. 10 b)
shows numerous irregular small contrast aggregates in several
of which are sharply demarcated radiolucent defects. This
patient was treated with an abdominal field of Cobalt 60 irradiation to 2650 rads with little evidence of improvement. He
continued to deteriorate over the next six months and succumbed to widely disseminated Hodgkin's disease.

Comment: Despite adequate contrast material in the
lymphangiogram, only small irregular lymph nodes and
faintly filling "ghost" storage patterns are demonstrated
at the site of lymphocyte depleted reticular Hodgkin's
disease.

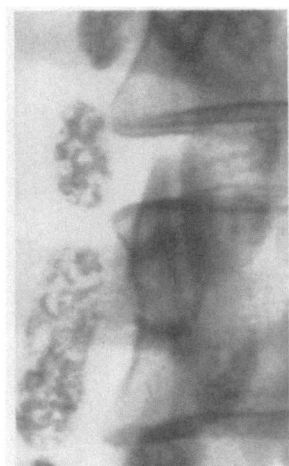

Fig. 11. Reticular Hodgkin's
disease. Aortic lymph node
— Simple   magnification —
Numerous sharply demar-
cated small filling defects
in nodes of normal size

Case 2: A woman, aged 22 years, complained of weight
loss, cough, and fatigue for six months. A small palpable node
in the right side of the neck was removed and showed a histological picture of Hodgkin's disease of reticular type. On the
chest radiographs, an extensive upper and mid mediastinal soft tissue mass without evidence
of lung infiltration was present. Lymphography showed numerous small lymph nodes in the

aortic regions of normal size with scattered irregular punched-out filling defects in the contrast pattern (Fig. 11). Liver function test were abnormal.

Comment: The histological and radiological findings are of an advanced type of disease in lymph nodes of normal size contiguous with extensive mediastinal lymphoma.

Atypical Lymphoma Patterns

Case 1: A female, aged 41 years, had noted a small swelling in the right supraclavicular region for six months. On examination, palpable lymph nodes were present in both sides of the neck. Chest radiography revealed some upper anterior mediastinal adenopathy, but no evidence of extensive intrathoracic disease. Biopsy of a neck node showed Hodgkin's disease of mixed cellularity type. Lymphography (Fig. 12 a) showed irregularity of the storage

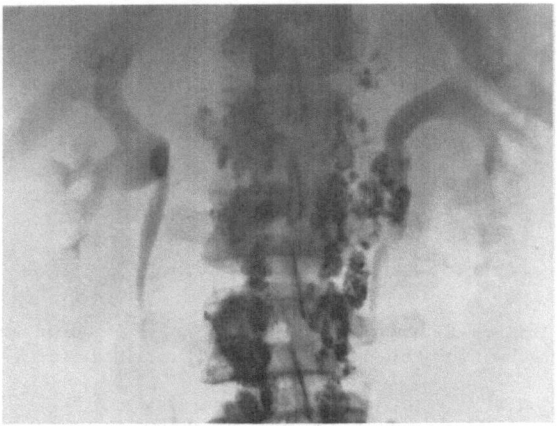

a

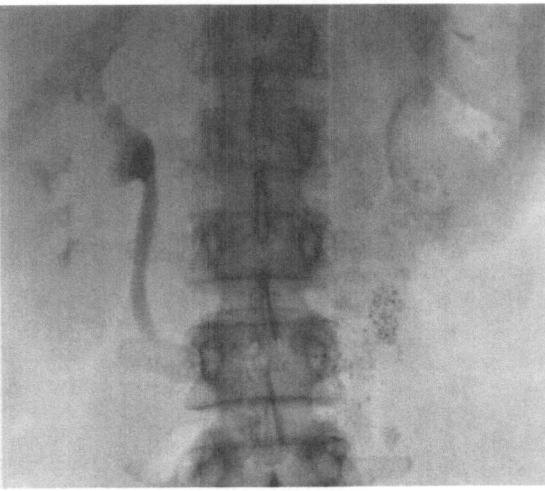

b

Fig. 12. "Atypical lymphoma" pattern. a Small irregular opaque nodes and adjacent irregular contrast residues. b Follow-up radiograph—Spreading of contrast residues pattern in nodes of normal size and numerous small irregular adjacent contrast aggregates in the aortic groups with normal appearances of the iliac nodes. This was considered an atypical lymphoma pattern. Following radiotherapy to the neck and mediastinum, this patient was apparently well for 14 months. Review film of the abdomen (Fig. 12 b) showed considerable spreading and lateral extension of the small amount of residual contrast material remaining in the aortic lymph nodes, indicating progressive enlargement. Despite further therapy to the abdomen, deterioration occurred with death from hepato-cellular failure. Autopsy revealed extensive involvement of all of the retroperitoneal lymph nodes by Hodgkin's disease with mixed features of diffuse fibrosis and reticular subtypes.

Comment: Multiple irregular storage patterns in small nodes and lymphoid aggregates are demonstrated 18 months prior to autopsy. Review radiograph after 14 months still showed enough contrast medium to indicate progressive node enlargement and architectural abnormality. The findings suggest that the atypical storage pattern was the first detected manifestation of lymphomatous infiltration of retroperitoneal nodes.

Case 2: An adolescent female had felt a small swelling in the right side of her neck for two months prior to diagnosis. Biopsy of a palpable lymph node in the right axilla revealed Hodgkin's disease of mixed diffuse type. On chest radiographs, extensive broadening of the superior mediastinum was noted and tomography confirmed bilateral paratracheal lymph node enlargement. The lymphographic storage pattern (Fig. 13 a and b) shows multiple small irregular confluent areas of contrast medium in both aortic regions consistent with numerous superimposed lymphoid aggregates. In addition, coarse granular lymph nodes of irregular size and shape are seen. The iliac glands showed normal radiographic appearances.

Comment: A more marked degree of architectural abnormality giving an "atypical" pattern in the aortic nodes is demonstrated in the presence of gross mediastinal adenopathy.

Multiple small irregular lymph nodes have been frequently seen in patients with extensive mediastinal disease presenting in the neck with the nodular sclerosing or mixed cellularity type of Hodgkin's disease. Of 11 such findings, only one patient was diagnosed by lymph node biopsy from the neck as having Hodgkin's disease with lymphocyte predominance. Atypical lymphographic storage patterns may be defined as those in which well formed lymph nodes are absent. Such appearances in minor departures from the normal range as classed as equivocal, and ancillary procedures including radiographic surveillance are recommended.

Ancillary Procedures

Minor flow abnormalities, such as stasis of the contrast medium within vessels at 24 hours, may provide additional evidence of abnormality in doubtful cases. Deviations of lymph trunks icnluding the cisterna chyli may occur (Fig. 14 a and b). Inferior vena cavography is also useful in those patients in whom normal or atypical storage patterns occur and may detect disease adjacent to or above the aortic lymph nodes (Fig. 14 c).

Comparison of the radiographic patterns of opacified periclavicular nodes following lymphography with those in the aortic regions, which may be regarded as in direct communication via the thoracic duct, may be of value in the presence of doubtful radiographic appearances.

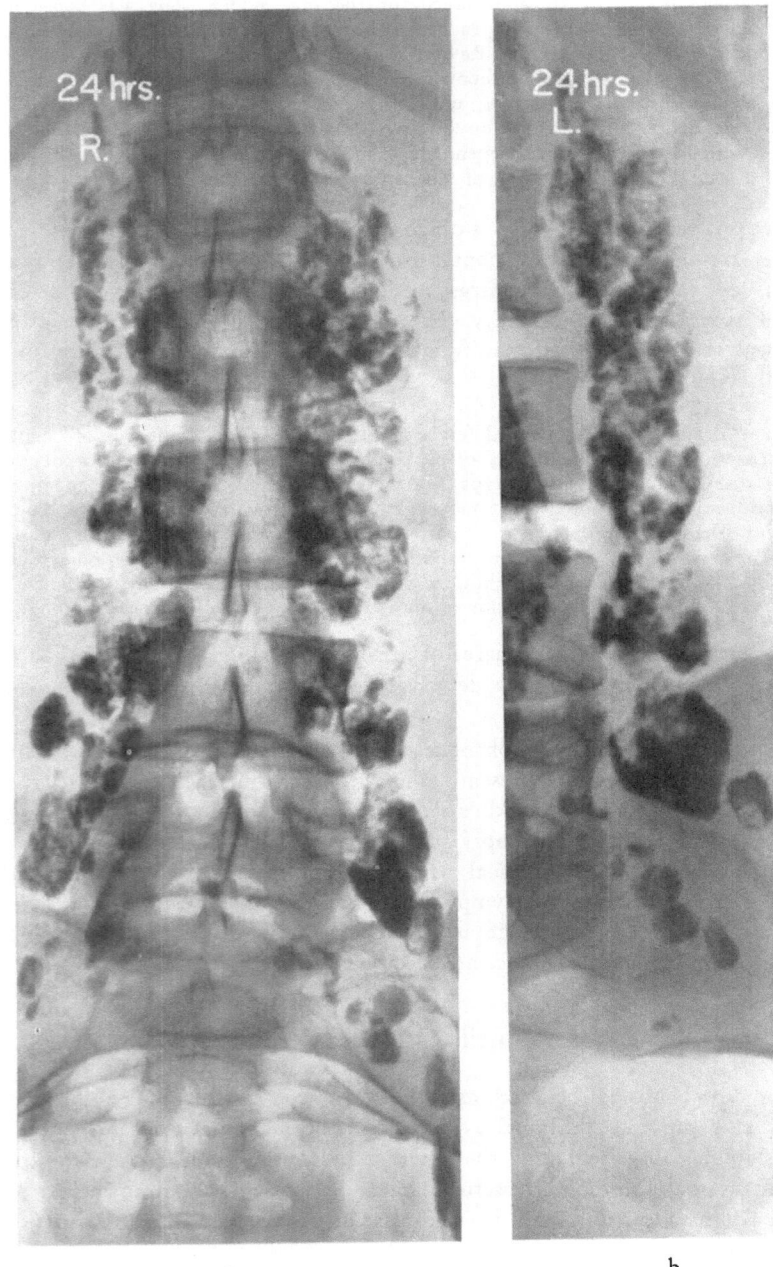

a   b

Fig. 13. Multiple irregular contrast filled lymphoid aggregates and confluent small nodes

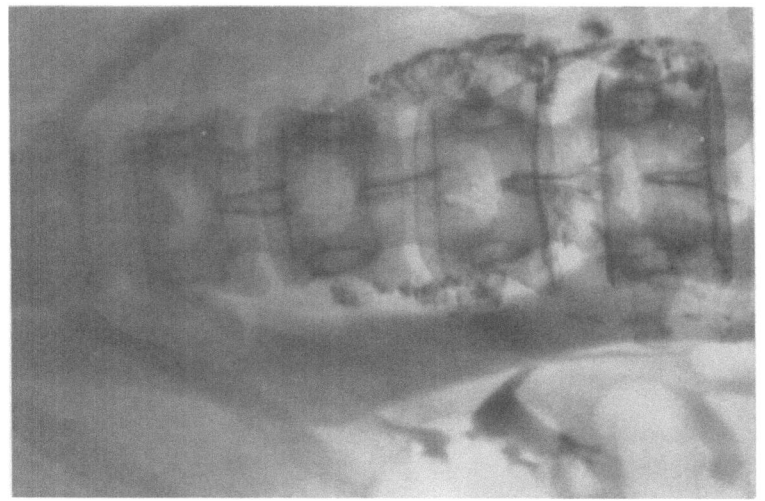

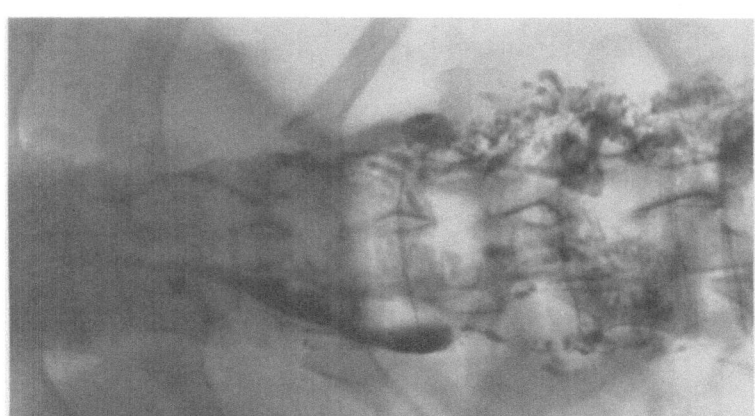

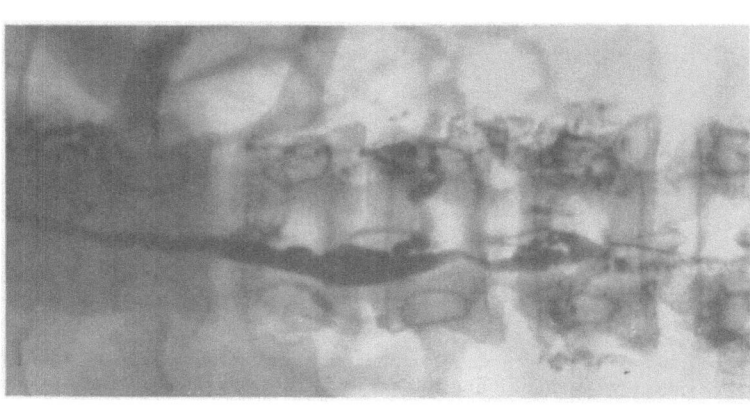

Fig. 14. Cisterna chyli deviation and inferior vena cavography. a Normal cisterna chyli. b Deviation of cisterna chyli to the right. c Displacement of opaque inferior vena cava at site of atypical lymph nodes

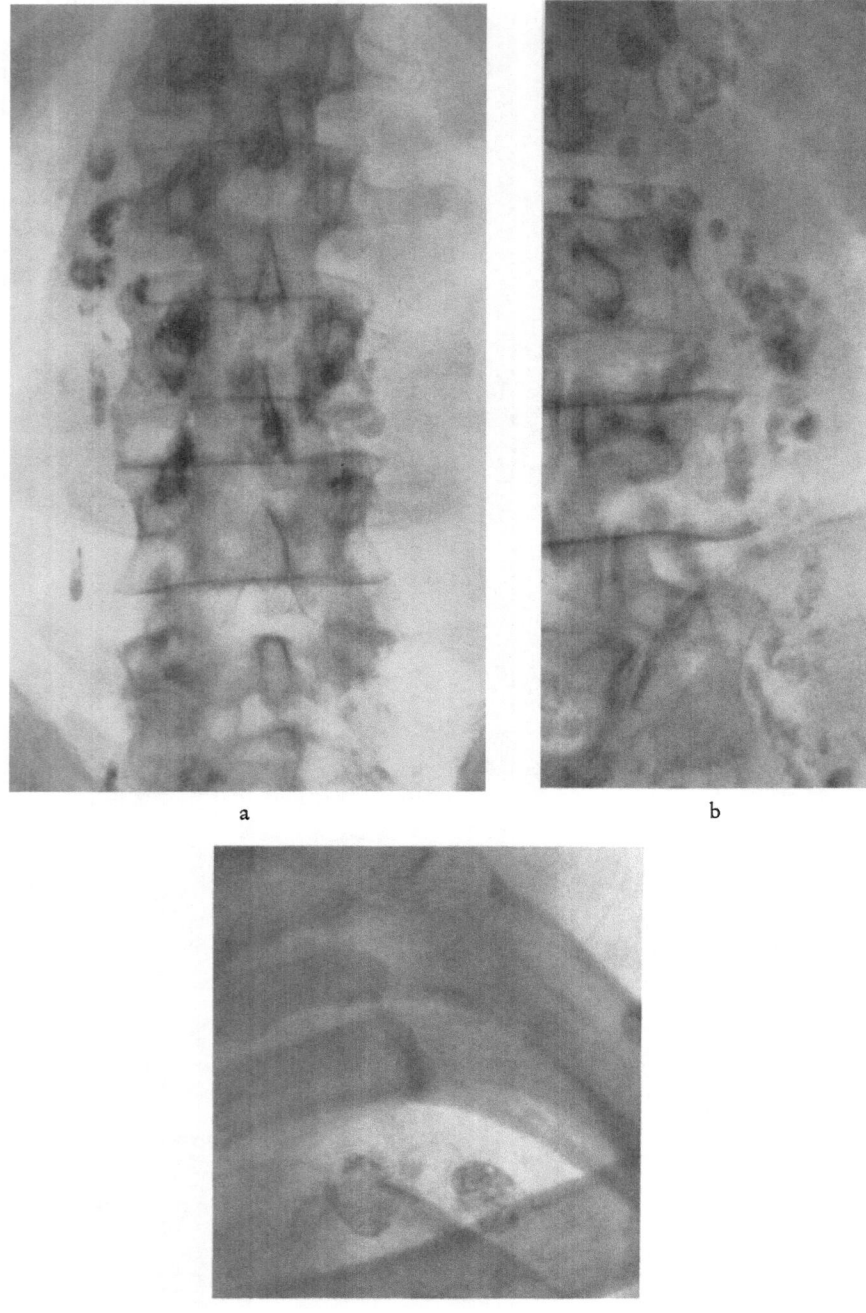

a   b

c

Fig. 15. "Scalene" node biopsy in small node—Lymphocytic and histiocytic disease. a and b Small irregular aortic nodes with faint filling defects. c Left periclavicular nodes—Coarse granularity and a few scattered 1 mm filling defects

Case Report: A 58-year-old male had been troubled with chronic skin irritation in the right axilla in which palpable lymph nodes had been present intermittently, for eight years. Biopsy showed diffuse lymphocytic and histiocytic proliferation throughout a lymph node with Reed-Sternberg cells, indicating Hodgkin's disease. Continuous oral steroid therapy had been administered during the previous six months. Lymphography (Fig. 15 a and b) showed small irregular aortic lymph nodes in which faint filling defects could be seen. Well opacified nodes adjacent to the left clavicle (Fig. 15 c) are of similar size to the aortic nodes and show a somewhat granular contrast pattern. On biopsy, one of these nodes was found to be infiltrated with lymphocytic and histiocytic Hodgkin's disease. Laparotomy was performed because of the clinical suspicion of more extensive intra-abdominal disease, and the aortic nodes of doubtful appearance were found to be infiltrated with lymphocytic and histiocytic Hodgkin's disease. In addition, unopacified infiltrated lymph nodes of larger size were noted in the mesentery and adjacent to the splenic hilum.

Comment: Suspected abnormality in lymph nodes of normal size in a patient following prolonged steroid ingestion was confirmed by biopsy of the scalene and aortic nodes to be due to lymphocytic and histiocytic Hodgkin's disease.

Radiographic Appearances in Terms of Pathology

Marked variability in post-lymphographic storage patterns of nodes infiltrated with Hodgkin's disease has been observed. Classic appearances of lymphomatous infiltration are well known [25, 27, 28] and vary from lace-like, coarse granular, or foamy patterns, to irregular filling defects in enlarged nodes. A marked increase in number of nodes of normal size, and "atypical lymphoma patterns" consisting of numerous irregular lymphoid aggregates have also been noted [10]. With extensive node replacement by fibrosis or tumour, "phantom" nodes demarcated by filling of marginal vessels, and lymphatic obstruction may ensue. Such macroscopic radiographic appearances reflect the architectural changes in lymph nodes by distortion, dilatation, or narrowing of intranodal sinusoids containing ultra-fluid Lipiodol, and total obliteration of sinusoids of varying degree occurs in areas of node replacement.

The significance of radiographic manifestations within individual nodes may best be evaluated by removal of radiopaque nodes following lymphography and comparison of storage patterns of ultra-fluid Lipiodol with the histology. Although second biopsies are seldom necessary in clinical practice, 10 such comparisons have been possible. Less valuable evidence may ensue from comparison of lymphographic storage patterns in areas adjacent to the site of previous lymph node biopsy, and this has been possible in 28 patients. In three of thirty-eight patients, false negative lymphographic studies occurred, and one equivocal lymphographic appearance was found due to lymphoma. Thus, lymphography has been extremely accurate in the detection of lymph node involvement, and the small number of false negative examinations confirms the expected limitation of the macroscopic method.

In Hodgkin's disease with lymphocyte predominance, node size and storage patterns may vary from normal to marked enlargement with a fine lace pattern. Slight enlargement of lymph nodes with a homogeneous coarse granular pattern has been shown to reflect diffuse cellular proliferation throughout the nodes. With lesser degrees of lymphocyte proliferation in nodes of normal size, no radiographic abnormality may be visible and a false negative examination will result. No detectable difference has been discernable on radiographs between nodular and diffuse forms of infiltration. In larger lymph nodes with diffuse cellular change, radiolucent areas in the storage pattern may be due to parenchymal replacement or to underfilling with contrast medium. The latter may occur despite optimal technique including demonstration of adequate flow on the lymphangiogram. Fine regular contrast filled sinusoids are usually visualized adjacent to such areas. A homogeneous distribution of the contrast medium regularly interspersed with 1 mm radiolucent filling defects is similar to the appearance of lacunar loosening and may also reflect diffuse lymphocytic and histiocytic proliferation. Thus, preservation of sinusoidal architecture has been a feature of infiltrations with lymphocytic predominance.

Increasing architectural abnormality and pleomorphism associated with the mixed form of Hodgkin's disease has been reflected by filling defects of irregular size and contour. Such changes may occur in small areas of a predominantly homogeneous storage pattern, or may be more prominent.

In more histologically advanced disease, increasing distortion of the storage pattern due to obliteration of sinusoids is seen as irregular or punched-out filling defects. Preservation of submarginal regions of the nodes has been a commonly noted feature, and may be demonstrated in nodes of very large size (Fig. 16). Small nodes with

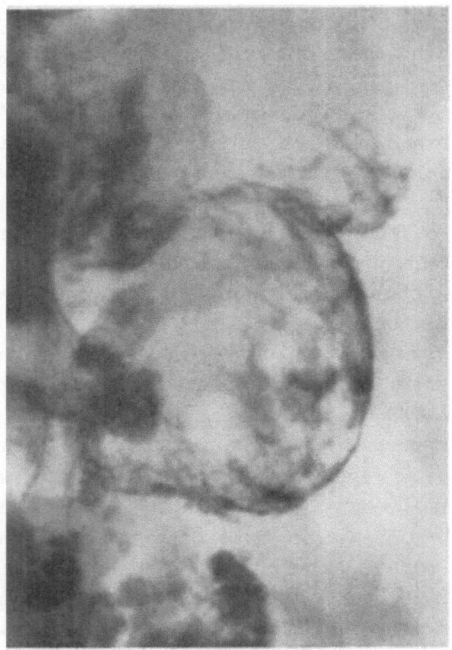

Fig. 16. Enlarged node showing marginal preservation and confluent contrast aggregates. At autopsy, diffuse fibrosis

regular or irregular punched-out radiolucent defects have been found in the aortic regions at autopsy in patients dying with advanced intrathoracic disease. Such changes of poorly preserved architecture with irregularly distributed filling defects in small or large nodes have reflected lymphocyte depleted forms of Hodgkin's disease.

Massive enlargement of lymph nodes has been demonstrated on reassessment lymphography in four patients in whom the original diagnosis was Hodgkin's paragranuloma or lymphocyte predominance. Contrast filled sinusoids throughout these nodes were demonstrated in one patient in whom an excellent response to radio-therapy was obtained. Three such patients died and at autopsy in one, massive node replacement with neoplastic and fibrous tissue was confirmed. In nodular sclerosis, small or moderately enlarged nodes have been common findings on reassessment lymphography.

Marked variability in the radiographic appearances may be noted in the same patient in adjacent lymph nodes or groups, and this may indicate the stage of evolution of the pathological process within individual lymph nodes. Lympho-graphic features of advanced abdominal disease in enlarged nodes may be found after presentation and biopsy of small neck nodes showing lymphocytic and histiocytic disease. Similarly, smaller abnormal nodes may be found in the upper aortic regions adjacent to gross mediastinal adenopathy in patients presenting in the neck with nodular sclerosis or mixed Hodgkin's disease. However, in the investigation of new patients, a fair degree of uniformity of storage patterns may frequently be found. Further experience of analysis of the radiographic patterns in Hodgkin's disease may provide useful information on its natural history if, as has been suggested, increasing immunological defects and induction of malignant neoplasia are reflected by the histological appearances.

Clinical Staging

The contribution of pre-management lymphography to clinical staging is shown in Table 6. All equivocal lymphographic appearances are classified as normal in the

Table 6. *Lymphography in Hodgkin's disease. Influence of lymphography in staging of 161 new patients*

Clinical stage	No. of patients	Abnormal	Normal and equivocal	Advanced to	
				Stage II	Stage III
I	62	24	38	11	11
II	73	31	42		30
III and IV	25	21	4		
Total	160	76	84	11	41

context of clinical staging, although further review by repeat radiography after an interval is advised. Fifty-two of 135 patients were found to have clinically occult disease in lymph nodes below the diaphragm with subsequent advance in staging. Abnormal lymphography has not advanced the staging in those patients in whom significant abnormality has been demonstrated by clinical examination or laboratory study.

Analysis of stage alterations due to lymphography in Stage I patients by present-ing sites is shown in Table 7. Eleven of 44 patients presenting in the neck or axilla were advanced to Stage III. No patient in whom Hodgkin's disease was discovered in the groin was found by lymphography to have disease above the diaphragm, but the majority had lymph node abnormalities extending to the aortic regions.

Similarly, in Stage II patients (Table 8), 30 of 72 patients with Hodgkin's disease above the diaphragm were found to have clinically occult involvement of aortic nodes. From Tables 7 and 8, it may be noted that in patients presenting in any region of the body, occult lympho-reticular abnormality may be present.

Stage alterations in those patients in whom the histology has been classified according to Lukes are shown in Table 9. The majority of patients with lymphocytic and histiocytic disease were initially thought to be in Stage I, while those with nodu-

Table 7. *Lymphography in Hodgkin's disease. Influence of lymphography on stage I patients*

Presenting site	No. of patients	Altered to Stage II	Stage III	No alteration
Low neck	23		7	16
High neck	11		1	10
Axilla	10		3	7
Groin	13	10		3
Other	5	1		4
Total	62	11	11	40

Table 8. *Lymphography in Hodgkin's disease. Influence of lymphography on stage II patients*

Presenting site	No. of patients	Altered to stage III	No alteration
Low neck	52	18	34
High neck	8	3	5
Axilla	8	5	3
Groin	1		1
Other	4	4	
Total	73	30	43

Table 9. *Lymphography in Hodgkin's disease. Stage alteration in the 3 main presenting subtypes of Hodkin's disease*

Subtype of disease	No. of patients	Stage	No. of patients	Abnormal	Normal and equivocal	Advanced to Stage II	Stage III
Lympho-cytic and histiocytic	37	I	26	14	12	5	8
		II	9	3	6		2
		III and IV	2	2			
Nodular sclerosis	32	I	3	1	2		1
		II	19	8	11		8
		III and IV	10	7	3		
Mixed	54	I	25	6	19	4	2
		II	23	6	17		6
		III and IV	6	6			
Total	123		123	53	70	9	27

lar sclerosis most frequently presented as apparent Stage II. Fifty-four patients with mixed Hodgkin's disease presented in almost equal numbers in Stages I and II. A similar incidence of clinically occult disease in the aortic nodes has been demonstrated in each of these three main subtypes.

Surveillance and Reassessment

In about 10% of patients with Hodgkin's disease, minor irregularities in the storage patterns of lymph nodes may be indistinguishable from normal multiple lymphoid aggregate patterns. Slight regional or individual node enlargement may also be of unknown significance. In such lymphograms, to distinguish normal appearances from early change associated with lymphomatous infiltration, review by repeat radiographs at one month and three monthly intervals and comparison with the original storage pattern may be a useful addition.

Case 1: A middle-aged woman was found to have mixed nodular Hodgkin's disease on biopsy of a lymph node from the left side of the neck. Lymphography (Fig. 17 a) showed storage patterns of normal appearance in aortic lymph nodes. Minor irregularities in contour in the upper left aortic nodes and granularity were noted. On repeat radiographs five months later, sufficient contrast was present within the nodes to indicate enlargement during the interval (Fig. 17 b). Spreading of the contrast residues in the storage pattern has occurred indicating change in the nodal architecture. These appearances suggested progressive lymphomatous infiltration, and as the patient's clinical condition had deteriorated during the interval, a further course of irradiation to the abdomen was advised.

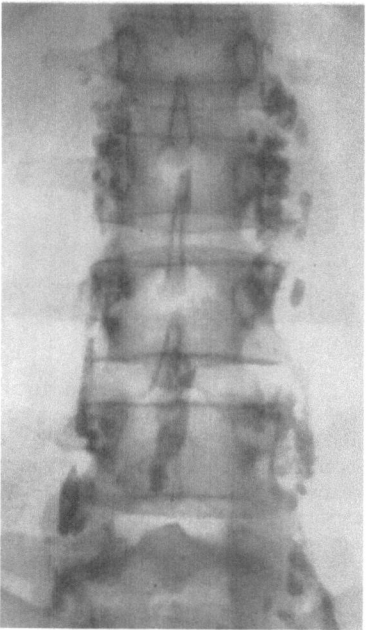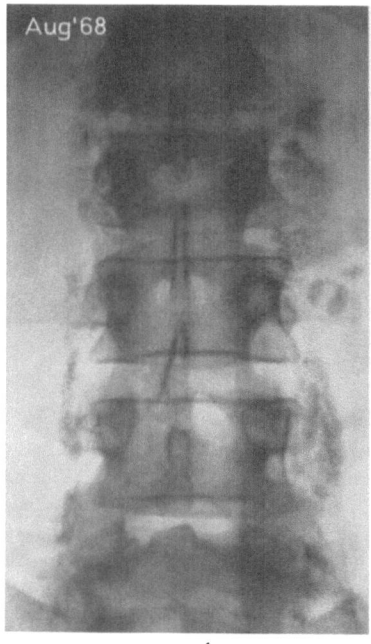

a   b

Fig. 17. Surveillance. a Normal lymphadenogram with small irregular nodes. b Five months later, spreading of residual contrast medium

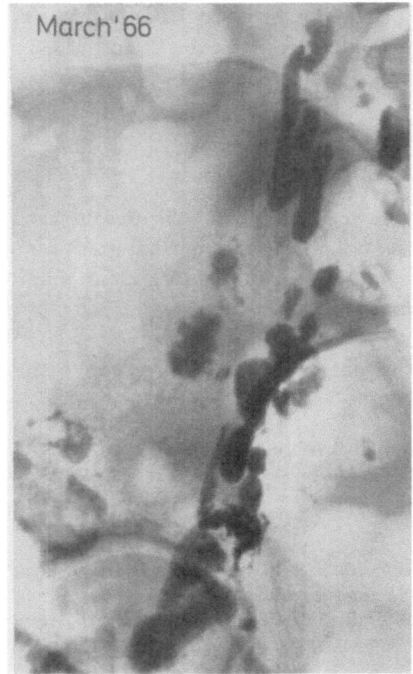 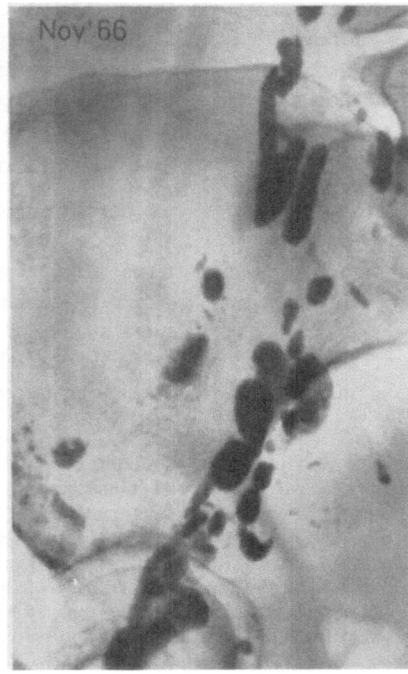

a   b

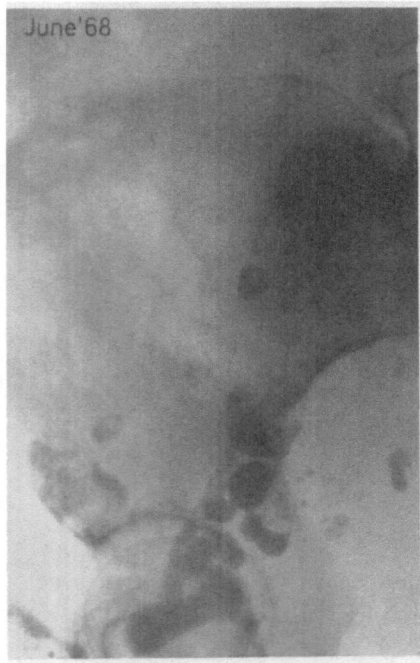

Fig. 18. "Second-look" lymphography in Hodgkin's disease. a Numerous well filled nodes of normal size in right iliac chains. b Second lymphogram—No change in normal appearances. c Third lymphogram—Gross replacement with "ghost" outlines in common iliac region—active lymphomatous disease

Comment: Detection of progressive change in the storage pattern of previously opacified nodes enables recognition of progressive disease at an early stage. Sufficient ultra-fluid Lipiodol may persist within the lymph nodes to yield useful diagnostic information for approximately one year after lymphography. However, if most of the contrast material has disappeared, and active disease is suspected, repeat or "second-look" lymphography is indicated.

Case 2: A 50-year-old female presented with a swelling in the neck, which on biopsy proved to be a lymph node infiltrated with nodular sclerosing Hodgkin's disease. Lymphography (Fig. 18 a) showed well filled, slightly irregular lymph nodes of normal size in the pelvic and aortic groups. Enlarged nodes were demonstrated at the left lung hilum on chest radiograph, and a small adjacent lesion in the lung parenchym was revealed. Radical radiotherapy to the entire thorax and both sides of the neck achieved a satisfactory response.

Eight months later because of generalized pruritus, a second lymphogram was performed as insufficient contrast residues remained in the abdominal nodes (Fig. 18 b). No significant change was present in the lymph node appearances, and further radiographs at three months' intervals were normal, although the patient continued to suffer from intermittent pruritus and sweats.

A third lymphogram, nineteen months later (Fig. 18 c), revealed a striking change in the aortic and iliac lymph nodes. Only faint residues of contrast medium with occasional marginal sinuses are seen in the common iliac region, indicating extensive replacement. Increase in size and granularity of nodes at a lower level is noted.

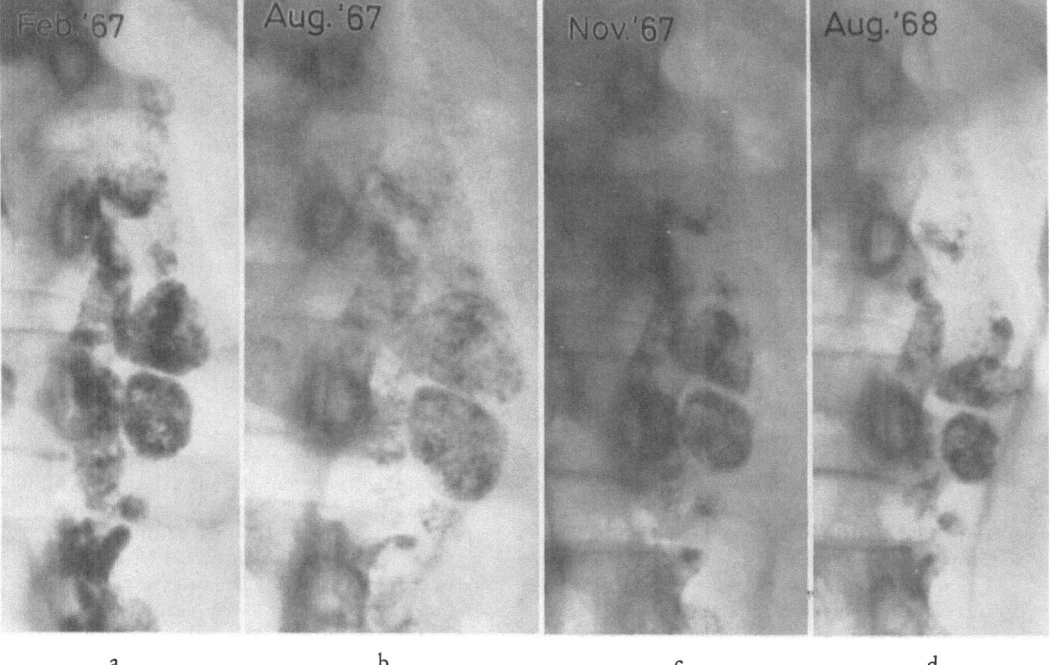

a   b   c   d

Fig. 19. Surveillance. a Reassessment lymphogram six years after radiotherapy to the upper trunk showing granular nodes. b Six months later—No therapy during the interval—Nodes enlarging with spreading of contrast residues. c VLB and Prednisone—Decrease in node size indicating response. d Further shrinkage indicating maintained response

Comment: Three lymphograms in a patient with uncontrolled disease have demonstrated, by continuing surveillance, progressive infiltration of iliac and aortic lymph nodes in the absence of clinical indications of sites of involvement. Such management may be of value in monitoring response to chemotherapy (Fig. 19 a—d).

In those with clinical breakdown at an interval following a previous course of therapy, lymphograms have been classified as reassessment studies. Ninety-two such investigations in 142 patients who had previous radiotherapy to the upper trunk have disclosed abnormal lymph nodes below the diaphragm. This may be of value in planning further therapy and recording response to treatment (Fig. 20).

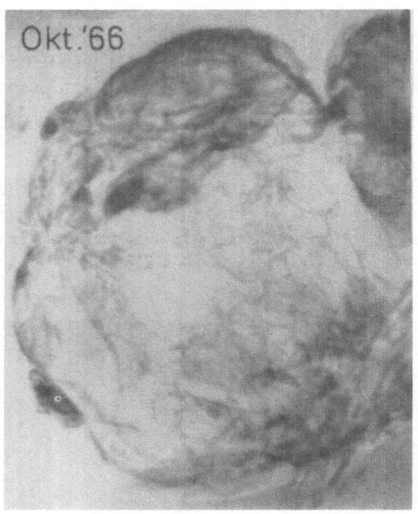 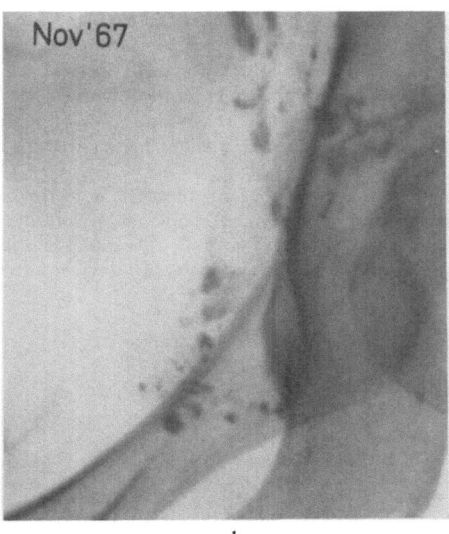

a   b

Fig. 20. Response to therapy. a Reassessment lymphogram. Huge iliac node in patient previously treated for L. & H. Hodgkin's disease. Note sinusoids in area of filling defects. b Marked shrinkage in same node following radiotherapy

Inferior vena cavography may prove useful in surveillance and reassessment following previous lymphography in those patients in whom intrathoracic disease precludes further use of intralymphatic ultra-fluid Lipiodol.

Case Report: A 17 year-old boy had been treated to the neck following biopsy diagnosis of Hodgkin's disease of mixed cellularity type. Initial lymphography showed normal appearances of the iliac and aortic nodes, and this was confirmed on repeat examination (Fig. 21 a and b) within a year. Chest X-ray a short time later showed a low density soft tissue lesion in the left lung field. A good response was obtained to radiation of the left lung lesion, but further circumscribed opacities were noted in the right lung. Chemotherapy was, therefore, commenced and surveillance as an out-patient was maintained. One year later to confirm a clinical suspicion of intra-abdominal disease, inferior vena cavography was performed (Fig. 21 c). Gross indentation of the posterior aspect of the inferior vena cava with displacement anteriorly and to the right is noted at L 1—2 level. A small amount of residual contrast material insufficient for diagnosis is present. Death occurred from progressive lung infiltration after a further eight months. At autopsy, infiltration of the aortic nodes by Hodgkin' disease was demonstrated with a large localized mass indenting the inferior vena cava at the site of the radiographic abnormality.

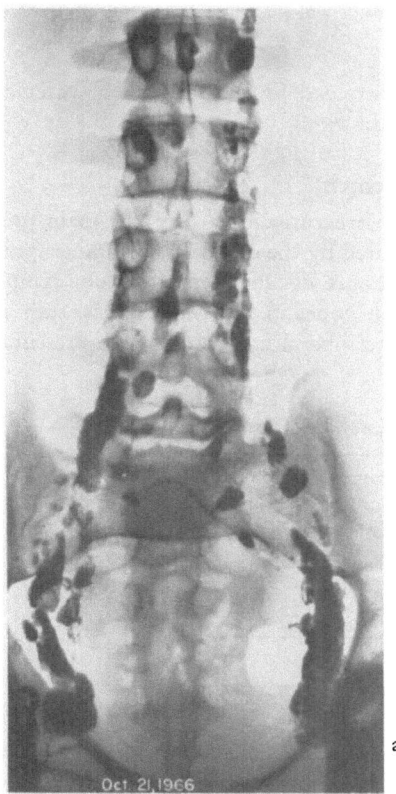

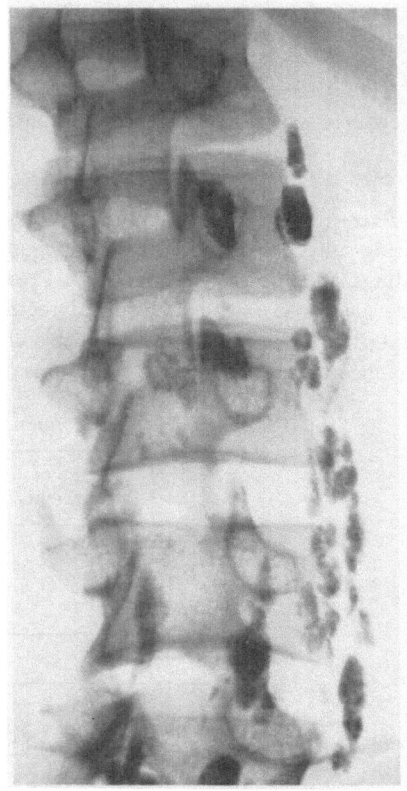

a b

c

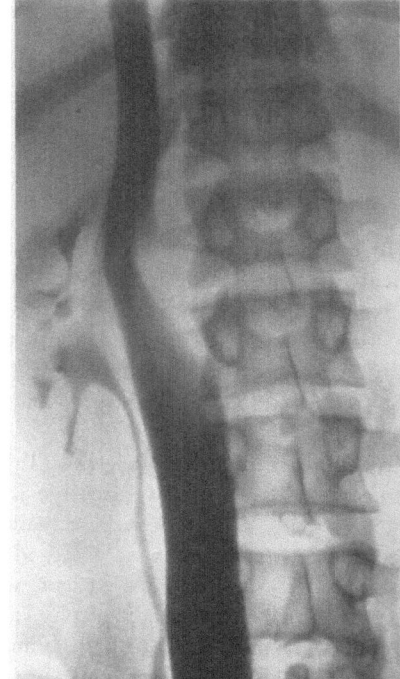

Fig. 21. Inferior vena cavography in surveillance. a and b Normal lymphogram. c Inferior Vena Cavagram—Extrinsic indentation of left side and anterior bowing by soft tissue mass. Faint contrast residues in adjacent nodes

Comment: Surveillance may be usefully maintained by supplementary vascular ,
procedures when lymphography is contraindicated.

Patterns of Involvement

Patterns of involvement of lympho-reticular structures in each of the main presenting subtypes of Hodgkin's disease may be elicited by the clinical and radiographic
findings, including lymphography. Presenting sites are documented to include lymph
node groups in broad anatomical regions. Lymph nodes in superficial areas, such as
the axilla, groin, and upper neck are classed as peripheral in site. Systemic presentation encompasses those with symptoms only.

Table 10. *Lymphocyte predominance. Sites of involvement in 37 new patients*

Presenting site	No. of patients	Mediastinal disease	Abdominal disease
Low neck	13	5	7
Peripheral	23	3	10
Abdomen	1	0	1
Total	37	8	18

Table 11. *Nodular sclerosis. Sites of involvement in 32 new patients*

Presenting site	No. of patients	Mediastinal disease	Abdominal disease
Low neck	25	21	9
Peripheral	3	3	2
Mediastinal	2	2	2
Systemic	2	2	2
Total	32	28	15

In Hodgkin's disease with lymphocyte predominance (Table 10), the majority of
patients presented in peripheral sites, and following investigation, a significant number were found to have involvement of aortic lymph nodes. Mediastinal disease was
less commonly detected, and in only three patients could be regarded as extensive.
Thus, palpable enlarged lymph nodes in a peripheral site or in the low neck was the
most frequent mode of discovery, and clinically occult involvement of aortic nodes
was common.

By contrast in nodular sclerosis (Table 11), lymph node enlargement at the base of
the neck was adjacent to extensive mediastinal disease, and again in a significant
number, occult retroperitoneal disease was present following investigation. In all
three patients presenting with enlarged lymph nodes in peripheral groups, mediastinal
disease was discovered. Four patients were seen to have nodular sclerosing Hodgkin's
disease following chest radiography, and of those, two had non-specific symptoms.
All four were discovered to have lympho-reticular involvement in the aortic region.

Of 54 patients with Hodgkin's disease of mixed cellularity type (Table 12), two main patterns of involvement were apparent. The majority presented with palpable nodes at the base of the neck and were found to have extensive mediastinal disease Occult retroperitoneal node infiltration was present in eight of thirty-three such patients. A second group of 18 patients was noted each of whom had presented with palpable lymph nodes in a superficial group. Half of these patients had occult abdominal lymphoma, and a small number mediastinal involvement.

Distribution of the sites of disease in each of the histological subtypes is recorded for comparison in Table 13. Two distinct patterns appear to be present corresponding to lymphocyte predominance and nodular sclerosis respectively. Hodgkin's disease of mixed cellularity type was the most frequent diagnosis on presentation and showed two main patterns of distribution similar to lymphocyte predominance, and nodular

Table 12. *Mixed cellularity type. Sites of involvement in 54 new patients*

Presenting site	No. of patients	Mediastinal disease	Abdominal disease
Low neck	33	20	8
Peripheral	18	4	9
Mediastinal	2	2	0
Systemic	1	0	1
Total	54	26	18

Table 13. *Sites of involvement on presentation in 129 patients with Hodgkin's disease by histological subtypes* (LUKES [12]) [a]

Subtype	High neck	Axilla	Groin	Abdomen	Mediastinum	Low neck	Systemic	No. of patients
Lymphocyte predominance (Lymphocytic and histiocytic)	7	7	9	1	0	13	0	37
	8	12	9	18	8	18	0	
Nodular sclerosis	3				2	25	2	32
	5	10		15	28	29		
Mixed	5	7	6	0	2	33	1	54
	6	21	7	18	26	41		
Lymphocyte depletion (Diffuse fibrosis and reticular)	1	0	0	2	0	3		6
	2	1	0	5	3	3		
Total	16	14	15	3	4	74	3	129
	21	44	16	56	63	91	0	

[a] Upper figures = presenting sites. Lower figures = involved sites.

sclerosis. It is possible that with increasing immunological defect and progressive neoplasia, progression from these two types to a common histological picture, namely mixed cellularity, may occur. Of six new patients with lymphocyte depletion, a finding more common at autopsy than on presentation, five were discovered to have extensive retroperitoneal involvement.

Prognosis

Although clinical staging has proven of particular value in prognosis, it has been noted that rapid transition from a favourable presentation of advanced disease and death may occur in unpredictable fashion. Evaluation of the post-lymphographic storage patterns in individual lymph nodes in patients with known Hodgkin's disease may prove of value in mapping the stage of evolution of the pathological process in individual lymph nodes in the areas opacified. Using the combined information from a histological diagnosis at biopsy, the lymphographic distribution of disease within aortic and iliac lymph nodes, and the radiogrpahic morphology, certain patterns emerge. Homogeneous distribution of the post-lymphographic storage pattern within lymph nodes appears to be associated with lymphocytic proliferation, disease confined to the lympho-reticular system, a favourable response to therapy, and a good prognosis. Filling defects and distortion of contrast filled sinusoids may reflect more advanced disease, lymphocyte depletion, the likelihood of extra-nodal disease, and poor prognosis. In 45 patients alive 5 to 22 years from the time of diagnosis of Hodgkin's disease, aortic lymph nodes with a homogeneous storage pattern were present, although in several patients these were of large size or adjacent to nodes displaying extensive replacement. Filling defects were present in the contrast pattern of all but 6 of 42 patients who died within 3 years of lymphography, and those 6 patients with normal storage patterns succumbed to extensive intrathoracic disease. Thus, lymphographic studies may have some value in predicting the course of patients with Hodgkin's disease, and response to current methods of therapy.

Unusual Clinical Circumstances

Three patients in whom early pregnancy was suspected have been found on biopsy of enlarged groin nodes to have Hodgkin's disease. Useful demonstration of the status of the lymph nodes to the diaphragm has been achieved with a two-film technique and a lead shield over the pelvis.

Case Report: A 31 year-old woman complained of a small swelling in the left groin which had increased in size over the past four months. Amenorrhea and symptoms of pregnancy had been noted for three months. Biopsy revealed a lymph node infiltrated with Hodgkin's disease of lymphocytic and histiocytic type. Lymphography (Fig. 22 a) showed a diffuse storage pattern of the contrast medium in slightly enlarged nodes adjacent to the site of biopsy with larger irregular granular nodes in the left aortic region. Termination of pregnancy and irradiation of the lymph node areas below the diaphragm was considered the optimal management. Response was confirmed by subsequent radiography (Fig. 22 b and c).

Comment: Lymphographic changes during and following pregnancy have been interpreted with caution. In one patient, enlarged nodes demonstrated in the puerperium were found to regress spontaneously without therapy.

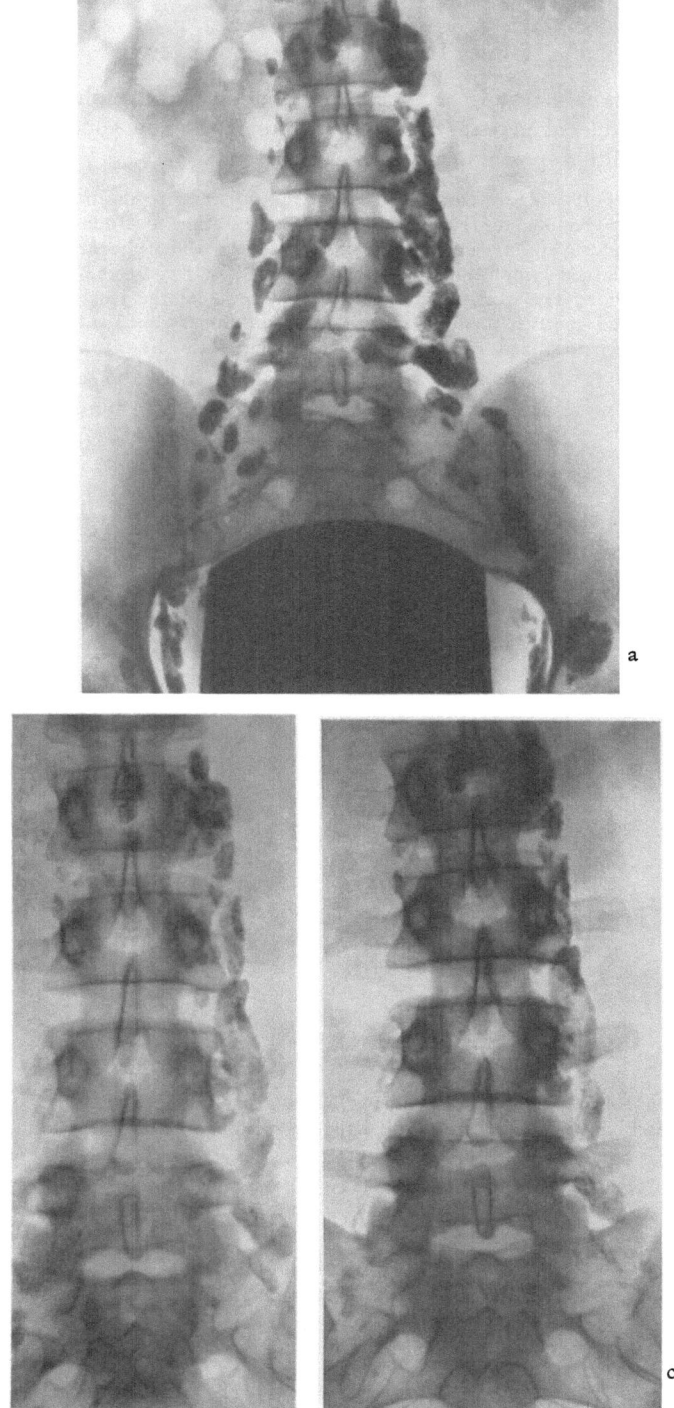

Fig. 22. Hodgkin's disease in pregnancy. a Lymphogram—Larger granular nodes in the left iliac and aortic groups. b and c Repeat radiographs at two and six months following radiotherapy show shrinkage of the lymph nodes

Upper Extremity Lymphography

Axillary nodes are readily accessible to palpation, and lymphographic study has rarely been considered necessary. However, axillary lymph nodes may be usefully opacified in conditions precluding accurate palpation.

Case Report: Following extensive courses of radiotherapy to the neck, mediastinum and both periclavicular regions for Hodgkin's disease, induration and edema around the right axillar were noted on follow-up. A lymphogram from the right arm (Fig. 23) showed early filling of enlarged lymph nodes and flow in fine vessels down the right chest wall with faint dermal backflow. The storage pattern confirmed node enlargement with filling defects in diffusely distributed contrast medium in several of the nodes consistent with lymphomatous infiltration. Further localized radiotherapy was given with clinical and radiographic improvement.

Comment: Useful evaluation of the lymph node status in lymphoedema has been achieved.

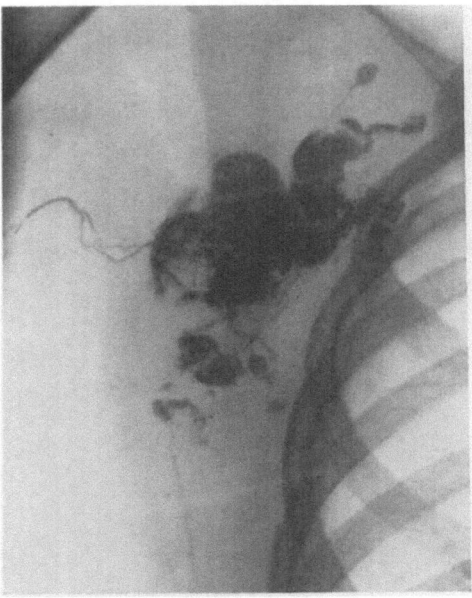

Fig. 23. Lymphoedema in Hodgkin's disease. Right arm lymphogram—Early filling in large nodes fine vessels down lateral chest wall irregular confluent filling defects in several nodes

Lymphosarcoma

Of new patients with lymphosarcoma, the majority examined were found to have apparently localized lymph node enlargement in the neck or groin. In such patients, bilateral lower extremity lymphography may be used as in the clinical staging of Hodgkin's disease, to more accurately define the extent of lympho-reticular disease. Abnormal lymphographic findings in diffuse lymphosarcoma are well known [26]. Generalized lymph node enlargement with alteration in the storage patterns due to diffuse abnormal proliferation of lymphocytic elements may be readily identified.

Presentations of lymphosarcoma outwith the lympho-reticular system are classed as extra-nodal, and staging concepts based on the extent of detected lymphomatous infiltration in lympho-reticular structures, are recent additions to pre-management appraisal [18]. The results of lymphographic study of 107 patients (Table 14) show no significant differences between each histological subtype in initial and reassessment lymphograms. Findings are discussed in terms of radiographic appearances, clinical staging, patterns of disease, and the value of lymphography in management.

Table 14. *Lymphography in lymphosarcomas*

Subtype of lymphosarcoma	No. of patients	No. of lymphograms			Lymphography		
		Initial	Reassess-ment	Repeat	Abnor-mal	Normal	Equi-vocal
Undifferentiated	20	13	7	1	13	8	0
Differentiated	47	33	14	1	32	14	2
Unclassified	40	16	24	1	26	12	3
Total	107	62	45	3	71	34	5

Lymphographic Appearances

Case 1: A 59 year-old woman complained of a slowly increasing swelling in the left sub-mandibular region of three months' duration. Palpable lymph nodes up to 2 cms in diameter were present in both posterior triangles of the neck and axillae. No further abnormality was detected on physical examination. Biopsy from the left submandibular region revealed a lymph node in which complete replacement of normal structures by densely packed masses of differentiated, but atypical, lymphocytes was present. The histology was subclassified as a differentiated, diffuse, lymphocytic malignant lymphoma. Lymphography (Fig. 24 a) shows normal flow of the contrast medium to both inguinal regions. Above this level, displacement of lymph trunks and marginal vessels around grossly enlarged nodes with early filling intra-nodal sinusoids is seen. No evidence of lymphatic obstruction was present. At 24 hours (Fig. 24 b), contrast filled marginal sinuses and branching irregularly dilated intranodal sinusoids are displayed. These are distributed homogeneously throughout the enlarged nodes separating irregular confluent 1 to 3 mm radiolucent areas. In the largest nodes (Fig. 24 c), dilated coarse sinusoids are most prominent in the peripheral parenchyma with preservation of a filled marginal sinus. Extensive confluent radiolucent areas may indicate more advanced disease or relative underfilling with contrast medium in the central areas of grossly enlarged nodes. In moderately enlarged nodes (Fig. 24 d), preservation of the sharply demonstrated marginal and radial sinusoids is depicted by the "spoke wheel" linear distribution of contrast material throughout the nodes. All of the lymph nodes opacified above the inguinal region are abnormal in size storage pattern.

Comment: The lymphographic findings below the diaphragm advance the clinical stage to III. In the presence of dense proliferation of differentiated lymphocytes, the storage pattern indicates increased size of intranodal structures with relative preservation of sinusoids. This gives generally distributed linear or floccular appearances of the contrast material in all of the lymph nodes opacified.

Case 2: A 48 year-old woman complained to her doctor of a painless swelling in the right groin which had been present for four months. Biopsy revealed a lymph node with alteration in its architecture due to numerous follicular collections of atypical lymphocytes surrounded by rims of small mature lymphocytes. The histological classification is of a well

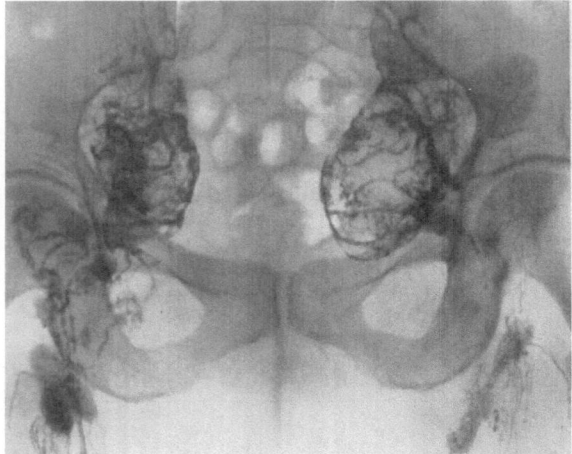

a

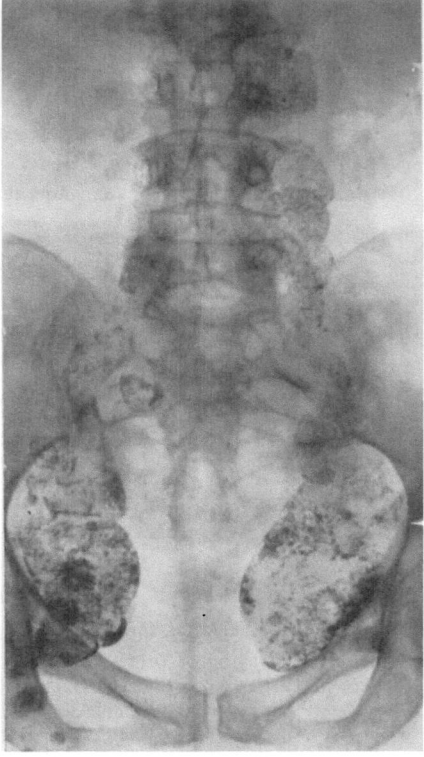

b

Fig. 24. Diffuse differentiated lymphocytic malignant lymphoma. a Lymphangiogram—Filled marginal vessels around grossly enlarged iliac nodes—Early filling intranodal sinusoids. b Lymphadenogram—All nodes visualized are abnormal. c Localized projection with simple magnification—Dilated irregular coarse contrast filled spaces giving floccular appearance. d Marginal and radial sinusoids sharply demarcated with regular arrangement

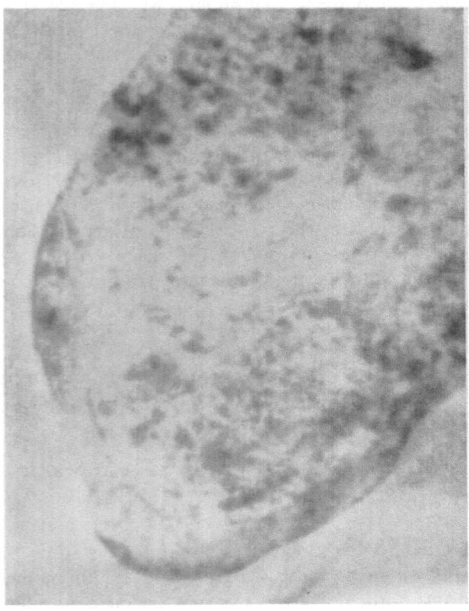

c

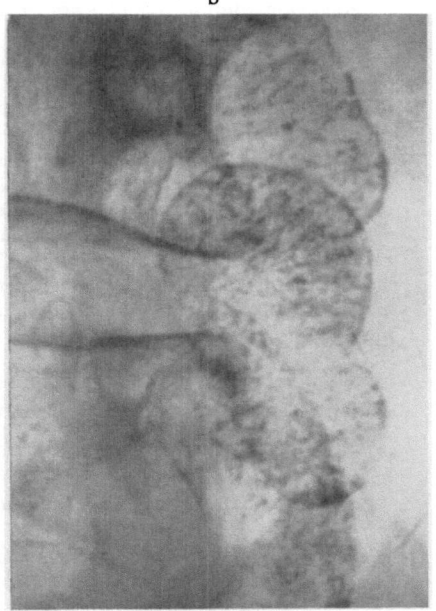

d

differentiated, nodular, lymphocytic malignant lymphoma. Lymphography (Fig. 25 a) demonstrates varying degrees of enlargement in lymph nodes which show a diffusely distributed increase in granularity. Uniformity of the radiographic pattern in all of the nodes visualized is present. Localized projection with magnification (Fig. 25 b) confirms the homogeneous reticular pattern in all of the visible nodes. A radiopaque, slightly granular, left "scalene" node of normal size was visualized on chest radiographs following the lymphogram. Using image intensification fluoroscopy, this node was removed and radiography (Fig. 25 c) showed a homogeneous distribution of contrast material in fine sinusoids throughout the parenchyma. Histologically, this node was extensively replaced by differentiated, nodular, lymphocytic malignant lymphoma. A histiocytic reaction around the lipid vacoules of ultra-fluid Lipiodol was noted.

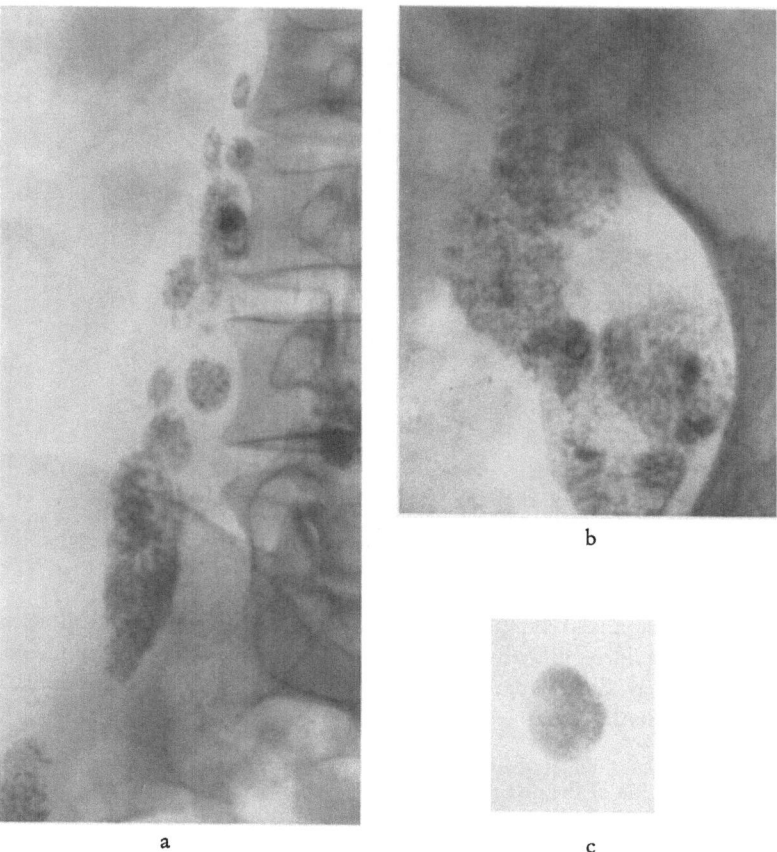

a   b   c

Fig. 25. Nodular differentiated lymphocytic malignant lymphoma. a Lymphadenogram—Coarse granular pattern in all opacified nodes. b Simple magnification—Homogeneous distribution of coarsened contrast pattern. c "Scalene" node—Minimal increase in granularity

Comment: Lymphographic demonstration of generally distributed lymph node abnormality follows a localized presentation. The histological subclassification in this patient replaces the well known term "giant follicular lymphoma". It may be noted that with the lesser degree of abnormality present in the "scalene" node, a normal storage pattern has occurred in the presence of diffuse lymphoma. In patients with

follicular differentiated lymphosarcomas, uniformity of the storage pattern throughout all of the nodes visualized has been a striking feature.

Case 3: A 16 year-old boy with a history of a swollen node in the right side of the neck
of two months' duration was found by biopsy of this node to be suffering from a poorly
differentiated, diffuse, lymphocytic malignant lymphoma. Clinical examination revealed
grossly enlarged nodes in both sides of the neck, both axillae, and groins. Lymphography
confirmed gross generalized enlargement of all of the opacified lymph nodes in inguinal,
iliac and aortic groups. Preservation of marginal sinuses and homogeneous distribution
of radial sinusoids of varying calibre extending to the medulla of the enlarged lymph nodes
are apparent (Fig. 26 a and b).

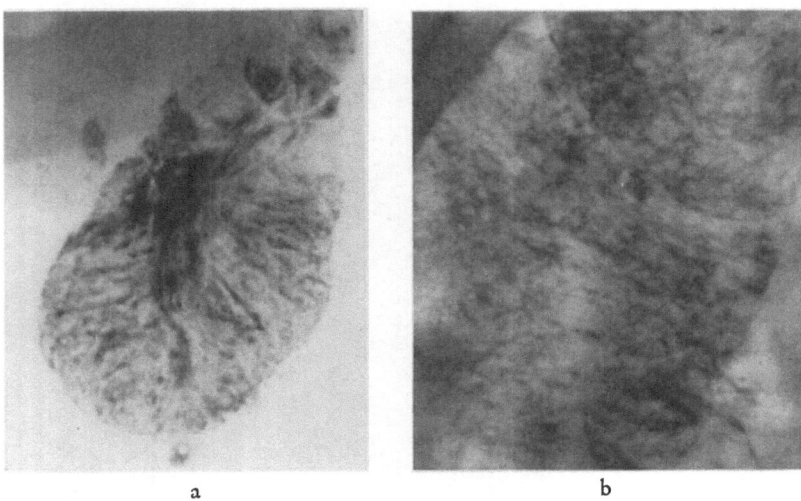

a   b

Fig. 26. Diffuse poorly differentiated lymphocytic malignant lymphoma. Regular sinusoidal
arrangement. a Femoral node. b Iliac nodes

Comment: Generalized lymph node enlargement with regular architectural arrangement of irregularly dilated radial sinusoids, interspersed with confluent radiolucent areas, depicts diffuse parenchymal abnormality in a patient with a poorly
differentiated lymphosarcoma.

Case 4: An adolescent male had been treated five years previously with Cobalt 60 irradiation to the right side of the neck following biopsy of a lymph node showing lymphoblastic
lymphosarcoma. He remained in apparent good health until one month prior to reassessment
lymphography at which time he noticed a small swelling behind the left clavicle. No
further evidence of enlarged nodes was elicited on physical examination. On the lymphangiogram (Fig. 27 a), an adequate amount of contrast material is seen in the aortic vessels.
At 24 hours (Fig. 27 b), moderate enlargement of several lymph nodes is seen with scattered
filling defects in a fairly homogeneous coarse granular or reticular background. A left paravertebral mass at the level of D 10—11 consisting of partially opacified lymph nodes with
marginal preservation was more clearly demonstrated on tomographs (Fig. 27 d) and spot
films (Fig. 27 e). Simultaneous opacification of the inferior vena cava and excretion urography (Fig. 27 c) outlined a more extensive soft tissue mass adjacent to the opacified lymph
nodes. Irregularity in the contrast pattern adjacent to the deviated left ureter indicates failure
to fill of many intranodal sinusoids due to underfilling indicated by diversion of flow at this
level on the lymphangiogram.

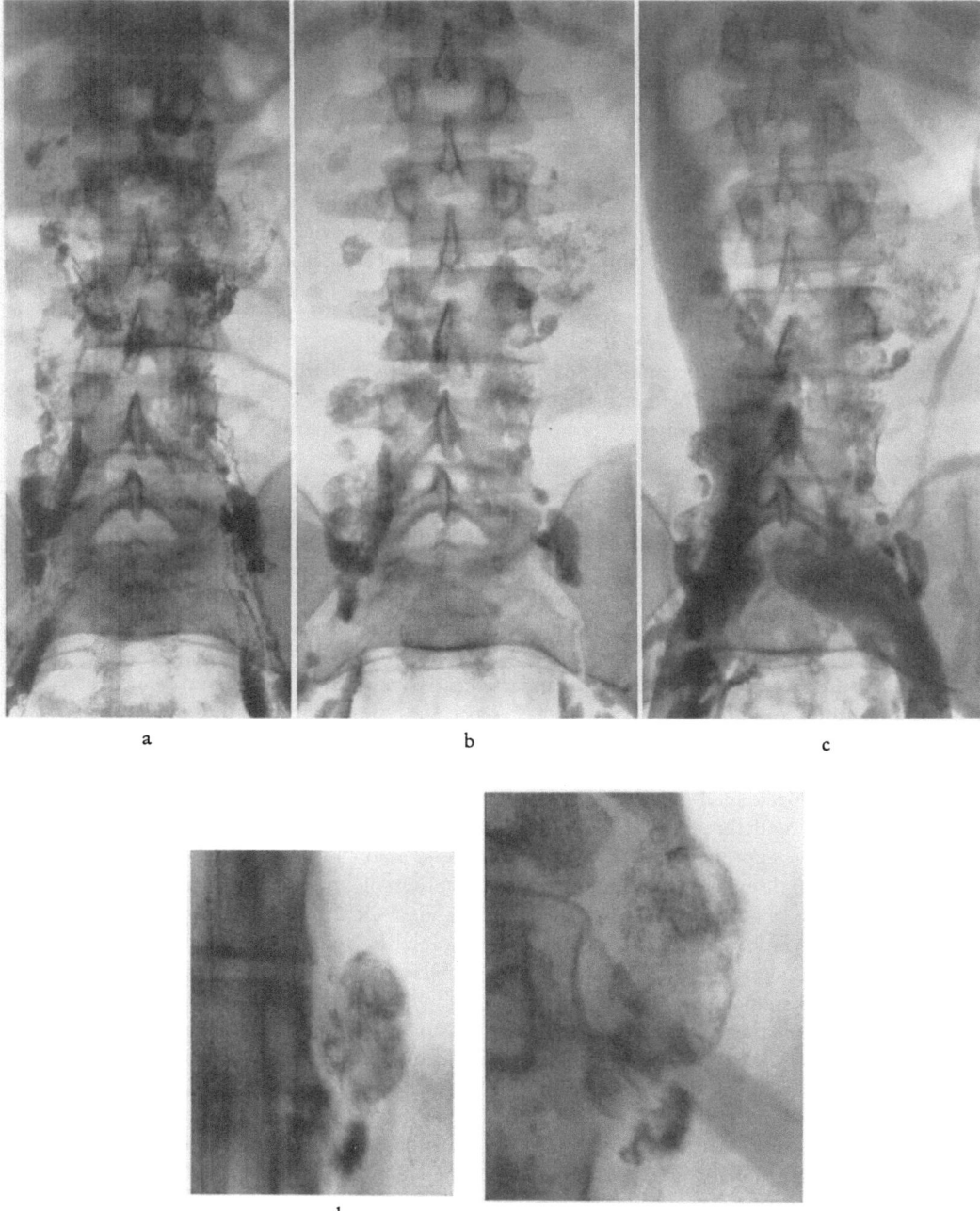

Fig. 27. Lymphoblastic Lymphosarcoma. a Lymphangiogram—Vessel displacement and early filling nodes. b Clearly demarcated filling defects in many nodes—underfilling left aortic region. c Deviation of the inferior vena cava and left ureter by extensive non-opacified soft tissue mass. d Tomograph—Opacified left paravertebral node. e Simple magnification left paravertebral node showing marginal preservation and faint homogeneous distribution of contrast material

Comment: Reassessment lymphography has demonstrated extensive clinically occult intra-abdominal and mediastinal disease in a patient with lymphoblastic lymphosarcoma. Following further radiotherapy, marked shrinkage of all of the opacified lymph nodes was seen with return to normal position of the left ureter.

As in Hodgkin's disease, sequential radiography of opacified lymph nodes allows surveillance by repeat radiographs when equivocal changes are present, and may also monitor response to therapy. Two of our patients have shown unilateral obstructive uropathy due to enlarged lymph nodes, and this has been seen to regress following irradiation.

Radiographic Appearances

A spectrum of radiographic appearances ranging from slight coarsening of the storage pattern in nodes of normal size to gross enlargement with irregular dilated intranodal sinusoids separated by confluent small radiolucent filling defects his been present in lymphosarcoma. Minor degrees of stasis in lymph vessels adjacent to or deviated by enlarged nodes has only occasionally been noted in new patients with lymphosarcoma. Severe lymphatic obstruction has occurred in only three patients with advanced previously treated disease. A generalized distribution in all of the opacified nodes of homogeneous architectural abnormality has been the most frequent finding in both initial and reassessment lymphograms. However, confluent irregular filling defects in the centres of the largest sized nodes and smaller lacunar filling defects have occurred in several of our patients.

No differentiation between lymphoblastic and lymphocytic lymphosarcomas has been possible, and there has been no difference in storage patterns of nodular and diffuse histological subtypes. Patients in the leukemic phase have shown similar appearances to those described. Further experience of reassessment lymphography in patients with prolonged survival may confirm a suggestion of an increased frequency of lacunar filling defects and flow abnormalities.

Despite the expected limitation of macroscopic study in comparison with histology, biopsy and autopsy studies confirm the accuracy of lymphography as a method of identifying abnormality within the lymph nodes. Of 20 new patients in whom histology of lymph nodes adjacent to those examined by lymphography is available, only one false negative diagnosis has occurred. Fifteen abnormal lymphograms were found to correspond to lymphosarcomatous involvement, and four normal lymphograms in patients with lymphosarcoma reflected normal lymph nodes. Autopsy study in 12 of 18 patients who died within two years of positive lymphography showed diffuse lymphosarcomatous infiltration in all but one patient who died of intercurrent infection following extensive chemotherapy. Thus, it appears that lymphography is a reliable practical method of identifying lymphosarcomatous nodes. In comparison with Hodgkin's disease, a much more homogeneous abnormality within individual lymph nodes is apparent, and this has commonly affected all of the demonstrated lymph nodes.

Clinical Staging

The influence of lymphographic studies in 62 new patients on clinical staging by the usual method (Table 2) is shown in Table 15. In 20 of 51 patients, abnormal lymph nodes have been demonstrated which were not detected on physical examination with subsequent advance in the pre-management stage. As in Hodgkin's disease, patients with more advanced disease than Stage II, have been less frequently examined. As anticipated, the majority of such lymphograms are grossly abnormal.

Further analysis of Stage I and II patients presenting with lymphosarcoma in various sites is demonstrated in Table 16. Of 24 patients presenting with enlarged cervical or axillary nodes, 13 were found to have clinically occult abdominal disease with alteration to Stage III. In 11 such patients, no lymphographic abnormality was detected. Only five of fourteen patients presenting in one groin showed evidence of additional disease extending to the aortic lymph nodes and in the remaining nine, the abnormality was localized to the area of clinical detection. Other lympho-reticular sites include the tonsil, mediastinal nodes and spleen. In one of two patients diagnosed following tonsillectomy, generalized adenopathy was found.

Table 15. *Lymphography in lymphosarcoma. Influence of lymphography in staging of 62 new patients*

Clinical stage	No. of patients	Abnormal	Normal and equivocal	Advanced to Stage II	Advanced to Stage III
I	37	20	17	7	8
II	14	7	7	0	5
III and IV Lympho-reticular	11	10	1	Not advanced	
Total	62	37	25	7	13

Table 16. *Lymphography in lymphosarcoma. Influence of lymphography on clinical stages I and II by presenting site*

Presenting site	No. of patients	Altered to Stage II	Altered to Stage III	No alter-ation
Neck	19	0	11	8
Axilla	5	0	2	3
Groin	14	5	0	9
Other lympho-reticular sites	4	0	1	3
Extra-nodal	9	2	0	7
Total	51	7	14	30

Nine patients in whom lymphosarcoma was discovered in extra-nodal tissues, mostly in the alimentary tract at laparotomy, have been examined. In only two such patients, has additional lymph node abnormality in several groups of nodes on the same side of the diaphragm been detected. The majority have shown normal lower extremity lymphograms.

Patterns of involvement in 46 new patients with lymphosarcoma are depicted in Tables 17 and 18. The most frequent finding in those with differentiated lympho-sarcoma was clinically localized adenopathy in the anterior or posterior triangles of the neck as a manifestation of generalized lymph node disease.

Of 20 such patients presenting in the neck or axilla, 13 were found to have diffuse distribution of abnormal lymph nodes below the diaphragm. In only one of nine patients with a differentiated lymphosarcoma presenting in the groin was there radiographic evidence of nodal abnormality in opacified periclavicular nodes. The majority of patients with clinically localized undifferentiated lymphosarcomas were found to show no lymphographic evidence of abnormality. Only four of thirteen patients were shown to have generalized disease.

Table 17. *Lymphosarcoma-differentiated. Distribution of disease in 33 patients at time of initial assessment*

Presenting site	No. of patients	Lympho-reticular disease	
		Local	General
Low neck	14	4	10
Peripheral—High neck	3	2	1
Peripheral—Axilla	3	1	2
Peripheral—Groin	9	8	1
Other lympho-reticular sites	2	1	1
Extra-nodal	2	2	0
Total	33	18	15

Table 18. *Lymphosarcoma-undifferentiated. Distribution of disease in 13 patients at time of initial assessment*

Presenting site	No. of patients	Lympho-reticular disease	
		Local	General
Low neck	1	1	0
Peripheral—High neck	2	0	2
Peripheral—Axilla	1	1	0
Peripheral—Groin	4	3	1
Other lympho-reticular sites	2	1	1
Extra-nodal	3	3	0
Total	13	9	4

Thus, although the number of patients examined in each of the histological subtypes has not yet proved sufficient for significant appraisal, further analysis in this respect may be of value in gauging patterns of distribution in the early stages of lymphosarcoma.

Mycosis Fungoides

A 67 year old man suffered from recurrent itchy red macular lesions on the back, buttocks, and legs for two years. In the month prior to presentation, exacerbation of his skin condition occurred with spread to other areas. Physical examination revealed a 1 cm lymph node on the right side of the neck below the angle of the mandible. Similar palpable nodes were present in both axillae and in both groins. Biopsy of one of the skin lesions was interpreted as Mycosis Fungoides. Lymphography showed enlargement of superficial and deep inguinal nodes (Fig. 28), with wide sinusoids and homogeneously distributed 2 mm filling defects throughout the entire nodes. The iliac and aortic lymph nodes showed normal appearances.

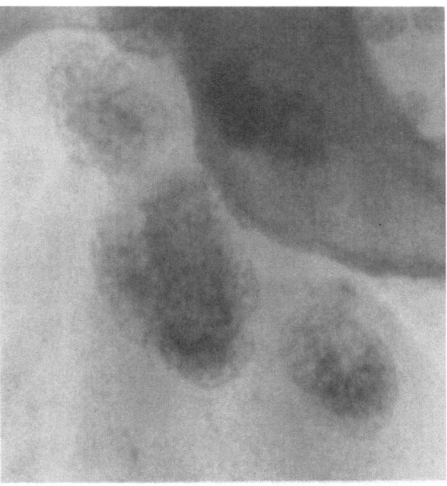

Fig. 28. Mycosis Fungoides—Preservation of marginal sinus and sinusoids with homogeneous distribution of contrast material

Comment: Two identical lymphographic patterns have been seen in elderly patients with Mycosis Fungoides. Biopsy of one of these opacified inguinal lymph nodes showed diffuse cellular proliferation interpreted as lymphoblastic lymphosarcoma. The absence of architectural abnormality in the iliac and aortic nodes suggests that this lymphoblastic lymphosarcoma may be confined to those nodes regional to the cutaneous lesions.

Conclusion

Radiographic appearances following lymphography are of value in detecting lymphosarcoma in clinically occult areas. Lymphographic studies appear to be of similar value to those in Hodgkin's disease in pre-management staging of new patients and in the detection of patterns of involvement of lympho-reticular structures. In patients with clinical breakdown at an interval following previous therapy, lymphographic study may prove a useful addition to subsequent management.

Reticulum Cell Sarcoma

A smaller proportion of patients with reticulum cell sarcoma have presented with enlarged peripheral lymph nodes, and first discovery of this condition outwith lympho-reticular structures has been common. In the former, clinical staging is similar to Hodgkin's disease. No widely accepted system of staging in extranodal presentations is yet available. However, Stages I, II, and III depending on the extent of lymph node involvement in the regional drainage of the affected organ, with Stage IV for multiple extra-nodal sites or widespread systemic disease, is a practical method of documenting lymphographic findings.

Bilateral lower extremity lymphography is now frequently performed prior to clinical staging of both localized lympho-reticular and extra-nodal presentations. Results of lymphograms in each histological type of reticulum cell sarcoma (Table 19) are discussed in terms of radiographic appearances, clinical staging, and patterns of disease.

Table 19. *Lymphography in reticulum cell sarcoma*

Subtypes of reticulum cell sarcoma	No. of patients	No. of lymphograms			Abnormal	Normal	Equivocal
		Initial	Reassessment	Repeat			
Stem cell	5	5	0	0	1	3	1
Histiocytic	31	29	2	1	18	9	5
Unclassified	41	27	14	0	24	16	1
Total	77	61	16	1	43	28	7

Lymphographic Appearances

Case 1: A 74 year-old lady in previous good health complained of a painless swelling in the left groin of one month's duration. On physical examination, a 1 cm discrète lymph node was palpable below the left inguinal ligament. Biopsy showed this node to be infiltrated with a diffuse histiocytic malignant lymphoma. During introduction of the lymphographic contrast medium (Fig. 29 a), early filling of dilated branching sinusoids is demonstrated without evidence of lymphatic obstruction. Later, pooling of the oily medium in numerous dilated sinusoids throughout enlarged lymph nodes is demonstrated in the external iliac region above which are lymph nodes of normal size and contrast pattern (Fig. 29 b).

At 24 hours (Fig. 29 c), dilated saccular contrast-filled sinusoids throughout enlarged irregularly shaped nodes are seen. No circumscribed filling defects are present in the areas of maximal contrast filling, and fine branching linear radiolucencies separate the dilated sinusoids. A normal homogeneous storage pattern was demonstrated in the remaining iliac and aortic nodes.

Comment: Dilated saccular sinusoids have channelled the ultra-fluid Lipiodol into the node parenchyma without filling of the marginal sinuses in an "early" case of diffuse histiocytic malignant lymphoma. Regular sinusoidal arrangement without evidence of a marked disturbance in the remaining elements of the node parenchyma are seen. The clinical stage is unaltered by this investigation, but radiotherapy fields may be more accurately applied and the response to radiation monitored by sequential films.

Case 2: A woman, aged 43 years, who complained of left chest discomfort was found to have a chylous effusion in the left pleural cavity. No enlarged peripheral lymph nodes or abnormal findings on examination of the abdomen were detected. Lymphography (Fig. 30 a) shows early filling of intranodal sinusoids in both iliac regions and stellate branching sinusoids in the left aortic region. The thoracic duct of normal calibre is outlined in the lower dorsal region. At 24 hours (Fig. 30 b), enlarged lymph nodes in both aortic regions with multiple small filling defects in the storage pattern are present. Contrast material in afferent and marginal vessels of normal calibre is seen. Above the well filled lymph nodes, numerous dilated branching sinusoids of irregular calibre within partially filled lymph nodes are demonstrated, more marked on the left side. Excretion urography confirms, by displacement of the left renal collecting system and ureter, a bulky soft tissue mass adjacent to the partly filled nodes. Mediastinal lymph nodes of smaller size with coarsening of the sinusoidal storage pattern and small irregular filling defects in the node parenchyma (Fig. 30 c) are visualized, consistent with lymphomatous infiltration. At mediastinoscopy, a lymph node was removed and histology revealed diffuse histiocytic reticulum cell sarcoma. Following radiotherapy to the abdomen and mediastinum, regression of the chylothorax occurred and this patient remains in good health one year later.

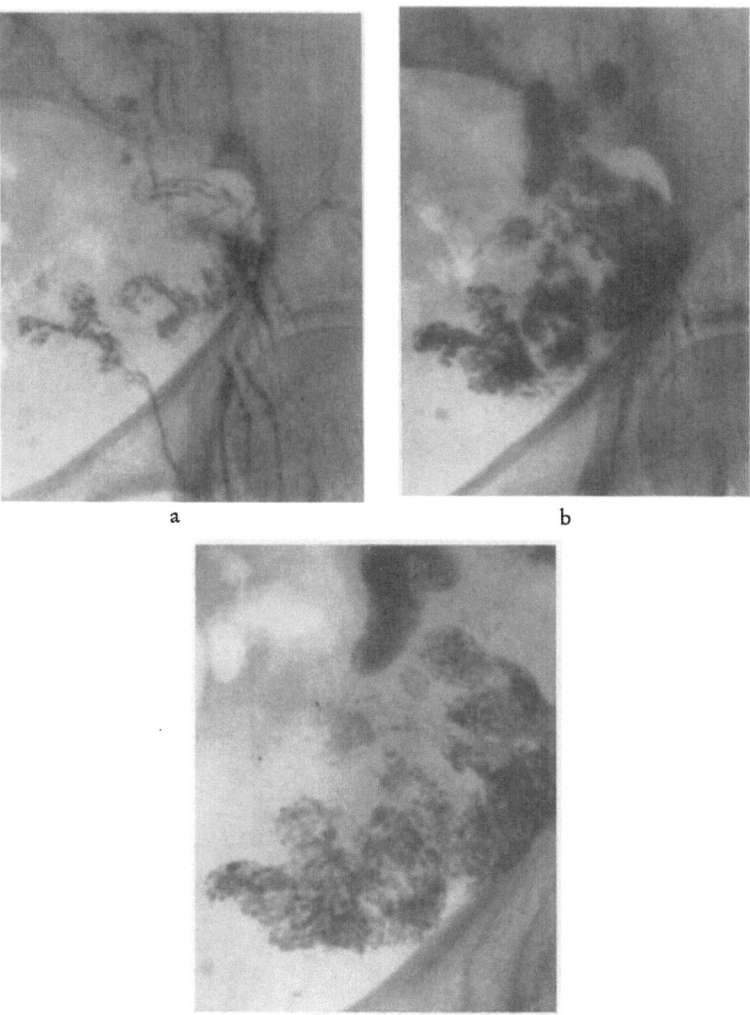

a   b

c

Fig. 29. Diffuse histiocytic malignant lymphoma. a Lymphangiogram—Early filling intranodal sinusoids. b Post-injection—Lack of filled marginal sinus—dilated contrast filled sinusoids in cortex of nodes. c At 24 hours, saccular dilated contrast filled spaces in cortex of nodes

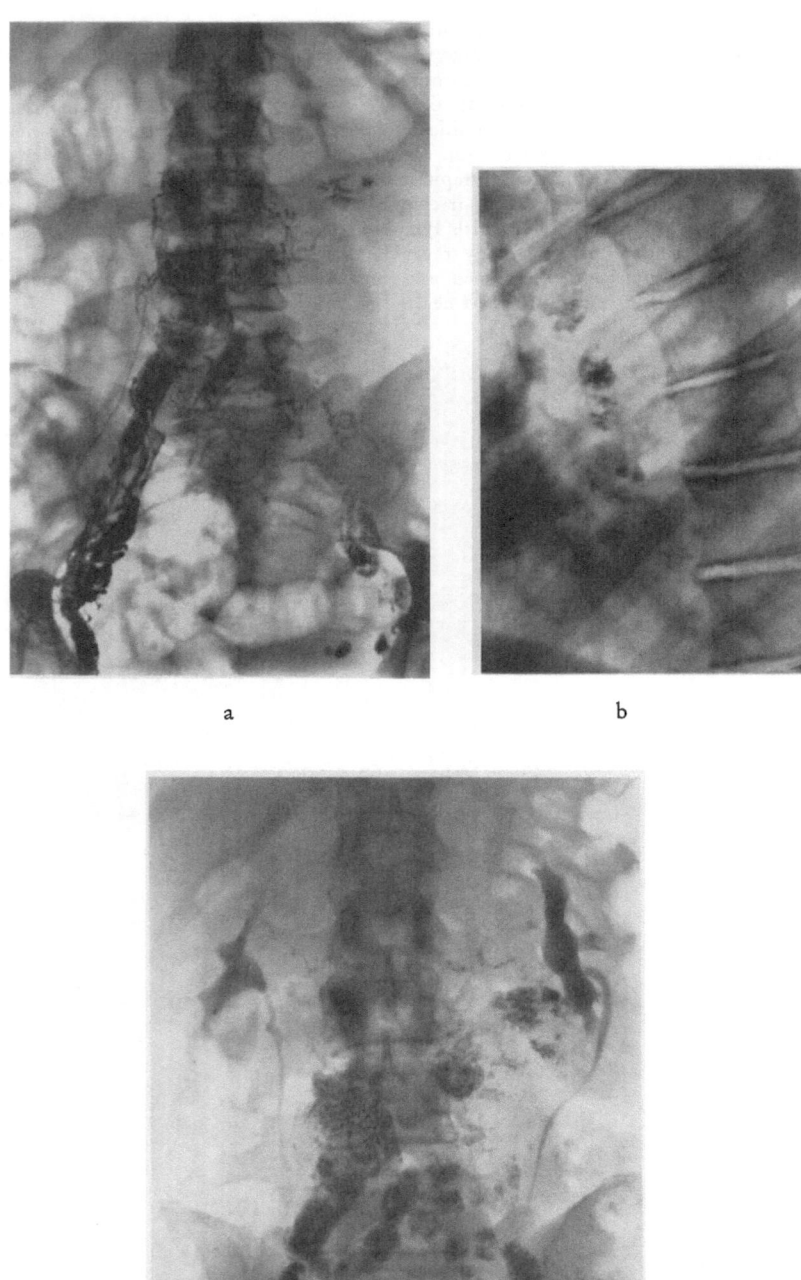

a

b

c

Fig. 30. Reticulum cell sarcoma. a Lymphangiogram—Early filling nodes and stellate sinusoids. b Opaque mediastinal nodes. c Excretion urogram—Deviation of left collecting system and ureter, adjacent to partially opacified lymphoma

Comment: Lymphography, in addition to indicating a suitable area for diagnostic lymph node biopsy, indicates advanced lympho-reticular disease compatible with diversion of lymph drainage at thoraco-abdominal level giving chylothorax. This patient may be regarded as having primary occult lympho-reticular disease with an extra-nodal presentation.

Case 3: An elderly lady complained of increasing backache with radiation down the anterior surface of both legs of three months' duration. Radiographs of the lumbar spine showed lytic destruction with partial collapse of the second lumbar vertebral body suggesting metastasis. Percutaneous biopsy of the paravertebral soft tissue adjacent to L-2 revealed malignant lymphoma of stem cell type. Lymphography (Fig. 31 a) demonstrated an enlarged lymph node adjacent to the skeletal lesion. Spot magnification projection (Fig. 31 b) shows preservation of the marginal sinus and irregularly dilated branching sinusoids throughout the node parenchyma. Confluent radiolucency is noted in the upper pole of the node. Similar changes are noted in the normal sized adjacent nodes, and stasis of contrast material in vessels adjacent to normal sized iliac nodes were noted on the left side. Small nodes of similar pattern were outlined in the mediastinum and periclavicular region.

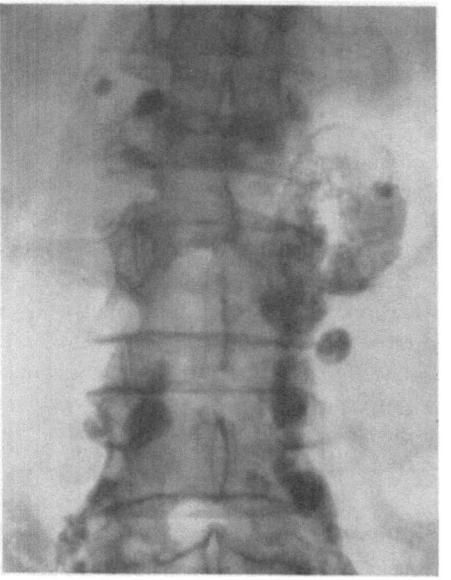 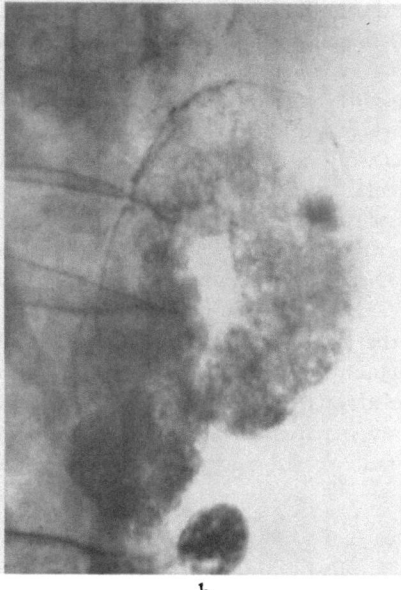

a   b

Fig. 31. Reticulum cell sarcoma. a Lytic destruction of L-2 with loss of height and adjacent opacified large node. b Spot film with simple magnification—Diffuse distribution of granular contrast material in parenchym—filled marginal sinus

Comment: A true extra-nodal presentation in which lymphography has demonstrated extensive lympho-reticular abnormality in retroperitoneal and mediastinal nodes. This patient provides a good example of the contribution of lymphography to understanding the patterns of involvement of skeletal and lymphatic structures by reticulum cell sarcoma. Skeletal abnormalities adjacent to advanced lymphomatous infiltration of lymph nodes has also been demonstrated in three of our patients with Hodgkin's disease. Such patterns of involvement may influence future concepts of clinical staging and indicate the need for a comprehensive system of assessment of both lympho-reticular and extra-nodal presentations.

Radiographic Appearances

The spectrum of storage patterns in reticulum cell sarcoma has varied from no detectable radiographic abnormality to the commonly recognized appearances of enlarged nodes with early filling dilated branching sinusoids throughout the parenchyma. The most commonly recognized abnormality in new patients has been node enlargement with coarsening of the normal granular storage pattern. In such "early" involvement, minor alterations in the flow of contrast medium, such as stasis, have been present in several examinations, and indicate a need for surveillance in those patients in whom lymph node changes are regarded as equivocal. Early filling of affected nodes during introduction of the contrast medium has been commonly observed but has not proven useful evidence of abnormality. Gross lymphatic obstruction has been present in four patients, two of whom had unilateral leg lymphoedema.

Preservation of regular sinusoidal arrangement has been noted by many observers both in large and small nodes, although marked variability in calibre of these branching sinusoids is seen. In grossly enlarged lymph nodes, defects of the storage pattern may be due to failure of contrast material to reach the more central areas. Conversely filling of a small number of irregular, branching 1 to 2 mm calibre intranodal sinusoids may be the sole evidence of advanced disease. In reassessment lymphograms in which prolonged disease and previous therapy have been given, irregular radiolucent filling defects of variable size due to partial or total replacement of lymphoreticular parenchyma have indicated more gross architectural disturbance. Storage patterns in the small number of patients with stem cell lymphomas, showed no difference from the larger numbers with histiocytic and unclassified reticulum cell sarcomas.

Distribution of the extent of involvement within the lymph node groups visualized may give further important diagnostic information. Generalized abnormality in all of the lymph nodes visualized has been the most frequent finding in patients with reticulum cell sarcomas, indicating diffuse disease. Opacification of periclavicular or intrathoracic nodes showing similar storage patterns to aortic nodes has occurred in seven patients. Such findings prior to histological diagnosis are of particular importance in allowing selection of the most accessible site for biopsy.

Accuracy

Surgical biopsy and histological diagnosis has frequently preceded lymphography, and some useful appraisal of the latter may be made from those patients in whom the site of biopsy is adjacent to opacified lymph nodes. Biopsy of nodes previously opacified by lymphography gives direct comparison and, although second biopsies are rarely necessary in clinical practice, five such instances have occurred in this series. Of 11 lymphograms showing abnormal architecture in enlarged nodes, all have been diagnosed histologically as reticulum cell sarcoma in nodes from adjacent sites. In one patient in whom lymphographic appearances were regarded as equivocal, diffuse reticulum cell sarcoma was found on biopsy of the opacified nodes. Of four patients in whom lymphadenograms showed normal appearances, two on biopsy were found to have diffuse reticulum cell sarcoma in the normal sized lymph nodes under consideration. Thus, although lymphography may define architectural abnormalities corresponding to diffuse reticulum cell sarcoma in both superficial and clinically occult sites, false negative diagnoses are not infrequent in early infiltration. In two of our patients in whom lymphograms had been regarded as normal, autopsy within one year revealed generalized diffuse lymphomatous infiltration in all of the moderately enlarged iliac and aortic nodes.

Nine of eleven patients with positive lymphograms died within one year, and in one instance, autopsy allowed direct confirmation of diffuse reticulum cell sarcoma in all of the nodes opacified by the lymphogram. In "early" lymph node involvement lymphograms may be negative, but as the disease advanced, characteristic diffuse changes become apparent.

Clinical Staging

In 61 new patients, lymphography has been used in determining the clinical stage (Table 20). As in Hodgkin's disease, in the context of clinical staging equivocal lymphograms are classified as negative, although surveillance by repeat radiographs

Table 20. *Lymphography in reticulum cell sarcoma. Influence of lymphography in staging of 61 new patients*

Clinical stage		No. of patients	Abnormal	Normal and equivocal	Altered to	
					Stage II	Stage III
Lympho-reticular	I	13	7	6	3	4
	II	9	2	7	0	1
	III and IV	13	11	2	0	0
Extra-nodal	I	18	8	10	7	1
	II	2	1	1	0	1
	III and IV	6	5	1	0	0
Total		61	34	27	10	7

to detect alteration in the position or storage patterns of suspicious lymph nodes is routinely advised. In eight of 22 patients with lympho-reticular disease presenting in clinical Stages I or II, demonstration of additional disease had advanced the stage. It should be noted that one of the abnormal lymphograms in a Stage II patient caused no alteration as palpable abnormal nodes were present in both groins. It is of particular significance that in four of thirteen patients in whom clinical examination had revealed only one or more adjacent groups of enlarged nodes, lymph node abnormality on the opposite side of the diaphragm was demonstrated by lymphography. Thus, in reticulum cell sarcoma presenting as localized adenopathy, further experience of lymphography in clinical staging may prove of similar value to that in Hodgkin's disease.

Demonstration of lympho-reticular abnormality in patients in whom reticulum cell sarcoma is discovered in other tissues has occurred in 14 of 26 patients. Eighteen of our patients were considered to be in extra-nodal Stage I because of presentation outwith the lymph system, and no evidence either clinical or at laparotomy, of disease in lymph nodes other than those immediately adjacent to the lesion was demonstrated. In seven instances, lymphography revealed more widespread abnormal lymph nodes on the same side of the diaphragm. One patient was found to have abnormal lymph nodes on the opposite side of the diaphragm with alteration to Stage III. Thus, following surgical appraisal at laparotomy of intra-abdominal nodes, lymphography may prove a useful supplement prior to consideration of further management. In six patients, abnormal lymphography contributed no further useful information, as extensive disease had already been diagnosed on examination of the presenting lesion.

Patterns of Disease

Alterations of staging in patients presenting with reticulum cell sarcoma in different sites (Table 21) allows appraisal of distribution of the disease process. It has been noted that with apparently localized abnormal neck or axillary lymph nodes,

Table 21. *Lymphography in reticulum cell sarcoma. Alteration of clinical stages I and II according to presenting site*

Presenting site		No. of patients	Lympho-graphy positive	Altered to		Not altered
				Stage II	Stage III	
Neck		10	3	0	3	7
Axilla		3	2	0	2	1
Groin		5	5	3	0	2
Other lympho-reticular sites		4	0	0	0	4
Extra-nodal	Alimentary tract	11	3	3	0	8
	Other	9	6	4	2	3
Total		42	19	10	7	25

abnormal aortic and/or iliac nodes may be found. Disease localized to inguinal and iliac nodes, following both clinical and lymphographic study, was revealed in two instances, while in a further three patients, inguinal adenopathy directed attention to the lymph node abnormalities involving all of the iliac and aortes nodes visualized. In four patients presenting with tonsillar or mediastinal disease, recorded as "other lympho-reticular sites", no evidence of generalized lymphoma was demonstrated.

Of 11 patients discovered at laparotomy to have a primary reticulum cell sarcoma involving the alimentary tract or mesentery, three were shown to have abnormal aortic lymph node architecture. Thus, the majority of intra-abdominal extra-nodal reticulum cell sarcomas have been considered localized. Other extra-nodal presentations occurred in the nasal cavity, skin, bone, kidneys, testes, muscle, and dura of the spinal cord, and of these, three were found to show no lymphographic evidence of abnormality.

Surveillance and Response to Therapy

As abnormal cellularity within lymph nodes showing normal size and architecture on the lymphadenogram will not be detected, follow-up studies are of considerable value in clinical management. Repeat radiographs at three months' intervals may prove a valuable addition, and should insufficient contrast material remain to permit adequate assessment of the lymph nodes, a "second-look" lymphogram [14] is performed.

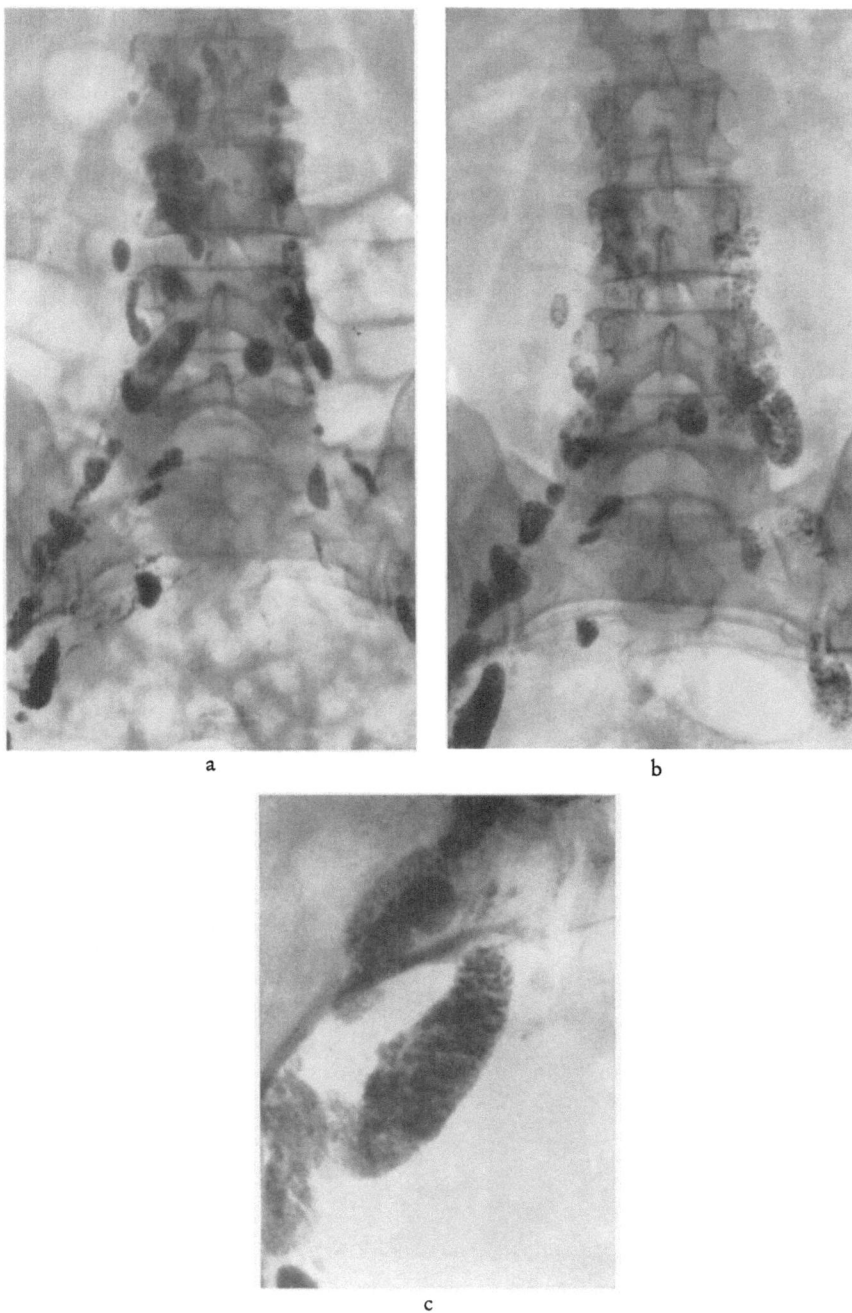

Fig. 32. Histiocytic malignant lymphoma. a Suspicious lymphadenogram—larger nodes right aortic region and contrast residues in iliac vessels at 24 hours. b Enlarged lymph nodes with coarse granular linear sinusoidal pattern in all of the aortic and iliac nodes. c Spot magnification showing coarse texture—right iliac nodes

Case Report: A 71 year-old woman was found on physical examination to have several discrete enlarged lymph nodes in the left anterior and posterior triangles of the neck. Biopsy disclosed a lymph node diffusely infiltrated with a histiocytic malignant lymphoma. The lymphogram (Fig. 32 a) showed residual contrast medium in vessels in the right common iliac region and lymph nodes of irregular size in the right aortic chains. The remaining nodes were within normal limits in appearance. The findings were regarded as suspicious of abnormality and repeat radiography in one month advised. Following local radiotherapy to the neck, the patient was discharged in good health until one year later when slight swelling in the right parotid gland was noted. As insufficient contrast material was present in the abdominal lymph nodes for satisfactory review radiographs, a "second-look" lymphogram (Fig. 32 b and c) was performed, and showed a marked generalized alteration in nodal architecture consistent with diffuse reticulum cell sarcoma.

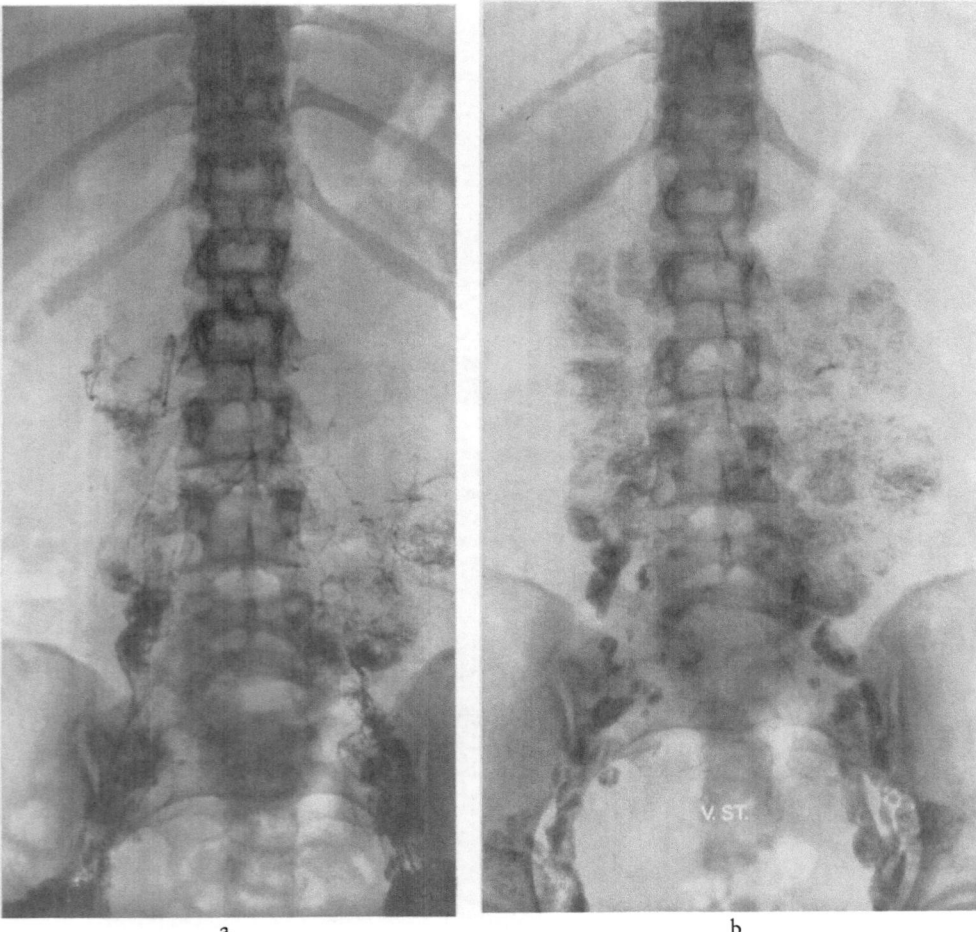

a   b

Fig. 33. Diffuse histiocytic malignant lymphoma. a Lymphangiogram—Early filling in large nodes and displaced lymph trunks. b Lymphadenogram—Huge aortic nodes with homogeneously distributed fine contrast pattern. c Review two weeks after radiotherapy showing shrinkage. d Review five months after therapy showing marked decrease in the size indicating satisfactory response

Comment: Stasis of contrast medium and irregular node enlargement in the right peri-aortic region on the initial lymphogram is good evidence of "early" lymphomatous infiltration. Node enlargement and architectural alteration demonstrated by repeat examination one year later shows the rate of progression of the disease process.

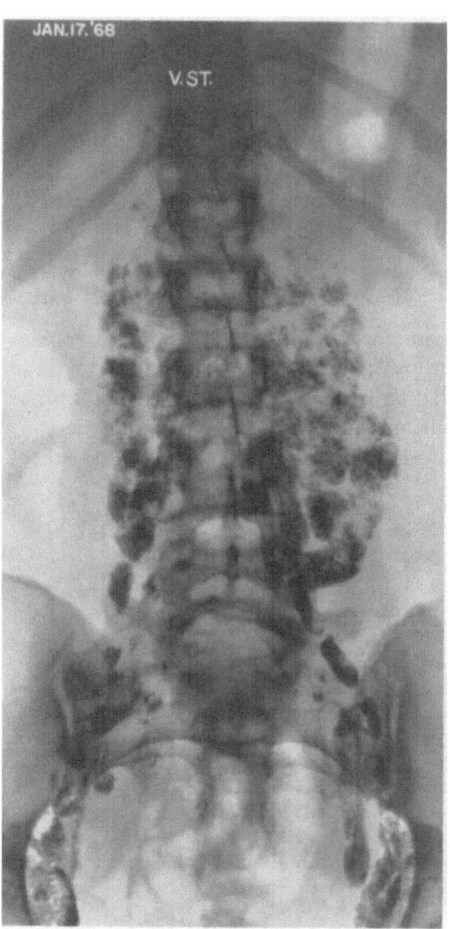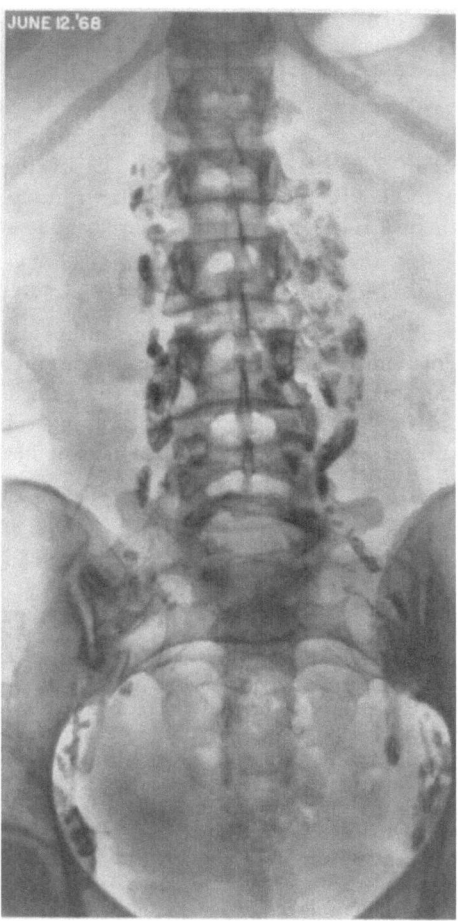

c   d

Response to Therapy

The status of lymph nodes following radiotherapy or chemotherapy may be usefully gauged by comparison of node size and architecture on repeat radiographs with the original lymphogram. Such monitoring may give additional accuracy in the timing of changes in therapeutic management.

Case Report: Having complained frequently of tiredness for several months, a female, aged 26 years, consulted her doctor because of a palpable swelling below the right side of the mandible. Biopsy revealed a diffuse histiocytic malignant lymphoma. Physical examination disclosed markedly enlarged lymph nodes on the right side of the neck forming a mass 6×7 cms in diameter. Several smaller nodes were palpable in the neck below this level.

Axillae were normal, but on palpation of the abdomen, an irregular nodular mass was felt in the left side of the abdomen. The liver edge was 3 cms below the costal margin, and the spleen palpable on deep inspiration.

Lymphography (Fig. 33 a) shows displacement of fine lymph vessels and early filling sinusoids within enlarged nodes in the aortic regions.

At 24 hours (Fig. 33 b), grossly enlarged lymph nodes are visualized showing areas of filling of marginal sinuses and numerous irregular sized radial sinusoids with confluent filling defects depicting gross architectural abnormality. At a lower level, a coarse granular pattern is noted in smaller lymph nodes.

Comment: Response to radiation is shown by repeat radiographs at two weeks (Fig. 33 c) and at five months (Fig. 33 d) by marked shrinkage of the intra-abdominal nodes. The rapid decrease in size of the grossly enlarged aortic nodes following radiotherapy might be consistent with a more favourable outcome than in patients in whom little change in the abnormal node architecture is seen after treatment.

Conclusion

Bilateral lower extremity lymphography in patients with histologically proven reticulum cell sarcoma has been a useful method of appraisal of the status of iliac and aortic lymph nodes, with the occasional bonus of visualization of mediastinal and periclavicular nodes. In evolving suitable methods of clinical staging, demonstration of patterns of involvement of both lympho-reticular and extra-nodal structures, is a useful addition.

"Lymphoma-Like" Conditions

"Burkitt-Type" Lymphoma

Case Report[1]: A boy, aged 5¹/₂ years, was found on physical examination to have an extensive soft tissue mass in the left side of the abdomen and a small discrete 1¹/₂ cm swelling on deep palpation in the left retroclavicular area. Surgical biopsy of the latter revealed a lymph node in which the normal architecture was replaced by an undifferentiated type of lymphocytic lymphoma. Cellular features including the non-specific "starry-sky" appearance of isolated phagocytic histiocytes were considered suggestive of "Burkitt lymphoma". Lymphography showed normal appearances of the iliac and aortic lymph nodes. However, lymph nodes of unusual appearance were opacified in the upper mediastinum and at the root of the neck on both sides, adjacent to an upper mediastinal soft tissue mass. Lacunar submarginal filling defects within a coarse granular storage pattern were present in irregular shaped lymph nodes (Fig. 34).

Comment: Although the significance of these findings is unknown, further experience of similar cases may be of importance in documenting the natural history of such subtypes of lymphoma.

Skin Lesions

In a patient with diffuse generalized *Kaposi's sarcoma*, lymphography (Fig. 35) showed an increase in size and granularity of axillary lymph nodes. At autopsy within one month, the histological picture was similar to a well differentiated lymphocytic lymphosarcoma.

Two cases of *Mycosis Fungoides* have been described with the lymphosarcomas.

---

[1] This case has been fully reported in the J. Canad. Ass. Radiol. **19**, 121—125 (1968).

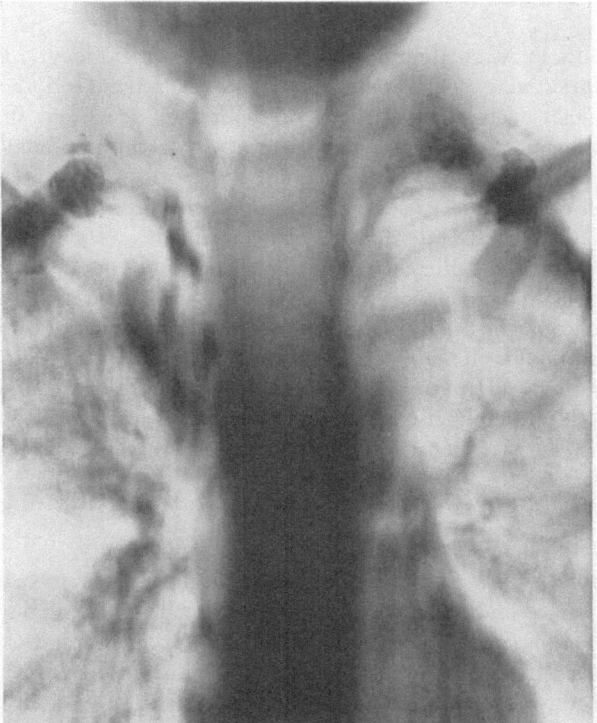

Fig. 34. "Burkitt-Type" Lymphoma. Tomograph showing opacified nodes in both periclavicular groups and upper mediastinum. Tracheal deviation to the right by a soft tissue mass is noted. Irregular contrast filling and submarginal radiolucent areas in several nodes

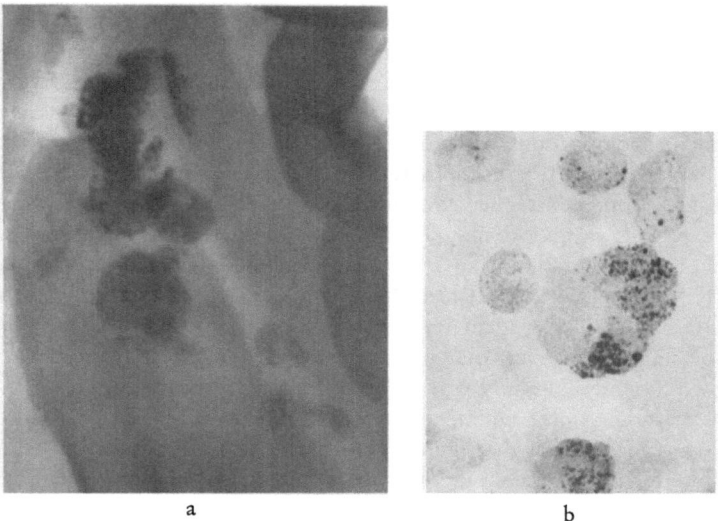

a   b

Fig. 35. Lymphography in Kaposi's sarcoma. a Axillary node with coarse granular contrast pattern. b Autopsy radiograph showing coarse sinusoidal pattern with filling defects

Reticuloendothelioses

In two patients in whom lymph node biopsy showed histiocytic lymphoma, the histological features were considered to be those of reticuloendothelioses. Diffuse architectural changes were demonstrated in moderately enlarged iliac and aortic nodes. In both patients, a coarse granular pattern with occasional small filling defects was noted in several of the nodes, and similar appearances were present in the left scalene node of one of these patients. At autopsy within one year in one case, the diffuse nature of the lymph node changes was confirmed to be similar to the original biopsy, and in view of the clinical course, lymphographic findings and histology, a final diagnosis of malignant histiocytosis ensued. Second biopsy from the neck in our surviving patient confirms the diffuse nature of the changes shown by lymphography in the iliac and aortic lymph nodes.

Occasional serious difficulties are encountered in histological interpretation of lymph node biopsies. Lymphographic studies in such patients may be useful indicators of optimal sites for further biopsies and of patterns of progression in lympho-reticular structures.

Discussion

As recent more widely accepted classifications of malignant lymphomas stress predominant cell types and morphological cell patterns within lymph nodes, the main contribution of lymphography lies in definition of the presence and extent of disease following diagnosis by lymph node biopsy. The value of macroscopic changes in lymphatic structures depicted by ultra-fluid Lipiodol is to provide information complementary to the histological diagnosis by allowing precise examination of whole chains of lymph nodes in clinically occult regions. In each of the malignant lymphomas, such in vivo examination has added a further dimension to appraisal of their natural history.

The increased precision of clinical staging resulting from lymphography, and the accuracy of detection of lymphomatous infiltration in opacified nodes has been similar to experience in other centres [1, 11, 24]. A small number of false negative examinations reflect the expected limitation of an indirect and macroscopic method of investigation in comparison with histological study. Although much useful information may be gained by examination of all of the nodes visualized following both lower and upper extremity lymphography, extensive disease in lymph nodes outwith the regions displayed may remain undetected by present methods. Nevertheless, it is of particular significance that in Hodgkin's disease, lymphosarcoma, and reticulum cell sarcoma, 39 of 114, 13 of 24, and 5 of 13 new patients presenting in the neck or axilla had clinically silent lymph node involvement below the diaphragm. It has yet to be shown, however, that treatment by current methods of occult involvement disclosed by lymphography will influence long term survival.

Analysis of radiographic findings following lymphography and mediastinal tomography supports the concept that the nodular sclerosing form appears to be a regional expression of Hodgkin's disease in the mediastinum. By contrast, Hodgkin's disease with lymphocyte predominance has, in new patients, more frequently involved lymph nodes in superficial groups and retroperitoneal regions. Both of the above patterns of distribution may be seen in Hodgkin's disease of mixed cellularity type. Such radiographic findings in conjunction with clinical, surgical and autopsy studies have enabled description of the mediastinal and retroperitoneal patterns of progression [16, 21] with particular inplications for future concepts of clinical staging and therapy. These distributions may reflect immunologic functions [8] resulting in regional differences in susceptibility to induction of the neoplastic process. It is to be anticipated that with further experience, lymphography will contribute to the identification of distinctive patterns of involvement in other lymphomas.

The lymphographic diagnosis of primary malignant lymphatic disease is still in its infancy. Many pertinent facts have already been elucidated based on experimental or clinical investigations, and on histological findings. With further experience, progressive improvement of the diagnostic possibilities ought to be achieved.

References

[1] ABRAMS, H. L., M. TAKAHASHI, and D. F. ADAMS: Usefullness and accuracy of lymphangiography in lymphoma. Cancer Chemotherapy Reports 52, 157 (1968).

[2] BAUM, S., K. M. BRON, L. WEXLER, and H. L. ABRAMS: Lymphangiography, cavography, and urography: Comparitive accuracy in the diagnosis of pelvic and abdominal metastases. Radiology 81, 207 (1963).

[3] DOLAN, P. A.: Lymphography. Brit. J. Radiol. 37, 405 (1964).

[4] DORFMAN, R. F.: Childhood lymphosarcoma in St. Louis, Missouri. Clinically and histologically resembling Burkitt's tumor. Cancer 18, 418 (1965).

[5] EASSON, E. C.: Long-term results of radial radiotherapy in Hodgkin's disease. Cancer Res. 26, Part I, 1244 (1966).

[6] —, and M. H. RUSSELL: The cure of Hodgkin's disease. Brit. med. J. 1963 I, 1704.

[7] FUCHS, W. A.: Lymphographic pattern of Hodgkin's disease, p. 166. Progress in lymphology. Stuttgart: Georg Thieme 1967.

[8] GOOD, R. A., and J. FINSTAD: The association of lymphoid malignancy and immunologic function. Proceedings of the International Conference on Leukemia—Lymphoma. C. J. D. ZARAFONETS. Philadelphia: Lea and Febiger 175, 1968.

[9] JACKSON, H., and F. PARKER: Hodgkin's disease. II Pathology. New Engl. J. Med. 231, 35 (1964).

[10] KOEHLER, P. R., and R. B. SALMON: Lymphographic patterns in lymphoma, with emphasis on the atypical forms. Radiology 87, 623 (1966).

[11] LEE, B. J.: Correlation between lymphangiography and clinical status of patients with lymphoma. Cancer Chemotherapy Reports 52, 205 (1968).

[12] LUKES, R. J., and J. J. BUTLER: The pathology and nomenclature of Hodgkin's disease. Cancer Res. 26, 1063 (1966).

[13] — —, and E. B. HICKS: Natural history of Hodgkin's disease as related to its pathologic picture. Cancer 19, 317 (1966).

[14] PEREZ-TAMAYO, R., J. R. THORNBURY, and R. J. ATKINSON: "Second-Look" lymphography. Amer. J. Roentgenol. 90, 1078 (1963).

[15] PETERS, M. V.: A study of survivals in Hodgkin's disease treated radiologically. Amer. J. Roentgenol. 58, 299 (1950).

[16] — Gordon Richards Memorial Lecture. Presented at The 31st Annual Meeting of the Canadian Association of Radiologists, Quebec City, March 1968.

[17] —, R. E. ALISON, and R. S. BUSH: Natural history of Hodgkin's disease as related to staging. Cancer 19, 308 (1966).

[18] —, R. HASSELBACK, and T. C. BROWN: The natural history of the lymphomas related to the clinical classification. Proceedings of the International Conference on Leukemia—Lymphoma. C. J. D. ZARAFONETS. Philadelphia: Lea and Febiger, 357, 1968.

[19] RAPPAPORT, H.: Tumors of the hematopoetic system. Armed Forces Institute of Pathology, Washington, D. C., 1966.

[20] ROSENBERG, S. A.: Report of the committee on the staging of Hodgkin's disease. Cancer Res. **26**, Part I, 1310 (1966).
[21] — Contribution of lymphangiography to our understanding of lymphoma. Cancer Chemotherapy Reports **52**, 213 (1968).
[22] —, and H. S. KAPLAN: Evidence for an orderly progression in the spread of Hodgkin's disease. Cancer Res. **26**, Part I, 1225 (1966).
[23] SMITHERS, D. W.: Hodgkin's disease. Lancet **1968 II**, 7573, 876.
[24] TAKAHASHI, M., and H. L. ABRAMS: The accuracy of lymphangiographic diagnosis in malignant lymphomas. Radiology **80**, 448 (1967).
[25] VIAMONTE, M., JR., D. ALTMAN, R. PARKS, E. BLUM, M. BEVILACQUA, and L. RECHER: Radiographic-pathologic correlation in the interpretation of lymphangiograms. Radiology **80**, 903 (1963).
[26] WALLACE, S.: Lymphangiographic interpretation. Radiol. Clin. N. Amer. **3**, 467 (1965).
[27] —, L. JACKSON, B. SCHAFFER, J. GOULD, R. GREENING, and A. WEISS: Lymphangiograms: Their diagnostic and therapeutic potential. Radiology **76**, 179 (1961).
[28] WILJASALO, M.: Lymphographic differential diagnosis of neoplastic disease. Helsinki-Helsingfors, 1965.

Supplemental Bibliography

ARVAY, N., J. D. PICARD et M. BABINET: La lymphographie dans la maladie de Hodgkin. Presse méd. **74**, 24 (1966).

BISMUTH, V., S. BERNAGEAU, J. P. DESPREZ-CURELY et R. BOURDON: La place de la lymphographie dans la maladie de Hodgkin. Sem. Hôp. 2311 (1964).

BRICKNER, J. T., C. W. BOYER, and R. H. PERRY: Limited value of lymphangiography in Hodgkin's disease. Radiology **90**, 52 (1968).

BOURDON, R., V. BISMUTH, M. DANA, and P. MASKOVITS: Incidence de la lymphographie sur la classification clinique de la maladie de Hodgkin. N. Rév. franç. Hémat. **47**, 32 (1966).

CHASSARD, J. L., et J. PAPILLON: Lymphographie et maladie de Hodgkin. A propos de 100 observations. J. belge Radiol. **58**, 295 (1965).

COOK, P. L.: The role of lymphography in the diagnosis and management of malignant reticuloses. Brit. J. **1966**, 561.

DANA, M., J. P. DESPREZ-CURELY, V. BISMUTH et R. BOURDON: Radiothérapie des hemopathies malignes. Intérêt de la lymphographie. J. Radiol. Electrol. **47**, 804 (1966).

DESPREZ-CURELY, J. P., V. BISMUTH, and R. BOURDON: Study on the extension of malignant lymphoma. Progress in lymphology. Stuttgart: G. Thieme 1967.

FARREL, W. J.: Lymphangiographic demonstration of lymphovenous communication after radiotherapy in Hodgkin's disease. Radiology **87**, 630 (1966).

FUCHS, W. A., and M. P. HÄRTEL: Die Prognose des Morbus Hodgkin auf Grund der Lymphknotenstruktur im Lymphogramm. Fortschr. Röntgenstr. 553 (1968).

GROS, C., R. KEILING, L. VROUSOS et S. SCHRAUB: Intérêt de la lymphographie dans l'extension de la maladie de Hodgkin et dans l'orientation thérapeutique. Radiol. clin. biol. **35**, 281 (1966).

JING, B. S., and J. P. McGRAW: Lymphangiography in diagnosis and management of malignant lymphomas. Cancer **19**, 565 (1966).

LAMARQUE, J. L., A. PAGES, H. PUJOL, J. F. GINESTIE et C. CAUBES: Anatomie radiologique et valeur sémiologique des images ganglionnaires en lymphographie. J. Radiol. Electrol. **48**, 253 (1967).

LEE, B. J.: Evaluation of the patient with lymphoma by means lymphangiography. Comments on importance and complications. Progress in Lymphology. Stuttgart: G. Thieme 1967.

— Lymphangiography in Hodgkin's disease. Indications and contraindications. Progress in Lymphology. Stuttgart: G. Thieme 1967.

—, J. H. NELSON, and G. SCHWARZ: Evaluation of lymphangiography, inferior venacavography and intravenous pyelography in the clinical staging and management of Hodgkin's disease and lymphosarcoma. New Engl. J. Med. **271**, 327 (1964).

MARCHAL, G., J. BERNHARD, G. ARVAY, G. BILSKI-PASQUIER, J. D. PICARD, G. MATHÉ et G. BRULÉ: La lymphographie dans la maladie de Hodgkin. Etude de 45 cas. N. Rev. Franç. Hémat. 2, 4 (1962).

PICARD, J. D., G. NACCHE, G. BILSKI-PASQUIER, J. DEBRAY et C. DÉBONNIÈRE: Contributions a l'étude clinique et lymphographique de la maladie de Brill-Symmers. Ann. Radiol. (Paris) 9, 685 (1966).

SCHWARZ, G., B. J. LEE, and J. H. NELSON: Lymphography, cavography and urography in the evaluation of malignant lymphomas. Acta radiol. 3, 138 (1965).

TRAPP, P., u. H. R. FEINDT: Zur Differentialdiagnose der malignen Lymphome aus dem Lymphogramm. Fortschr. Röntgenstr. 107, 336 (1967).

WEISSLEDER, H.: Retroperitoneale Lymphknotenveränderungen beim Morbus Hodgkin. Fortschr. Röntgenstr. 101, 449 (1964).

—, u. J. BAUMEISTER: Das lymphographische Bild der chronischen lymphatischen Leukämie. Fortschr. Röntgenstr. 105, 24 (1966).

—, H. RENNEMANN, und L. BAUMEISTER: Der diagnostische Wert lymphographischer Verlaufskontrollen. Fortschr. Röntgenstr. 104, 14 (1966).

—, u. A. STOPS: Morbus Hodgkin: Eine Gegenüberstellung klinischer und lymphographischer Untersuchungen. Fortschr. Röntgenstr. 106, 169 (1967).

Chapter 9

Special Clinical Applications of Lymphograhpy

W. A. Fuchs

With 4 Figures

Postlymphographic Control Roentgenograms

Analysis of the postlymphographic control roentgenograms is of great importance in detecting new, recurrent or progressive malignant disease in inguinal, iliac, aortic and even mediastinal and supraclavicular lymph nodes. The long period of time during which oily contrast material is retained by the lymph nodes after lymphography provides the possibility of performing serial radiographs over a period of months. In doubtful cases lymphographic diagnosis will be more accurate when comparing size and structure of suspicious lymph nodes at regular time intervals (BELTZ and THURN, 1966; FABIAN et al., 1966; TAKASHI and ABRAMS, 1967). Lymph nodes which were previously normal in appearance may enlarge and develop filling defects due to metastatic foci, as a first sign of recurrence or extension of the disease. Furthermore, the effect of treatment on lymph nodes can be verified.

Follow-up roentgenograms are routinely taken at intervals of 2 weeks to 6 months for periods as long as 2 years, depending on the nature of the malignant disease.

A slight but definite increase in size of normal lymph nodes following lymphography is observed, with a subsequent gradual decrease in size. Contrast material is lost from the nodes in greatest quantity during the first month and then more gradually during the succeeding months. An amount of contrast agent adequate for interpretation remains in most of the patients for at least one year, but may be retained for as little as 6 months or as long as 34 months.

Second-look lymphography by re-injection of contrast material becomes necessary if an inadequate amount of contrast material is present within the lymph nodes at the time of control.

Development of central and marginal filling defects, increase in size and displacement or separation of lymph nodes are lymphographic symptoms of new or recurrent metastatic lymph node involvement (Figs. 7/5, 7/30, 7/75). The same criteria apply for malignant lymphoma in which, additionally, the appearance of a typical lymphoma pattern is observed (Figs. 8/12, 8/17, 8/18). In case of uncertain diagnosis of lymph node metastases, changes in the size of filling defects within lymph nodes should be carefully evaluated. Because the original study is always available for comparison, inflammatory or fibrolipomatous changes may be identified as such.

The results of irradiation therapy or chemotherapy are followed by follow-up roentgenograms. Decrease in size of the nodes and disappearance of filling defects are objective parameters by which to judge the effectivness of the treatment (Figs. 7/14, 7/31, 8/19, 8/20, 8/22, 8/33). However, the persistence of nodal enlargement and filling defects does not imply residual malignant growth, because the malignant cells may be completely replaced by fibrous tissue. Lymphographic evaluation of tumor regression is more difficult in metastatic carcinoma than in primary malignant lymphoma, where lymph node enlargement is usually a prominant feature. Size reduction is easily seen and assessed. In metastatic carcinoma the filling defects in lymph nodes rarely reach similar dimensions, and obstruction of the lymphatic circulation with consequent non-filling of nodes occurs frequently. Consequently, evaluation of therapy may be extremely difficult and even impossible.

Growth rates of different histologic types of tumors are obtained by measuring the size of lymph nodes infiltrated by malignant tissue in successive roentgenograms. MacDONALD et al. (1968) conducted a study on the doubling times of enlarging nodes. The 47 cases investigated included Hodgkin's disease, lymphosarcoma, reticulosarcoma, carcinoma of the cervix and urinary bladder, and teratoma testis. The investigators concluded that the rate of growth of malignant foci in lymph nodes is comparable with the rate of growth of metastases in the lung, although measurement in the nodes is more difficult.

Similar observations have been reported in the chapters on tumor metastases and malignant lymphoma. The different growth rates of different types of malignant testicular tumors (Figs. 7/30, 7/34), the relatively slow growth rate of lymph node metastases in a case of carcinoma of the uterine cervix (Fig. 7/9), and the very fast increase in size of a supraclavicular lymph node metastasis in a case of solid scirrhous carcinoma of the stomach (Fig. 7/64) deserve particular attention. Through accumulation of data on the growth of different histologic types of tumor, a more detailed knowledge of them may be acquired. Thereby, prediction of the expected rate of growth is possible once the histologic classification has been established by biopsy.

Combined Lymphography, Cavography and Urography

The relative accuracy of lymphography, inferior vena cava cavography and urography for evaluation of malignant involvement of the retroperitoneal lymph nodes has been clearly established by BAUM et al. (1963), PUJOL and LAMARQUE (1964), MAHAFFY (1964), LEE et al. (1964). Disappearance of the psoas contours on abdominal roentgenograms does not yield conclusive diagnostic information (ELKIN and COHEN, 1962). Urography demonstrates stasis or dislocation of the ureters by compression or direct infiltration only in advanced metastatic disease within the retroperitoneal area (Figs. 7/5, 7/8, 7/16, 8/12b, 8/30b). In a series of 186 patients with malignant lymphoma investigated by LEE et al. (1964), false negative results of urography were obtained in 70%. However, it should be stated that urography is very valuable in detecting obstruction of the ureters in cases of malignant tumors of the urinary bladder (Fig. 7/51). Impairement of urinary flow following radiotherapy of tumors of the female genital tract is also easily recognized by urography.

Cavography demonstrates malignant involvement localized within the right latero-aortic and external and common iliac lymph nodes (Figs. 7/8, 7/18, 7/31b,

7/61, 8/14 c, 8/21 c). Pathologic enlargement of the other aortic node groups cannot be diagnosed because of the topographic-anatomic localization of the inferior vena cava (Fuchs, 1961, 1964; Pujol and Lamarque, 1964; Mahaffy, 1964).

In a series of 201 consecutive investigations of the author's case material including lymphography, cavography and urography, informative data on the actual diagnostic value of the combined investigative technique were obtained (Hopf and Fuchs, 1969). In 136 patients with epithelial tumors, 47% manifested pathologic changes in one or several of the 3 types of studies. Lymphography indicated metastatic spread to the regional lymph nodes in 30% and cavography in 18%. Urography showed impairment of flow in the ureter in 26%, a finding which was particularly frequent in the 28 cases of carcinoma of the urinary bladder. In 30% of the positive findings the accurate topographic-anatomic extension, of the disease could be determined only by combining the results of all three investigative methods.

Fifty-eight patients with primary malignant lymphoma were studied by combined lymphography, cavography and urography. Pathologic findings were observed in 67% of the cases, of which lymphography was abnormal in 60%, cavography in 33% and urography in 12%. In 33% of the pathologic cases combined evaluation of all 3 investigative methods was necessary to establish accurately the extent of malignant disease. The reliability of lymphography is evidently the highest, as this method directly demonstrates the pathologic changes within the lymph nodes. Inferior vena cava cavography and urography rely upon indirect radiologic signs. The same applies for axillary venography. However, the value of cavography as an additional method to lymphography has become more and more evident.

Demonstration of malignant metastatic spread to the upper aortic node groups is an important indication for cavography. Poor visualization of the right aortic node group is relatively common. As described in Chapter 5, the upper level of contrast-filled nodes of the right latero-aortic node group was only L 3 in 40%, whereas the nodes of the remaining cases did visualize up to that level. Malignant metastases to lymph nodes situated above this level are frequently observed in cancer of the testes, ovaries, and the uterine corpus, because these node groups represent the primary regional lymph nodes of these organs. Cavography is therefore an indispensable complement. Indirect signs such as compression and dislocation of the vein by metastatic aortic node groups will enable the correct evaluation of metastatic spread.

Preoperative Lymphography

Complete surgical excision of lymph nodes is more accurately achieved with the use of radiographic controls before closing the operation site (Figs. 1, 7/27, 7/66). In addition, staining of the lymphatics and lymph nodes by adding chlorophyll or elementary carbon (Lemmon et al., 1965; Ludvik and Kindl, 1966, 1968; Hartgill, 1966; Davidson et al., 1967; Gregl et al., 1968) to the contrast agent makes dissection and removal of lymph nodes an easier and more rapid procedure resulting in a minimum of unnecessary trauma. Other authors are not of the same facorable opinion, especially regarding the use of chlorophyll, because good staining was observed only in the primary regional lymph nodes (Mayor, 1966). Also fatty tissue obscured the pale green nodes in many cases (Jackson, 1968).

Obstruction of lymph flow caused by chlorophyll has been reported by LEMMON et al. (1966), DAVIDSON et al. (1967) and JACKSON (1968). Consequently, the use of this type of dye for preoperative staining of lymph nodes will be discontinued, most likely.

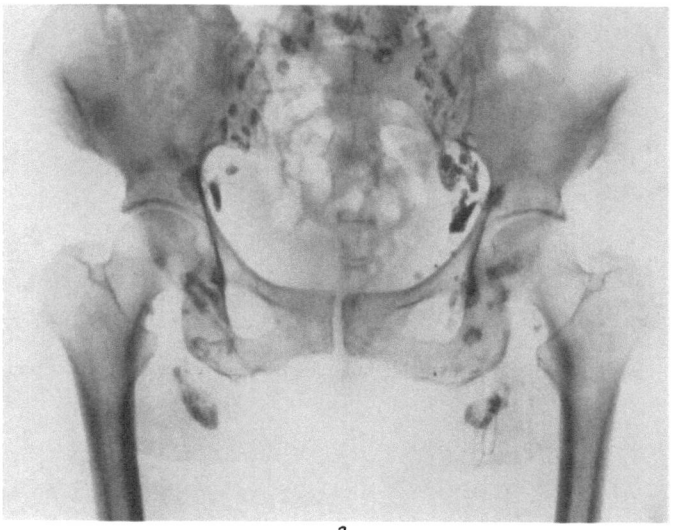

a

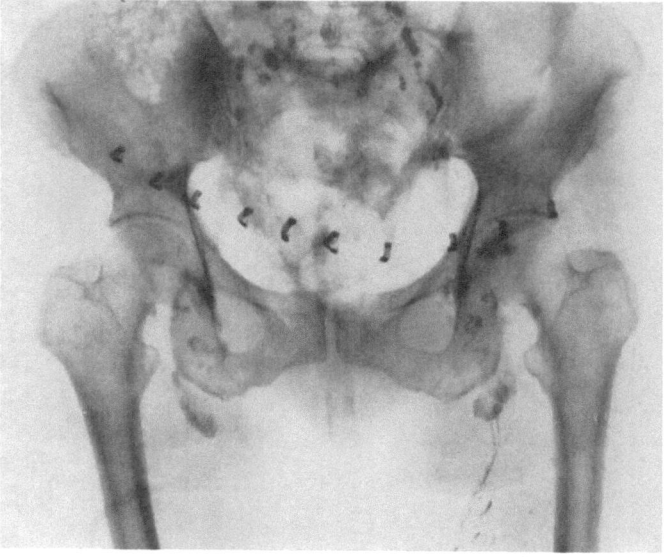

b

Fig. 1. Postoperative control following pelvic lymphadenectomy in a case of carcinoma of the uterine cervix. a Preoperative lymphogram. b Postoperative lymphogram. Complete excision of only the external iliac lymph nodes

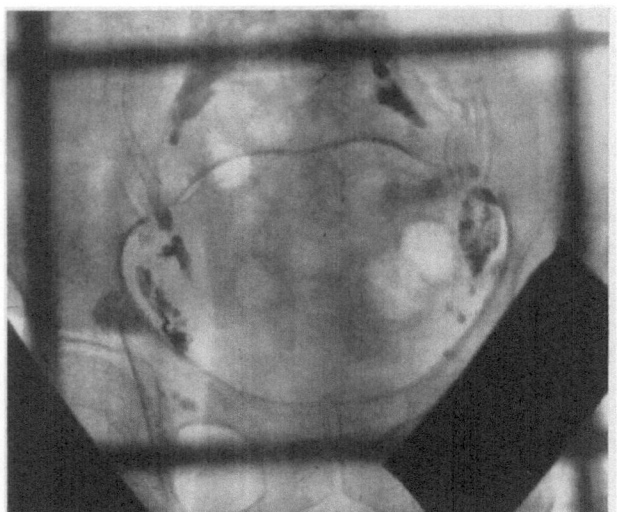

Fig. 2. Lead marking of iliac portal fields in a case of carcinoma of the uterine cervix

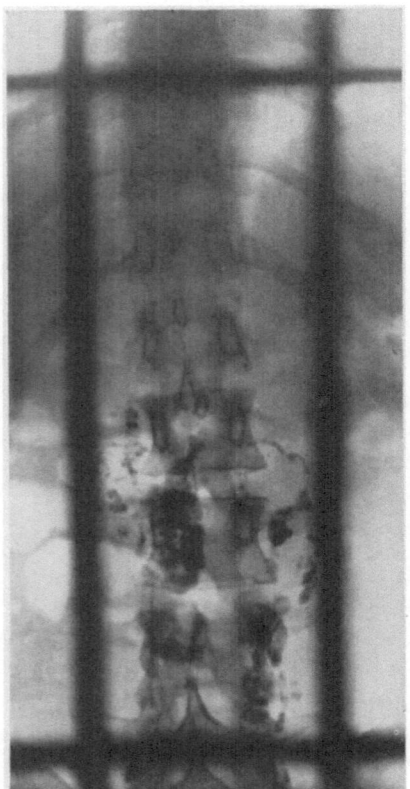

Fig. 3. Lead marking of aortic portal fields in a case of seminoma

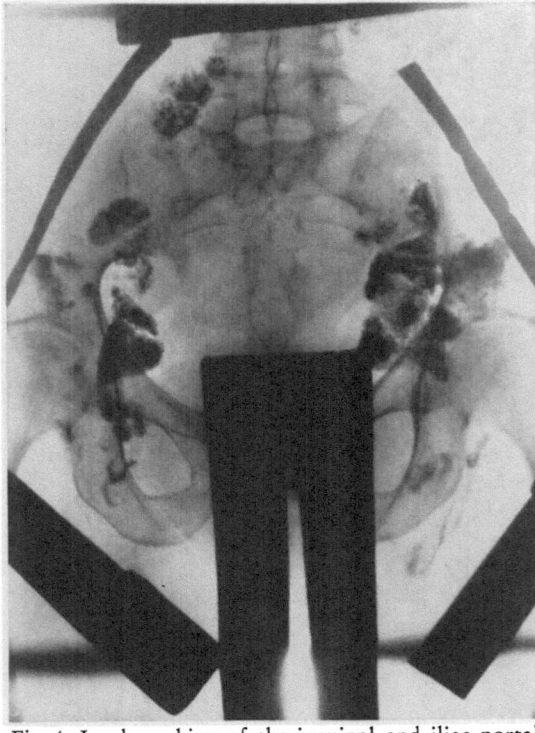

Fig. 4. Lead marking of the inguinal and iliac portal fields in a case of generalised lymphosarcoma

Planning of Radiation Therapy

In planning external irradiation of lymph nodes with malignant disease, the exact topographic-anatomic localization of the lymph nodes is of particular importance. Control roentgenograms in the simulated position of irradiation with lead markings of the portal fields ensure the accurate positioning of the irradiation area (Figs. 2, 3, 4). Thorough knowledge of the position of the lymph nodes in relation to the skeleton ensures detailed measurement of the radiation dose applied to a particular group of lymph nodes. In radium therapy of gynecological tumors, calculation of the radiation dose to the external and common iliac lymph nodes is established with exact measurement of the distance between radiation source and each lymph node group.

References

BAUM, ST., K. M. BRON, L. WEXLER, and H. L. ABRAMS: Lymphangiography, cavography and urography. Radiology 81, 207 (1963).

BELTZ, L., u. P. THURN: Zur Verlaufskontrolle des Lymphadenograms bei retroperitonealen Lymphknotentumoren. Fortschr. Röntgenstr. 104, 1 (1966).

DAVIDSON, J. W., E. A. CLARKE, and D. WALKER: Radiographic appearances in chromo-lymphadenography. J. Canad. med. Ass. 10, 316 (1967).

ELKIN, M., and G. COHEN: Diagnostic value of psoas shadow. Clin. Radiol. 13, 210 (1962).

FABIAN, C. E., E. J. NUDELMAN, and H. L. ABRAMS: Postlymphangiogram film as an indicator of tumor activity in lymphoma. Invest. Radiol. 1, 386 (1966).

FUCHS, W. A.: Der diagnostische Wert der Cavographie. Radiol. Clin. 30, 129 (1961).

— Lymphography. Ann. Rev. Med. 15, 287 (1964).

GREGL, A., M. EYDT, U. KRACK, and H. J. FICHTNER: Chromolymphographies of the upper extremities. Fortschr. Röntgenstr. 108, 565 (1968).

HARTGILL, J.: X-ray control during excision of lymph nodes. Progress in lymphology, p. 215. Stuttgart: G. Thieme 1967.

HOPF, M. A., u. A. W. FUCHS: Die Lymphographie-Cavographie-Urographie als Kobinationsuntersuchung. Radiologe 1969 (in print).

LEE, B. J., J. H. NELSON, and G. SCHWARZ: Evaluation of lymphangiography, inferior vena cavography and intravenous pyelography in the clinical staging and management of Hodgkin's disease and lymphosarcoma. New Engl. J. Med. 271, 327 (1964).

LEMMON, W. T., A. S. KETCHAM, J. D. MacLOWRY, and J. HERDT: Surgical applications of ethiodol with chlorophyll in lymphangiography: Histopathologic, radiographic and clinical disadvantages in 36 cases. Ann. Surg. 1, 114 (1966).

LUDVIK, W., u. H. KINDL: Präoperative Vitalfärbung von Lymphknoten im Rahmen der Lymphographie. Chir. Praxis 12, 1 (1968).

MacDONALD, J. S., A. LAUGIER, and M. SCHLIENGER: Observations on the growth of tumours in lymph nodes changing from normal to abnormal while remaining opacified after lymphography. Clin. Radiol. 19, 120 (1968).

MAHAFFY, R. G.: A comparison of the diagnostic accuracy of lymphography, cavography and pelvic phlebography. Brit. J. Radiol. 37, 422 (1964).

MAYOR, G.: Discussion note. Progress in Lymphology, p. 188. Stuttgart: G. Thieme 1967.

PUJOL, H., et J. L. LAMARQUE: Ilio-cavographie et lymphographie dans la recherche des adenopathies retropéritonéales. Paris: Masson & Cie. 1964.

TAKASHI, M., and H. L. ABRAMS: The accuracy of lymphangiographic diagnosis in malignant lymphoma. Radiology 89, 448 (1967).

Chapter 10

Isotope Lymphography

H. Rösler

With 9 Figures

Transport through the lymphatic pathways is an important mechanism in the spread of cancer. Colloidal sols when injected intralymphatically or even interstitially, follow the same course and are trapped in the lymph nodes. After they have been labeled with gamma emitting radioisotopes, these nodes can be visualized externally by scintigraphy. The radioactive substance fails to be taken up by lymphatic tissue which has been replaced by tumor. Therefore, the typical findings in radioisotope lymphography show disruption of normal isotope distribution as caused by a blockade of flow or a collateral flow bypassing an obstruction. Because the resolving power of the scintigraphic techniques in use today is poor, the pictures of isotope distribution do not exhibit the morphological detail obtainable in direct lymphography using radio-opaque contrast media. There are a number of aspects, however, which make radioisotope lymphography an important clinical method:

1. Radioactive sols, especially radio-gold, are chemically inert and non-toxic in the small amounts which are used routinely. Their transport mimics lymph flow affording a more faithful representation of physiologic conditions than does lipiodol.

2. *Indirect radioisotope lymphography* gives access to practically all regions of the body, including lymphatic systems of the neck, the mediastinum and pelvic organs.

3. The procedure requires no time-consuming punctures of lymph vessels.

4. There are no side effects or dangers inherent to this technique, thus patients in poor general condition may undergo the procedure without great concern, and follow-up studies may be performed at short intervals.

Functional studies in which radioisotopic material is injected directly into lymphatic vessels or lymph nodes are mostly of historical interest today, although they are well-suited to studies requiring quantitation of transport, storage and elimination data. Known as *direct radioisotope lymphography*, the study most commonly uses ^{131}I lipiodol as the tracer material. The direct technique is applied also for intralymphatic radiotherapy of primary tumors and metastases in the lymphatic system. In this technique the dose determination is based on the observed distribution of a small amount of tracer in a trial injection. Another method known as *direct tumor scintigraphy* makes use of isotopic substances which are taken up by tumor enabling positive delineation of abnormal tissue in the lymphatic system.

Methods
Radioactive Substances

Injected ^{131}I iodide and radio-iodide from labeled macroaggregated human serum albumin diffuse into the blood circulation from lymph vessels as demonstrated after intralymphatic application [22]. The rate of disappearance of ^{131}I human serum albumin (RIHSA) from the site of an interstitial injection was recommended as a measure of lymphatic drainage [27]. But significant amounts may enter the blood directly from the site of injection [50] or after a direct intralymphatic injection may fail to reach the first lymph node [22]. This substance is therefore of little use in the assessment of lymphatic function. For the same reason ^{131}I-fibrinogen, ^{131}I-iodinated polyvinyl pyrrolidone (^{131}I-PVP) or ^{51}Cr-human serum albumin (^{51}Cr-HSA) were found to be impractical for lymphographic studies [62].

HAHN and co-workers demonstrated that radioactive silver colloids were drained rapidly by the lymphatics of the lung when introduced by bronchoscope [18]. Their use on a diagnostic scale, however, is made impossible by technical difficulties in the production of a suitable isotope of silver. Addition of a dispersion of inactive silver to radioactive [198]Au gold colloids resulted in silvercoated particles, which were drained by the thoracic lymphatics within two to five days following interstitial administration [17, 19]. These observations could be confirmed by animal experiments [31]. Using HAHN's bronchoscopic technique HÖFER and BENZER injected commercially available colloidal gold into the submucosal layers of the bronchus. They demonstrated lymph node uptake scintigraphically within 3 hours. Exact comparative studies, using silvercoated as well as non-prepared particles have not been reported.

WALKER (1950) injected yttrium hydroxy citrate colloid into a trunk afferent to the popliteal node of the rabbit and then measured its retention in the popliteal and pelvic nodes. The popliteal node retained a major portion of the injected colloid; secondary or tertiary nodes usually contained far less activity and never as much as the primary node. Using two preparations, that with the larger particles was retained more completely in the primary nodes. Retention was the best when the fluid volume was the smallest [60].

These experiments demonstrated that, independent of the radioactive label, one specific chemical preparation has been most useful in lymphatic function studies. The substance is a suspension of particles stabilized by a sol such as gelatin, the size and metallic nature of the particles introduce phagocytic activity [52]. Colloidal [198]Au has the following characteristics making it a suitable particulate material for lymphographic studies:

1. Its gamma emission with a mean energy peak of 0.412 mev (95.8%) can be traced and measured with external measurement techniques using the equipment standard to a nuclear medicine department.

2. [198]Au has a short half-life of 2.7 days, short enough to prevent excessive irradiation.

3. Sufficient activity can be contained in a small volume, so that a possible volume effect is eliminated. There is no dilatation of lymph vessels caused by a large volume of fluid as seen with direct injection of radio-opaque contrast media.

4. It is readily available and the commercial product is standardized.

5. Gold is chemically inert and provokes little tissue reaction.

After interstitial application, all activity which leaves the site of injection enters the lymphatic system, and all of the colloidal gold follows the lymphatic pathways [50]. Measurements of the lymph dynamics and lymphatic morphology truly represent the physiologic and pathologic states studied. Using [198]Au-colloidal gold, continous or interrupted quantitative observations can be made *in vivo*. For double isotope techniques, another label is available, [199]Au, the main photo peaks of which, 0.158 mev (38.2%), 0.208 mev (9.4%) can be easily separated from that of [198]Au [17, 20].

In accordance with WALKER's findings in animals [60] GEST (1963) ascertained that of two commercially supplied preparations, one with smaller 3 μ particles was better suited for visualization of lymphatic structures in indirect lymphography than the other with particles averaging 30 μ in diameter [14] (Table).

Table

a) [198]Au		[199]Au	
Half-life = 2.70 d		Half-life = 3.15 d	
β = 0.29 mev	(1.2%)	β = 0.25 mev	(23%)
0.96	(98.8%)	0.30	(70%)
1.37	(0.025%)	0.46	(7%)
γ = 0.412 mev	(95.8%)	γ = 0.05 mev	(0.4%)
0.68	(1.0%)	0.158	(38.2%)
1.0	(0.2%)	0.208	(9.4%)

b) Colloidal suspension of metallic gold, stabilized with gelatin and sodium citrate. Optimal particle size: 50 Å

c) *Radiation exposure:* Lymph node: 1—5 rad/µCi
Whole body: 0.02 mrad/µCi
Liver: 0.1 mrad/µCi
(OESER and co-workers, 1969 [44])

a) Physical properties of radiogold: [198]Au and [199]Au
b) Chemical preparation of radiogold for radiolymphography
c) Radiation exposure of radiolymphography ([198]Au)

Ultrafluid lipiodol with ^{131}I-iodine label is used for simultaneous X-ray and radioisotope-functional studies and is used in doses sufficient for therapeutic effects [22, 23, 38, 64, 66, 67].

Substances capable of producing positive delineation of primary or secondary lymph node tumors are to be described separately in the last section of this chapter.

Instruments

Instrumentation was a matter of technical evoluation since HAHN and his co-workers measured the retention of therapeutically administered radio-gold in adjacent lymph nodes using GEIGER-MUELLER counters [17, 18, 19]. In this way WALKER measured the β-emission of ^{90}Y in lymph nodes which he had dissected one to nine days after application of Yttrium-colloid [60]. The distribution of radioactive material in tissues can be studied autoradiographically or by micro-autoradiographic method [51]. *In vivo*-external-countings became possible with the introduction of scintillation counters. Using lead shielding, regions of interest could be selected [50]. Corrections for geometric irregularities, for absorption, backscattering and background activity have been described in detail by SAGE [50] and by HULTBORN [29]. HULTBORN used a movable γ-sensitive directional shielded scintillation counter during operation [29].

Additional shielding of a scintillation detector makes it sensitive along a small channel (conic collimator) or along an arrangement of small channels (honeycomb type collimator). Manually measured impulse rates, point by point, are arranged in isoimpulse charts. This most reliable and consistently exact method in thyroid and brain tumor examination was not tested routinely in lymphography.

Scintigraphy utilizes an automatic device to move the collimated detector over a region of interest. The scanner simultaneously transforms the impulses which are registered from radioactive decay over each small region of view into electrical impulses which steer the printer or a photo cathode valve. Varying amounts of radioactivity, distributed regionally and three-dimensionally in the body region, are translated into a two-dimensional pattern of black dots which are printed in densities directly proportional to the amounts of radioactivity. Supplementary electronic circuits erase or subtract background activity. The clarity of scintillation scan images may be enhanced by recording in several contrasting colors, each representing a pre-chosen fraction of the maximal activity. The picture produced may be visually improved by using closed circuit television. Digital display of the radioisotope scan and statistical testing for the evaluation of count intensity fluctuations in neighboring areas brings greater objectivity and reliability to interpretations of a scan [56].

Modern scintiscanners with the most sensitive detectors (crystal diameters of 5 inches and more) retain the resolving power of small detectors when focused on a plane only a few millimeters thick at a given distance from the detector surface. This tomographic effect demands special attention in lymph node scintigraphy of the abdomen. Here the detector-to-target distance differs significantly over inguinal (short distance), iliac (large distance), and para-aortic lymph nodes. Only one group within the focus plane can be delineated sharply. For the same reason, counting efficiency depends highly on distance. Thus, comparisons of absolute impulse rates coming from different groups of nodes must be made with caution. In routine work the distance to the lymph nodes in the para-aortic region is selected [65].

With modern scintillation cameras the mechanical motion of the detector over a region of interest is replaced by electronic localization of decay events registered by a stationary γ-sensitive head with a diameter of 12 inches or more. The disintegrations are projected onto an oscilloscope. With a camera mounted in front of its screen, all scintillations within a pre-chosen time are integrated on film. Two types of collimators are available. One has a lead grid which presents a picture in parallel projection, i. e. without focusing. The other works like a pinhole camera in central projection mode whereby the region registered may be enlarged or reduced according to the distance between the hole and the target.

For lymphographic studies both types are useful. The screen type collimator is more sensitive but is restricted to the diameter of the area seen [64]. The pinhole collimated scintillation camera has better resolution for the high energy γ-emission of the ^{198}Au-peak but loses much of its inherent sensitivity. By varying the collimator-to-target distance a standard technique may be found to visualize e. g. the whole abdomen, from liver region to groin, with one adjustment. One must be aware, however, of geometric distortion inherent to the pin hole collimator.

Results

Direct Radioisotope Lymphography

Two years before KINMONTH [35, 36] introduced the direct puncture of lymph vessels as a routine technique for roentgenographic lymphography, WALKER (1950) injected radioactive yttrium-hydroxy-citrate colloids into lymph vessels afferent to the popliteal node in rabbits, measuring its retention by the popliteal and pelvic nodes [60]. His method of single, small volume injection is essentially unchanged today because disturbance of normal physiologic conditions is at a minimum. WAL-KER'S results in lymphatic function studies have proven fundamental to further investigations using direct as well as indirect lymphographic techniques with radio-isotopes:

1. The primary node retained a major portion of the injected colloid. Secondary or tertiary nodes consistently contained much less activity.

2. Of two colloidal preparations, that with the larger particles was more completely retained in the primary node, demonstrating a correlation between colloid particle size and retention.

3. The colloid retention was most complete when the volume injected was smallest.

FISCHER (1962) using radio-gold colloid for *in vivo* counting techniques observed an instantaneous increase of activity over the popliteal lymph nodes after injection into its afferent lymphatic. Subsequent saline injections displaced most of the activity to the next lymphatic filters, but the residual activity in the node remained above the pre-gold injection level. Newly injected tracer material was stored again in the first node [8]. Continuous infusion of radioactive colloidal chromium phosphate ($^{51}Cr^{32}PO_4$) or colloidal gold ^{198}Au in aqueous solution into a lymph vessel of the foot according to KINMONTH'S technique resulted in retention predominantly in the inguinal lymph nodes in man (HEINZEL and co-workers: 22, 23). But in agreement with FISCHER'S report, there was deposition within the lymphatic chain as far superior as the lymph nodes at the angulus venosus (Fig. 1). Retention of radioactive substances within the lymphatic system remained constant over several days and amounted to nearly 50% of the total body activity.

Overflow into the blood circulation was followed by extensive accumulation in the reticulo-endothelial elements of the liver [22]. When these colloids are administered immediately following diagnostic lymphography with non-radioactive lipiodol, then the distribution picture is quite different. Radioactivity is found consistently over the inguinal lymph nodes. The height to which the colloid is distributed is a function of the amount of aqueous carrier given. The previously administered lipiodol apparently blocks further spontaneous transport. The distribution of the colloidal substance between the inguinal and pelvic lymph nodes remains constant from the 2nd to the 14th day [22]. Over the liver there is no activity measurable for as long as 14 days after lymphography [23]. For therapeutic purposes in cancer this modified application seems to be advantageous.

Ultrafluid lipiodol can be followed from a punctured lymph vessel to transient deposition in the lung by X-ray examination. Quantitative studies of its distribution and surveys on the later disposition of the iodinated contrast medium can be conducted more easily after labeling with radioiodine. After a typically performed X-ray lymphography with ^{131}I-lipiodol in dog experiments, KOEHLER and co-workers recovered 35% of the iodine in the urine from the first to the 17th day. An average

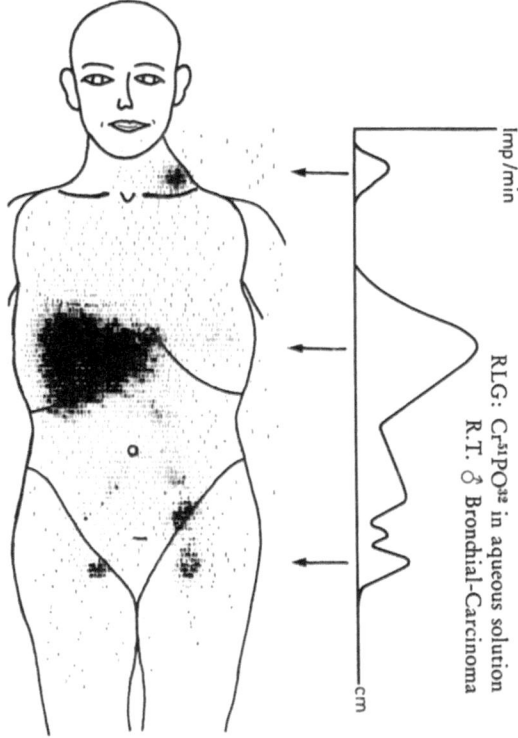

Fig. 1. Direct radiolymphography using chromium phosphate (^{51}Cr^{32}PO$_4$) in aqueous solution. (HEINZEL, RÖSLER et al. 1968 [23])

of only 25% of the injected medium was retained in the lymphatics at the end of 3 days, but 50% was recovered from the lung [38]. Radioiodine lipiodol, administered with greater amounts of ^{131}I activity for therapeutic purposes is eliminated more quickly. Using whole-body-counting, ZUM WINKEL found nearly 50% retention after 2 days [67]. Thirty-nine to seventy-eight percent of the total retained activity was found in the retro-peritoneal lymph nodes, leaving them with an effective half-life of 2—8 days [68]. Up to 9.7% of the total activity might be trapped by the thyroid gland [67]. Spillover of ^{131}I-lipiodol to the lung was followed under varied conditions by HEINZEL and RÖSLER [22]. Two days after administering 9 ml of ^{131}I-lipiodol via the foot, retention in the lungs reached a maximum of 50% of the total body activity falling to nearly 10% after 14 days. When ^{131}I-lipiodol was injected as a small volume of high specific activity immediately after a typical diagnostic quantity of non-labelled lipiodol, maximum lung retention of the radio-active material was only about 25% of the total activity distributed in the body, but was eliminated with a similar rate constant, as with larger amounts of active lipiodol. When, however, the injection of radioactive lipiodol precedes the non-radioactive lipiodol, the rate of elimination is faster although the maximum lung retention is the same [22], (Fig. 2).

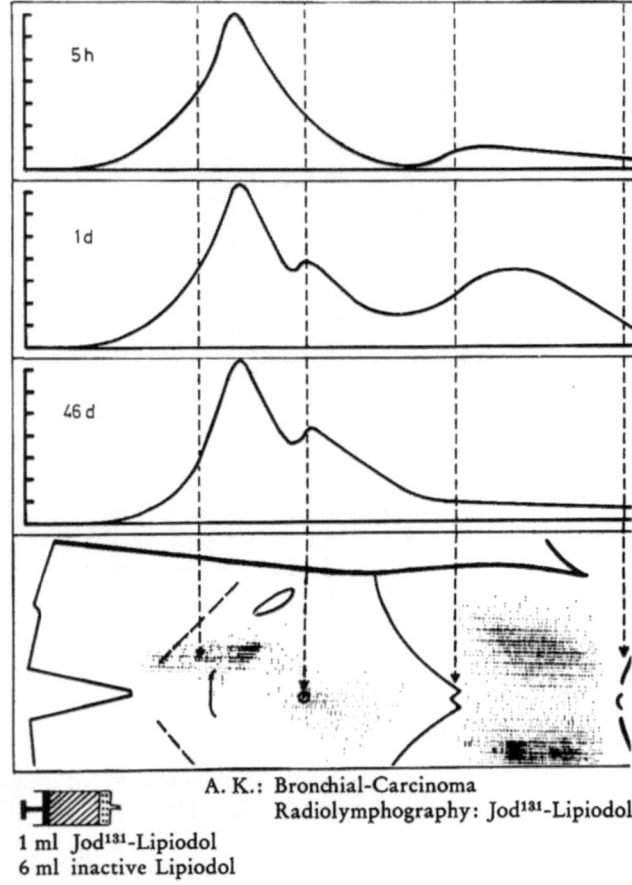

1 ml Jod^{131}-Lipiodol
6 ml inactive Lipiodol

A. K.: Bronchial-Carcinoma
Radiolymphography: Jod^{131}-Lipiodol

Fig. 2. Direct radiolymphography with ^{131}I-lipiodol, injected into the lymph vessels of the right foot. Only the initial portion of the injection (1 ml) was radioactive lipiodol, the following 6 ml were inactive. (HEINZEL and RÖSLER 1967 [22])

From the above data, it is apparent that the lymph system is usually overfilled with the large volumes of lipiodol administered during routine X-ray lymphography. The system behaves like an elastic chamber when overfilled, and for a number of days after injection the contrast material is slowly pressed from the lymphatics into the general circulation [23]. The resulting distribution pattern is a function of pressure and is not a consequence of normal lymph flow. The differing patterns observed in isotope and X-ray techniques are determined mostly by the volumes of contrast material used. For example, normal or increased retention by inflamed nodes is seen when using radio-gold, thus indicating for certain that the cause of lymph node enlargement is in fact inflammation [70]. Also comparative studies have shown that observation of filling-defects in tumorous nodes with non-radioactive lipiodol are preceeded by a filling of less active accumulation of radio-gold in the node [66].

Indirect Radioisotope Lymphography

1. Preliminaries

HAHN (1946) first reported drainage of radio-colloids by regional lymphatics after intrabronchial injection of carcinomas for therapeutic purposes [15, 17]. After additional experience with the use of colloidal gold in the treatment of superficial lesions in leukemia cutis, bladder tumors and prostate carcinoma [16], HAHN commenced systematic studies of the lymph node uptake of "silvercoated radioactive gold colloids" in dogs following subcutaneous and intramuscular injection [17, 31]. Commercially available radio-gold, injected subcutaneously in the inguinal region or into the parametrium of rabbits during laparotomy is drained to the regional lymph nodes rapidly and effectively, as was HAHN's preparation [52]. Maximum tracer concentration in the nodes was attained within 3—6 hours of subcutaneous injection and within 6—10 hours of injection into the parametrium. The maximum concentration remained constant for 60 hours. Up to 0.04% per mg tissue of the injected dose was accumulated by the inguinal node and 0.008%/mg by the common iliac and pre-aortic nodes together (SHERMAN and TER POGOSSIAN 1953 [52]). SAGE and co-workers (1958) first used scintigraphic techniques and noticed a pick-up by primary lymph nodes within 15 minutes. One quarter of the total activity injected into the tongue was accounted for in the main upper jugular node by dissection and quantitative analysis of the radioactivity [47]. Thus, it has been demonstrated that most of the colloidal gold which leaves a site of injection enters the lymphatic system [50]. In normal human subjects the disappearance rate from a subcutaneous depot amounted to 18—39% in 24 hours. Between 80 and 100% of the colloidal gold disappearing from a site of injection is picked up by the lymph nodes within 6—12 hours, where activity remained at a constant level for a week, thus giving a measure of filtration function of the node. The disappearance rate is a measure of lymph flow (SAGE and co-workers: 50). A decreased rate generally indicates incompetence of lymphatics as in primary diffuse lymphedema precox or severe lymphedema secondary to cancer, trauma or surgery [50]. An increased disappearance rate is an indication for the presence of lymphatic shunts. Early overflow into the circulation with accumulation in the liver can be seen regularly after radiation therapy of lymphatic chains. But as SCHEYBANI and co-workers warn, full use cannot be made of this finding [57].

Disappearance in the course of the first four hours is the result of body movement [50]. There is no detectable transport of the tracer material via the lymphatic system when injected under general anaesthesia [62]. The spreading effect of hyaluronidase may enhance resorption of the colloid from the infiltrated tissue [16, 61].

In agreement with FISCHER's results, SAGE and co-workers found 88—100% of the colloidal gold from the afferent lymphatics to be in the supernatant lymph after dissection and centrifugation, indicating that phagocytosis alone is not responsible for active accumulation of radioactive colloid in lymph nodes [50].

2. Methods, Risks and Complications

In principle, radioactive gold-colloid may be injected at various sites in the body. The procedure is nearly painless, but local anaesthesia, when desirable for extremely anxious patients, has no negative effect on the distribution of the radioactive material. Dosages recommended are 100 to 250 microcuries (μCi). Higher doses of 0.5 to 1.0 millicurie (mCi) have been used without local acute or late radiation reaction at the site of injection. Even intralymphatic application of therapeutic doses is not typically followed by general reactions, and these are never seen after small diagnostic amounts of radio-gold. In case of local or generalized cancer the radiation burden of the whole body might be regarded as a matter of secondary interest. Radiation to the critical organ, the liver, is never critical in radioisotope lymphography (Table).

3. Results in Cancer

a) Non-standardized Techniques

HULTBORN and co-workers (1955) studied lymph drainage from the breast to the axillary and para-sternal lymph nodes with the aid of colloidal [198]Au [28]. Regardless of the site of injection, colloid was transported to the axillary nodes; in most cases only a very small portion was transported to the para-sternal lymph nodes. The method was unsuitable for quantitative studies in mammary carcinoma, as some lymph vessels were blocked by primary tumors. After infiltration of extensive areas of the breast with colloidal radio-gold a few days before radical mastectomy, a movable γ-sensitive directional scintillation counter was used to detect lymph nodes in the axilla, finding nodes in two cases after dissection of the axilla had been considered complete [30]. Similarly SEAMAN and POWERS injected radiocolloid into normal breast tissues adjacent to tumor masses in women prior to radical mastectomy for carcinoma [51]. Activity trapped in the residual lymphoid tissues could be measured in only 20 of 64 cancer-containing lymph nodes. Pre-surgical diagnostic approaches for examination of the radio-colloid distribution became available after the introduction of scintiscanners. SAGE and GOZUN (1958) followed the radioactivity for as long as 14 days scintigraphically and observed that distribution was dependent on the physiologic lymphatic pathways regardless of whether the injection was made into the mucosal, submucosal or deeper layers of the lip, tongue, cheek, palate, tonsil or skin [47, 48, 49]. Injection into tissues adjacent to tumors of the head in a position avoiding superposition of the activity onto the lymphatic structures was preferred by GEST (1963) and FERNHOLZ (1967) [6, 14]. Application into or beneath the tumor is necessary when investigating the lymphatic drainage of bronchogenic carcinoma (HÖFER and BENZER 1966 [26]). But routine radio-lymphography requires standardized techniques which take into account typical lymphatic morphology and physiology.

b) Standardized Techniques

α) *Inguinal-abdominal Lymphatics.* Inguinal and intra-abdominal lymphatic pathways are visualized after subcutaneous injection of radio-colloid into the first interdigital space on the dorsum of the foot.

If subsequent X-ray lymphography is intended a few days later, an alternate site of injection may be chosen at the space between the 2nd and 3rd toe. The total administered dose should be divided into 2 or even 3 injections. Scanning may be started after 30 minutes if the leg is exercised, but routinely, scanning is performed after 24 hours. For evaluation of the deeper intra-abdominal lymph nodes, the prone and supine positions present similar results, but the supine is more comfortable and thus preferable [64].

According to MALEK and co-workers (1960) several lymphatic pathways may be differentiated in the leg, merging into one deep system of the thigh [42]. The deep systems of the leg may be visualized by injection into the sole of the foot or into the gastrocnemius muscle [20]. Occasionally a popliteal lymph node is seen [42].

Lymph chains identical with those seen in lipiodol lymphography are visualized scintigraphically (see Chapter 5) under normal conditions (Fig. 3). The appearance of activity in the liver is proof that the thoracic duct is patent. The deep inguinal

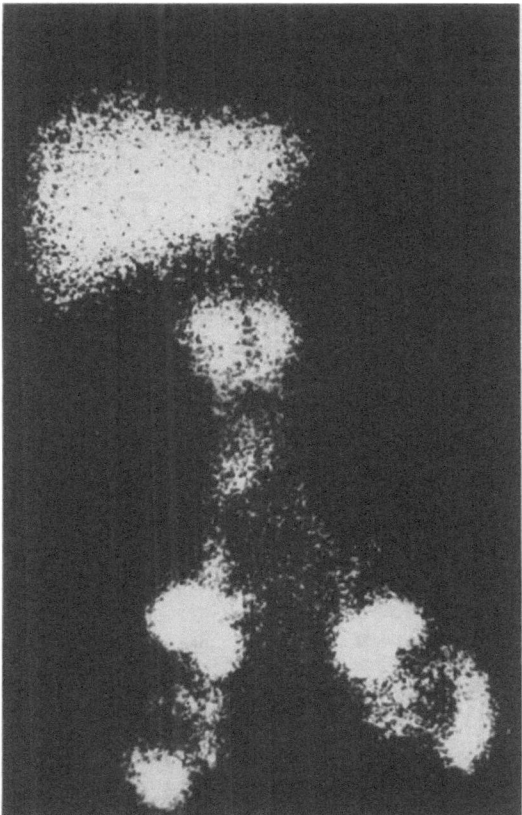

Fig. 3. Indirect radiolymphography with radioactive colloidal gold [198]Au. Normal inguinal and intra-abdominal lymphatics were visualized after subcutaneous injection into the first interdigital spaces of both feet. The figure was composed from two single exposures with the pin-hole-collimated scintillation camera

lymph nodes and the inferior superficial nodes are seen as one compact group. However, differentiation can be achieved by repeated scans in oblique projection. The external and common iliac lymph nodes are well separated, but trapped activity is less than 10% of that in the inguinal nodes, a factor which might cause the misinterpretation that an apparent interruption of the lymph chain exists. This is possible especially when maximum contrast in scintigraphic data processing has suppressed the normal activity in the few small nodes of this region [62].

The internal iliac lymph nodes, which are the primary regional lymph nodes for the bladder, rectum and anus as well as for the genital organs, are not visualized by this technique. Separation of the aortic lymph nodes in most cases is poor, even between the chains of both sides. Multiple individual variations in the distribution pattern are possible. Symmetry of both sides in number of delineated lymph nodes and concentration of activity affirms normality.

KROENERT and WOLF (1968) proposed a more descriptive classification of scintigraphically separated lymph nodes. In the groin, one, two or even a seldom three groups of nodes were counted on each side, along with three to four iliac, cranial and caudal groups.

Differentiated in addition were 3—6 groups in the cranial, iliac and aortic region. The area of each node averaged 3.8 ± 2.3 cm²; the area of all visualized lymph nodes on one side averaged 34 cm² [37].

Metastases cause discontinuity of a lymph node chain as well as partial or total defects in filling of some nodes, node dislocations or enlargements of node groups.

Defects less than 2 cm in diameter cannot be resolved by scintigraphic techniques [63], especially when they are solitary. Because tracer accumulation is diminished even by smaller metastases, a reduction in the radio-gold fixation, which is a functional alteration, is suspect of an early stage of metastatic destruction of lymphatic tissue (Fig. 4). The X-ray lymphadenogram will demonstrate partial fixation of lipiodol in these nodes and will delineate size and shape of the metastases

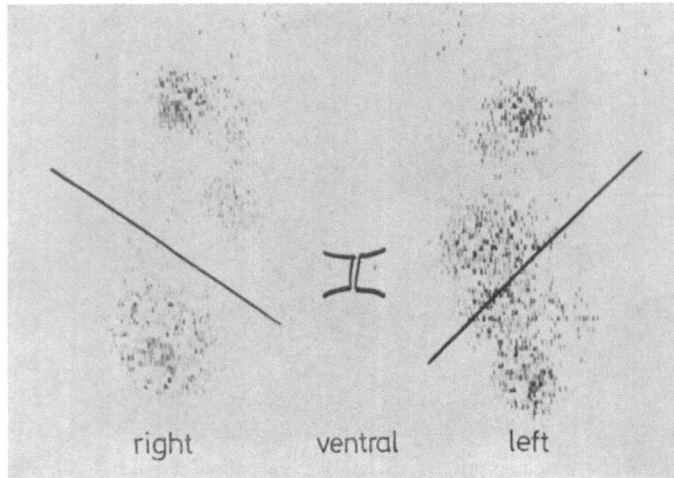

right   ventral   left

Fig. 4. Filling defects in superficial inguinal and iliac lymph nodes on the right side: metastases from penis carcinoma

much better. Blockage of transport of the radio-colloid is caused by complete metastatic destruction of one or several lymph nodes. The intensity of radioactivity within peripheral lymph nodes increases in these cases, but can be assessed only if function of the contralateral chain is not altered. These findings precede lymphedema as an early indication of obstruction of functionally efficient lymph nodes capable of fixation [57]. Collateral pathways are described [64] but are seldom seen.

Asymmetric dislocation of one node is caused by peripheral growth of metastases which have not blocked lymph passage totally. Partial involution of a few neighboring nodes results in a significant enlargement of a lymph node chain [62]. ZUM WINKEL and co-workers, however, stress that metastases of solid tumors, each of considerable size, may be found in X-ray lymphadenography [66].

In primary malignant lymphoma the single lymph nodes as well as chains of nodes are enlarged to 8.0 cm² and 80—84 cm² respectively [37]. The uptake is heterogeneous and decreased [37, 62, 66].

The contours of the single nodes are less sharp. With additional mediastinal involvement the passage to the thoracic duct is often slowed down [37].

In 37 patients with Hodgkin's disease, KROENERT and WOLF reported decreased activity retention in relatively enlarged lymph nodes with irregular contours and a heterogeneous distribution of radioactivity [37]. Only discrete defects may be found in spite of the wide-spread alterations seen in X-ray lymphadenograms [63]. However, SCHEYBANI and co-workers (1967) and MICHAILOY et al. (1968) described an increased uptake within broadened lymphatic chains [43, 57]. This combination is identified also in an earlier picture given by ZUM WINKEL [64]. The X-ray control adenograms demonstrated findings which FUCHS (1967) classified as reactive hyperplasia [10]. An increased avidity for radio-colloid [57] corresponds well to the comment of FUCHS and HAERTEL that these lymph nodes might be found particularly often adjacent to pathologically involved lymphatic structures, but that they are free of granulomatous destruction [10, 12]. According to their arguments a more extensive evaluation of both X-ray and radioisotope lymphography will improve the diagnosis of lymphogranulomatosis. For statistical evaluations, ZUM WINKEL (1967) separated groups with indifferent, dubious and pathologic findings. Among the 260 cases which he followed up, 85 (i. e. 33⁰/₀) were classified as dubious, 22 (26⁰/₀) of which were confirmed pathologic by X-ray lymphography. Only one case with a pathologic ethiodol lymphograph was found to have a normal scintigram; seven normal lipiodol lymphographs demonstrated pathologic scintigrams [65]. The author classifies radiolymphography of the abdominal lymph chains as a fair method in searching for metastases, but as a method which can supplement, not replace X-ray lymphadenography. This view is confirmed by others [26, 37, 57].

β) Head and Neck Lymphatics. X-ray lymphadenography requires the *direct* application of contrast media into lymphatic vessels. For visualization of the cervical lymphatics a special method, developed by FISCH [7], gives excellent pictures, but preparation of the retro-auricular lymph vessels is a troublesome technique not performed routinely. In contrast, *indirect* radiolymphographic studies require only an injection of radio-gold colloid subcutaneously over the mastoid process. The techniques have been standardized by SCHWAB and ZUM WINKEL, who scanned in anterior, posterior and lateral projections, strictly avoiding incorrect positioning of the patient [58, 59]. Normally, the total activity injected is taken up in the ipsilateral neck region. No colloid wanders into the circulation, and consequently there is no accumulation in the liver. Thirty to fifty percent of the applied activity is retained in the mastoid region: transport is directed caudally. In accordance with FISCH, zones of circumscribed, increased activity may be identified in association with nodes along the internal jugular vein and the accessory nerve, in the supraclavicular region and with the one or two nodes in contact with the trapezius muscle (Fig. 5) [59]. Lymph node metastases are suspect in areas of unilateral low activity, i. e. in "cold" areas not contralaterally symmetrical. However, asymmetrical tracer distribution may also reflect the increased accumulation by inflamed nodes (ZITA 1969 [70]), (Fig. 6). Very small metastases cannot be found by this method [59].

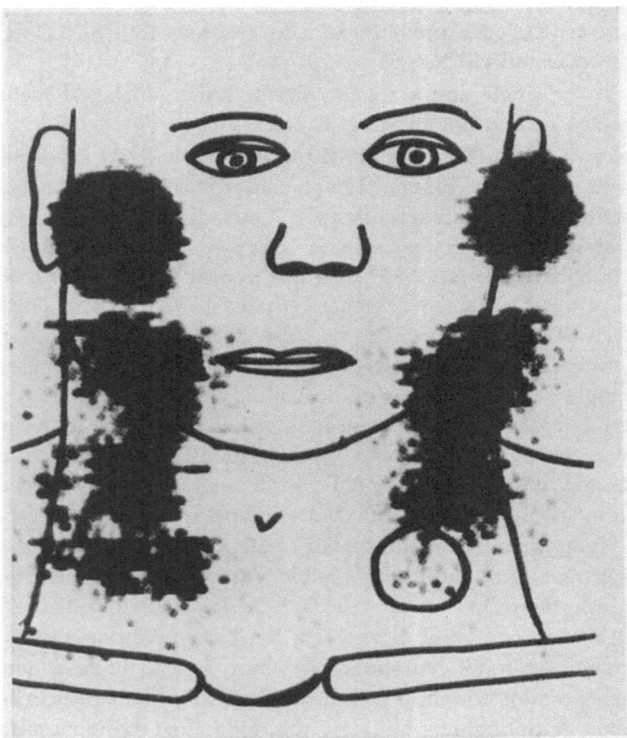

Fig. 5. Radiolymphography of the neck after subcutaneous injection of [198]Au colloid in the mastoid regions. Defect in trapping of a left cervical lymph node from a metastasis of a laryngeal cancer. (Courtesy of G. ZITA 1967 [70])

γ) *Lymph Drainage of the Breast.* Axillary lymph nodes may be visualized scintigraphically after the subcutaneous application of radio-gold into the dorsum of the hand. HEILMANN (1965) examined 56 patients after radical mastectomy and observed no decrease in the number of the accumulating nodes in the axillary and infraclavicular regions on the side not operated on but a decrease of 80 and 43% on the treated side respectively. Uptake by supraclavicular nodes was seen twice as often on the operated side as contralaterally [21].

Scintigraphy promised to be a good approach for the detection of lymph node metastases along the internal thoracic vessels. The technique of injecting radio-gold into the interstitial spaces below and behind the xiphoid process was proposed in 1966 by 3 groups simultaneously: DIETHELM [5], ROSSI and co-workers [46] and SCHENK [55]. The needle is directed towards both the right and left axillas during the injection. Routinely 150 units of hyaluronidase are mixed with the radio-gold injection, but the injection volume may not exceed 0.3 cc [55]. Normally, two or 3 lymph nodes are visualized para-sternally on both sides of the sternum, being found as a rule in the 1st and 2nd intercostal spaces and also with high frequency in the 3rd and 6th spaces. They are missing in the 4th and 5th ICS. Their size and the levels of activity accumulated by them vary within wide normal ranges. Sym-

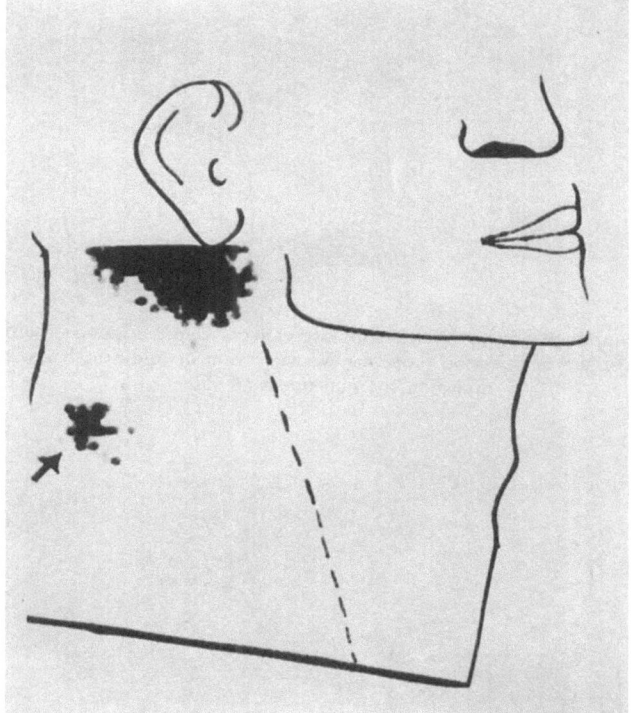

Fig. 6. Increased retention of radiocolloidal gold ^{198}Au in a nuchal lymph node in chronic laryngitis, visualized with background activity and normal lymphatics, electronically erased. (Courtesy of G. ZITA 1967 [70])

metric activity levels can be expected regularly. In almost 50% of the normal cases an additional uptake of gold in a lymph node group adjacent to the angulus venosus and transport to the axillary lymph nodes can be observed [45]. Accumulation in the liver is seldom seen. The deeper mediastinal nodes are not visualized (Fig. 7).

In pathologic conditions there is a decreased uptake of radioactivity on the diseased side with one or all lymph nodes not visualized, and there is evidence for collateral transport to the contralateral lymphatic chain as well as to the ipsilateral axillary or infraclavicular lymph nodes (Fig. 8). DAHL-IVERSON et al. (1955) [1] examined one hundred consecutive cases of breast cancers of all stages histologically after operation. One-third exhibited para-sternal lymph node metastases with the primary tumor lying in the medial half of the breast and one-tenth with the tumor originating laterally. The number of pathologic findings in scintigraphy of the para-sternal lymphatics is much higher [45]. To date no retrospective studies are available. In practice, diminished or entirely absent tracer uptake within parasternal lymph

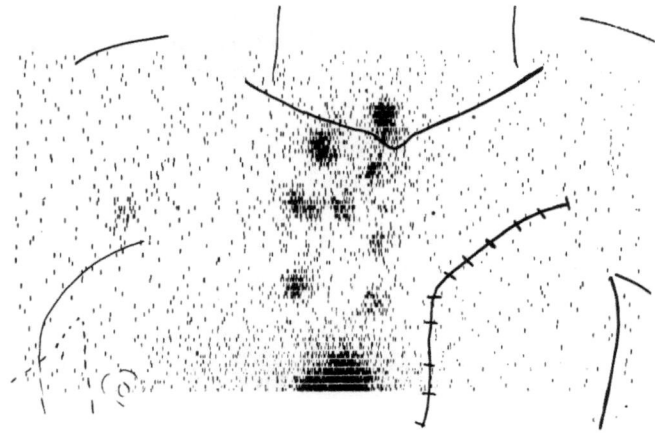

Fig. 7. Indirect lymphography in operated breast cancer. Depot of non-mobilized colloidal radiogold under the site of injection (bottom). Visualization of additional uptake by axillary nodes on the non-operated side

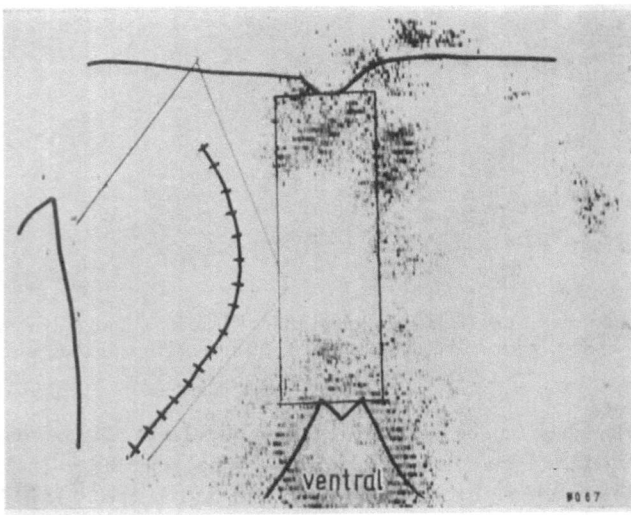

Fig. 8. Indirect lymphography of the parasternal lymph nodes with delineation of supra-clavicular and axillary nodes contralateral to the side operated on. There is no uptake in some para-sternal nodes on the operated side. The study was performed in order to demarcate the sternal field for post-surgical radiotherapy

nodes after surgery is indication for radiotherapy with therapeutic doses on both sides. The correct size of the field to be irradiated is determined from the radio-lymphographic findings.

δ) Visceral Lymph Drainage. MAGNENAT and DELALOYE (1964) published works on radio-lymphography of the liver, which may serve as a prototype for studies in lymph kinetics of other organs [3, 40]. Using a needle with openings in its side, 0.2—0.3 cc of colloidal ^{198}Au is injected transcutaneously into Glisson's capsule of the liver [41]. The procedure is painless and is tolerated well. The optimal time after injection for scintiscanning was found to be 6 hours. The tributary region includes anterior and posterior mediastinal lymphatic chains. There is no transport in carcinomatous lymphangitis. Blockage in one case of bronchogenic carcinoma of the right lower lobe of the lung was seen. No spread was observed in non-malignant diseases also, as in cirrhosis of the liver and sarcoidosis [3].

c) Externally Altered Lymph Kinetics

After roentgenographic lymphography the abdominal lymph nodes are blocked for one to two weeks with ultrafluid lipiodol [34, 64]. The blockage was substantiated in lymphokinetic studies with radio-colloid by HEINZEL and co-workers [22].

After surgery the disappearance rate for interstitial radio-colloid deposits is decreased. In secondary lymphedema after radical mastectomy, as an extreme situation, activity injected into the dorsum of the hand is found in the upper arm

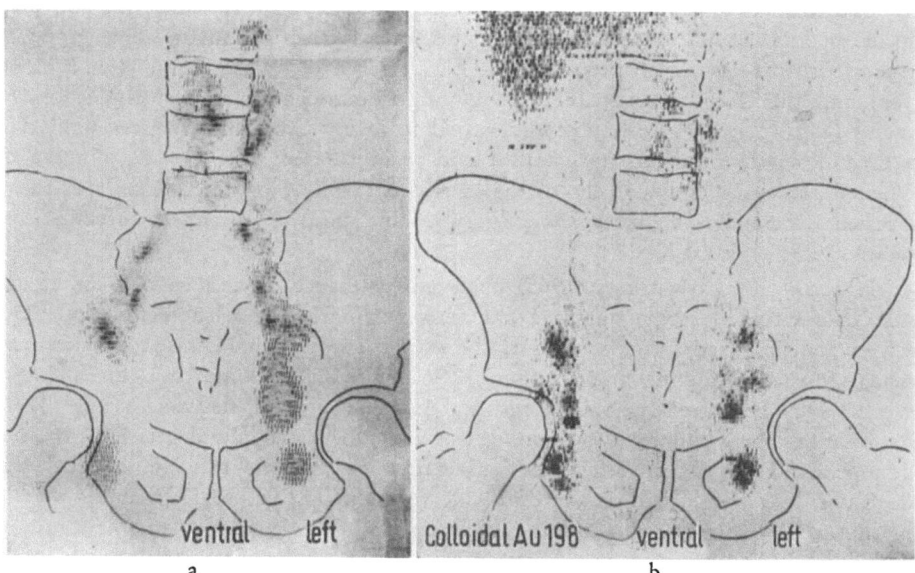

Fig. 9. a Distribution of ^{131}I-lipiodol administered therapeutically (35 mCi) for Hodgkin's disease stage II. b Indirect lymphography (^{198}Au colloid) nine months later: accelerated lymph flow with accumulation in the liver. Lymph nodes are missing in the deeper iliac region, and there is additional uptake by inguinal nodes on the right. (Courtesy of F. HEINZEL 1969 [24])

not bound to lymphatic structures [61]. After neck dissection transport on the ipsi-lateral side is blocked, and drainage via contralateral lymphatics is seen [4, 6, 57, 58, 59].

Lymph node function following *irradiation* was examined systematically in animals by DETTMANN et al. (1966) [4]. Irradiation did not entirely prevent the localization of colloidal gold in the popliteal lymph nodes in any case. After ir-radiation with doses of 2000 R no alteration of lymph kinetics was seen in com-parison with non-irradiated control animals. An increased lymph flow with addi-tional tracer accumulation in abdominal lymph nodes was induced after 6000 to 10 000 R, but these effects were delayed for 2 months after irradiation of the popliteal region, i. e. after fibrosis of the irradiated lymph nodes had been estab-lished. In correspondance with FISCH's results with direct lymphography, SCHWAB never saw complete lymph obstruction after radiotherapy, even after therapeutic doses in the neck region. Retention of radio-gold was decreased more or less, depen-dent on the doses given [58, 59]. In the case of primary malignant lymphoma, irradiated lymph chains lost their ability to accumulate radio-colloids [37], but transport was maintained [57] even after very high local doses of radioiodinated lipiodol [24]. Irregularities in colloid distribution are more pronounced in irradiated Hodgkin-lymphomas [63] (Fig. 9).

Positive Tumor Visualization

Extracranial tumors can be detected scintigraphically by the same method used to detect intracranial tumors employing the same apparatus and the same group of tracers (BONTE and co-workers, 1967) [2]. Presence of tracer in the tumor blood pool and the likely entrance of tracer into protein-containing spaces within the tumor (e. g. foci of necrosis) are understood to follow from disturbances similar to a breakdown in the function of the blood-brain barrier. The selective binding of labelled proteins by tumor cells or the increased turnover of biochemically essential labelled substances in malignancies may enable positive contrasts sufficient for scintigraphic registration.

HERRERA and co-workers (1965) observed by chance an abnormal focus of up-take in a lymphosarcoma during a pancreas scan with ^{75}Se selenomethionine [25]. Seven additional patients with clinically active disease demonstrated uptakes suf-ficient for scintiscanning at 30 minutes, 24 hours and in some cases as late as 2 weeks. However, non-lymphomatous malignancies yielded negative scans. These observations were confirmed by SPENCER et al. (1967) who found after intravenous administration of tagged selenomethionine to mice that the radioactive label was deposited in a trichloroacetic-acid-insoluble form in the tumor [54]. Binding could be blocked by actinomycin D and puromycin. In a comparative series the authors noted that lymphangiography results agreed with the results of ^{75}Se selenomethionine-scans in 10 of 13 cases. In a study of 50 patients with proven malignant lymphomas, 49 could be diagnosed by scintigraphy. Diagnosis was missed in the one case of Hodgkin's disease (JOVANOVIC, 1968 [3]). ^{75}Se administered intravenously as selenate or selenite entered mouse lymphomas also, but specificity was not as favorable as following ^{75}Se selenomethionine administration [54].

Uptake of these substance, however, is not specifically increased in systemic lymphomatoses. Liposarcomas [54] and various other cancers [33] give positive contrasts as well.

Sodee and co-workers (1965) localized malignant tumors by scanning, utilizing chlormerodin ^{197}Hg as the tracer, but stressed the unspecific accumulation in inflammatory processes also [53].

Use of tagged chlormerodin and HgCl$_2$-^{197}Hg by Wolf and Fischer (1966) gave positive scintigrams in Hodgkin's and chronic lymphatic leukemic lymphomas [69]. Even RIHSA exhibits selective uptake in malignancies [2]. But the critical evaluation of 85 scans by Bonte and co-workers classified only 4 as excellent and 14 as good results [2]. The normal blood pools often visualized scintigraphically in the pharyngeal mucosa, heart and great vessels, liver, spleen and kidneys and the uterine fundus are also factors affecting the quality of scans, as is increased uptake in inflammatory processes.

The correct differentiation of these normally labelled pools from adjacent tumors is often impossible. In addition poor contrast of small differences in radioactivity make detection of all but large tumors extremely difficult. Unequivically positive scintigrams may be expected only in malignancies of advanced stages. Small primary tumors and metastases, in spite of their slightly greater affinity for tracer substances, are not seen for technical reasons alone. Therefore, in its present form, scintigraphic visualization of tumors is better considered as a promising experimental technique than as a routine clinical diagnostic procedure.

References

[1] Andreassen, M., E. Dahl-Iversen, and B. Sørensen: Glandular metastases in carcinoma of the breast. Results of a more radical operation. Lancet **266**, 176 (1964).

[2] Bonte, F. J., Th. S. Curry III, R. E. Oelze, and A. J. Greenberg: Radioisotope scanning of tumors. Amer. J. Roentgenol. **100**, 801 (1967).

[3] Delaloye, B., et P. Magnenat: La lymphographie indirecte et son intérêt en oncologie. Medical radioisotope scanning. J.A.E.A. 227 (1964).

[4] Dettmann, P. M., E. R. King, and G. H. Zimberg: Evaluation of lymph node function following irradiation or surgery. Amer. J. Roentgenol. **96**, 711 (1966).

[5] Diethelm, L.: Elargissement du diagnostic de carcinome mammaire avec l'aide des isotopes. Sympos. Europ. Radiol. mammaire, Strasbourg 1.—3. Juli 1966.

[6] Fernholz, H. J.: Lymphoszintigraphie im Kopf-Hals-Bereich. Fortschr. Röntgenstr. **106**, 524 (1967).

[7] Fisch, U.: Lymphographische Untersuchungen über das zervikale Lymphsystem. Fortschr. Hals-Nasen-Ohrenheilkunde, Vol. 14. Basel-New York: S. Karger 1966.

[8] Fischer, H. W.: Intralymphatic introduction of radioactive colloids into the lymph nodes (Preliminary study). Radiology **79**, 297 (1962).

[9] Fuchs, P., F. Wolf u. H. J. Schmidt: Die Lymphknotendarstellung durch peritumorale Au-198-Kolloid-Infiltration bei Kiefertumoren. 4. Jahrestagung d. Dtsch. Ges. f. Nuklearmedizin, Oktober 1966, Kongreßbericht.

[10] Fuchs, W. A.: Lymphographic storage patterns in Hodgkin's disease. In: Progress in lymphology 9. Stuttgart: Thieme 1967, p. 165.

[11] —, and M. P. Härtel: Prognosis of Hodgkin's disease according to the radiographic pattern of lymph nodes. 2nd Int. Symp. on Lymphology, Miami Beach 1968.

[12] — — Die Prognose des Morbus Hodgkin auf Grund der Lymphknotenstruktur im Lymphogramm. Fortschr. Röntgenstr. **109**, 553 (1968).

[13] Herman, P. G.: Radiation effect on the barrier function of the lymph node. Radiology **91**, 698 (1968).

[14] Gest, J.: La lymphographie isotopique. Bull. Schweiz. Akad. med. Wiss. 19, 97—113 (1963).

[15] Hahn, P. F., and C. W. Sheppard: Lymphatic transport of radionuclides. Sth. med. J. (Bgham, Ala.) 38, 558 (1946).

[16] — Tumor therapy by direct infiltration of radioactive colloidal metallic gold. In: P. F. Hahn: A manual of artificial radioisotope therapy. New York: Academic Press 1951, p. 186.

[17] —, and E. L. Carothers: Radioactive metallic gold colloids coated with silver and their distribution in the lung and its lymphatics following intrapulmonary administration: therapeutic implications in primary lung and bronchiogenic tumors. Brit. J. Cancer 5, 400 (1951).

[18] —, G. Router, H. Brummitt, J. Moorehead, and E. L. Carothers: The drainage of radioactive silver colloids by the lymphatics following intrapulmonary administration in dogs. J. Lab. clin. Med. 39, 624 (1952).

[19] —, and E. L. Carothers: Lymphatic drainage following intrabronchial instillation of silver-coated radioactive gold colloid in therapeutic quantities. J. thorac. Surg. 25, 265 (1953).

[20] Haid, H., O. Lofferer, A. Mostbeck u. H. Partsch: Die Lymphkinetik beim postthrombotischen Syndrom unter Kompressionsverbänden. Med. Klin. 63, 754 (1968).

[21] Heilmann, H. P.: Lymphoszintigraphie der Axillarregion beim Mammakarzinom. In: K. E. Scheer in G. Hoffmann: Radioisotope in der Lokalisationsdiagnostik. Stuttgart 1967, S. 197 (1965).

[22] Heinzel, F., and H. Rösler: Quantitative investigation on the dynamics of intralymphatically applied substances, p. 248. Progress in lymphology. Stuttgart: Thieme 1967.

[23] — —, A. Rüttimann u. W. Wirth: Kinetische Untersuchungen nach intralymphatischer Applikation radioaktiver Substanzen. Ihre Bedeutung für die Diagnostik und für therapeutische Maßnahmen bei malignen Geschwülsten. Radiologe 8, 154 (1968).

[24] — Personal communication.

[25] Herrera, N. E., R. Gonzalez, R. D. Schwartz, A. M. Diggs, and J. Belsky: 75-Se-Methionine as a diagnostic agent in malignant lymphoma. J. nucl. Med. 6, 792 (1965).

[26] Höfer, R., u. H. Benzer: Die indirekte Lymphographie der Lunge. In: Radioaktive Isotope in Klinik und Forschung. Vol. VII, S. 410 (1966).

[27] Hollander, W., P. Reilly, and B. A. Durrows: Lymphatic flow in human subjects as indicated by the disappearance of I-131 labeled albumin from the subcutaneous tissue. J. clin. invest. 40, 222 (1961).

[28] Hultborn, K. A., L. G. Larsson, and J. Ragnkult: The lymph drainage from the breast to the axillary and parasternal lymph nodes studied with the aid of colloidal Au-198. Acta radiol. 43, 52 (1955).

[29] — — — A study of the lymph drainage of the lower limb with the use of colloidal radiogold (Au-198). Acta radiol. 43, 139 (1955).

[30] —, and L. J. Jonsson: The use of colloidal Au-198 for the detection of lymph nodes in radical excision of the breast. Acta radiol. 43, 132 (1955).

[31] Jackson, A. H., F. A. Staggers, and P. F. Hahn: Uptake of subcutaneous and intramuscular silver coated radioactive gold colloids by lymph nodes in dogs. J. Lab. clin. Med. 42, 739 (1953).

[32] Jovanovic, D.: 75-Se-selenmethionine uptake by malignant tumors. In: Radioactive Isotope in Klinik und Forschung, Vol. VIII. München-Berlin-Wien: Urban & Schwarzenberg 1968, S. 444.

[33] —, and A. Bonckaert: 75-Se-Selenomethionine as diagnostic agent. Clinical and experimental study. IAEA-Symposium on medical radioisotope scintigraphy. Salzburg 6.—15. 8. 1968 (SM.—108/132).

[34] Keiser, D. K. von, K. zum Winkel, H. J. Frischbier u. H. Müller: Vergleich zwischen röntgenologischer und szintigraphischer Darstellung des abdominellen Lymphsystems. Fortschr. Röntgenstr. 100, 557 (1964).

[35] KINMONTH, J. B.: Lymphangiography in man; a method of outlining lymphatic trunks at operation. Clin. Sci. 11, 11, 13 (1952).

[36] —, G. V. TAYLOR, and R. A. K. HARPER: Lymphangiography: Technique for its clinical use in lower limb. Brit. med. J. 1, 940 (1955).

[37] KRÖNERT, E., u. F. WOLF: Zur praktisch klinischen Bedeutung der Lymphknotenszintigraphie. In: W. KEIDERLING u. G. HOFFMANN: Radioisotope in Pharmakokinetik und klinischer Biochemie. Stuttgart: Schattauer-Verl. 1969 (in press).

[38] KOEHLER, P. R., W. A. MEYERS, J. F. SKELLY, and B. SCHÄFER: Body distribution of Ethiodol following lymphangiography. Radiology 82, 866 (1964).

[39] LEBORGUE, F. E., R. LEBORGUE, E. SCHAFFNER, and F. E. LEBORGUE JR.: Study of lymphatics of mammary gland with radioactive gold. Thorax 4, 233 (1955).

[40] MAGNENAT, P., et R. DELALOYE: La lymphographie hépatique isotopique. Radioaktive Isotope in Klinik und Forschung. Vol. VI, S. 420 (1965).

[41] —, and B. DELALOYE: Isotopic visceral lymphography, p. 253. Progress in lymphology. Stuttgart: Thieme 1967.

[42] MALEK, P., u. B. VAVREGN: Die Radiolymphadenographie, eine Methode der gezielten Untersuchung der funktionellen Dynamik des lymphatischen Systems. Fortschr. Röntgenstr. 92, 597 (1960).

[43] MICHAILOV, V., G. MITROV u. CHR. MLATSCHEKOV: Indirekte Isotopenlymphographie der parasternalen Lymphknoten mit radioaktivem Gold Au-198. Rad. biol. ther. 9, 299 (1968).

[44] OESER, H., W. SCHUMACHER, H. ERNST u. D. FROST: Atlas der Szintigraphie. Berlin: Walter de Gruyter & Co. 1969.

[45] RÖSLER, H.: Ergebnisse der sternalen Lymph-Szintigraphie beim Mamma-Carcinom (1969) (in press).

[46] ROSSI, R., e O. FERRI: La visualizzazione della catena mammaria interna con Au-198. Presentazione di una nuova methodica: la linfoscintigrafia. Minerva med. 57, 1151 (1966).

[47] SAGE, H. H., and B. V. GOZUN: Lymphatic scintigrams: a method for studying the functional pattern of lymphatics and lymph nodes. Cancer 11, 200 (1958).

[48] — — Methods for studying lymphatic function in intact man utilizing Au-198. Proc. Soc. exp. Biol. (N. Y.) 197, 895 (1958).

[49] —, B. SINKA, D. KIZILAY, M. MIYAZAKI, and G. SHAPIRO: Lymph node scintigrams. Amer. J. Roentgenol. 84, 666 (1960).

[50] — — —, and R. TOULON: Radioactive colloidal gold measurements of lymph flow and functional patterns of lymphatics and lymph nodes in the extremities. J. nucl. Med. 5, 625 (1964).

[51] SEAMAN, W. B., and E. W. POWERS: Studies on the distribution of radioactive colloidal gold in regional lymph nodes containing cancer. Cancer 8, 1044 (1955).

[52] SHERMAN, A. I., and M. TER POGOSSIAN: Lymph node concentration of radioactive colloidal gold following interstitial injection. Cancer 6, 1238 (1953).

[53] SODEE, D. B., R. R. RENNER, and B. DI STEFANO: Photoscanning for localization of tumors, utilizing chlormerodrin mercury 197. Radiology 84, 873 (1965).

[54] SPENCER, R. P., G. MONTANA, G. F. SCANLON, and O. R. EVANS: Uptake of selenomethionine by mouse and in human lymphomas, with observation on selenite and selenate. J. nucl. Med. 8, 197 (1967).

[55] SCHENK, P.: Szintigraphische Darstellung des parasternalen Lymphsystems. Strahlentherapie 130, 504 (1966).

[56] SCHERPAS, H., and C. WINKLER: An automatic scanning-system using a tape perforator and computer techniques. In: Proceedings of the symposium in medical radioisotope scanning. Athens, Greece, 1964, Vol. 1, 321.

[57] SCHEYBANI, M. SCH., V. KLEIN u. H. W. PABST: Die abdominelle Lymphknotenszintigraphie. Therapeutische Umschau 24, 425 (1967).

[58] SCHWAB, W.: Der lymphatische Transport von Radiokolloiden in die bestrahlte und unbestrahlte Halsregion. Z. Laryng. Rhinol. 43, 230 (1964).

[59] —, u. K. ZUM WINKEL: Der gegenwärtige Stand der Szintigraphie des zervikalen Lymphsystems. Nucl. Med. (Stuttg.) VI, 234 (1967).

[60] Walker, L. A.: Localization of radioactive colloids in lymph nodes. Z. Lab. 8, Clin. Med. 36, 440 (1950).

[61] Winkel, K. zum: Funktionsuntersuchungen des Lymphsystems mit radioaktiven Substanzen. In: Radioaktive Isotope in Klinik und Forschung. Bd. VI, S. 423 (1965).

[62] —, and K. E. Scheer: Scintigraphic and dynamic studies of the lymphatic system with radio-colloids. Minerva nucl. 9, 390 (1965).

[63] — Die Bedeutung der Szintigraphie in der Diagnose abdomineller Lymphknotenmetastasen. In: J. Becker / G. Hoffmann: Radionuklide in der klinischen und experimentellen Onkologie. Stuttgart 1965, S. 205.

[64] —, and H. Müller: Technik, Beurteilung und röntgenologische Kontrolle der abdominellen Isotopen-Lymphographie. Radiologe 5, 381 (1965).

[65] — Scintigraphie des lymphatischen Systems. In: K. E. Scheer u. G. Hoffmann: Radioisotope in der Lokalisationsdiagnostik. Stuttgart 1967, S. 172 (1967).

[66] —, J. Becker, E. Jahns, H. Scheurlen u. U. Herzfeld: Indikationsstellung und Dosimetrie bei der endolymphatischen Therapie mit Jod-131. Strahlentherapie 133, 2 (1967).

[67] — —, H. Scheurlen, M. Georgi, E. Jahns u. U. Herzfeld: Endolymphatische Therapie mit Radioisotopen. Die Therapiewoche 34, 1170 (1967).

[68] Wolf, R.: Die Szintigraphie (Grundlagen und Anwendungen). Der Radiologe 5, 345 (1965).

[69] —, u. J. Fischer: Tumorszintigraphie mit radioaktiven Quecksilberverbindungen (197-Hg Cl$_2$+197-Hg-Neohydrin). In: J. Becker u. G. Hoffmann: Radionuklide in der klinischen und experimentellen Onkologie. Stuttgart 1965, S. 223.

[70] Zita, G.: Beitrag zur zervikalen Lymphoszintigraphie. Fortschr. Röntgenstr. 107, 644 (1967).

Chapter 11

Intralymphatic Therapy

GEORGES JANTET

Introduction

Surgical excision, external irradiation and, in more recent times, regional or systemic administration of cytotoxic drugs form the basis of the treatment of primary or secondary malignant processes affecting the lymphatic system. Each of these methods has its limitations: surgical exision may be impossible or incomplete, external irradiation may be limited by skin tolerance and requires a prolonged course of treatment, many cytotoxic agents have severe side-effects and regional administration is associated with a fairly high degree of morbidity.

As an alternative to external irradiation attempts have been made to obtain internal irradiation of the regional nodes by administering radioactive substances by interstitial, intracavitary or intratumoral routes. One of the earliest reports was by MENVILLE and ANÉ (1932) who investigated methods of visualizing the lymph nodes and vessels with thorium dioxide injected into the subcutaneous and other tissues of animals; they suggested this might offer a method of treating malignant disease of lymph nodes. HARRIS (1932) showed that the nodes could be completely replaced by fibrosis in this way. However, the use of thorium was abandonned when its carcinogenic properties became known and no further progress was made in this field until the advent of the radioisotopes in clinical practice.

In 1950, WALKER conducted a series of animal experiments during which he injected colloidal suspensions of ^{90}Y compounds into the afferent lymphatic of the popliteal node in the rabbit. He found high concentrations of radioactivity in the popliteal nodes but also found that some of the administered dose localised in the liver. In 1954, KINMONTH developed the technique of clinical lymphangiography in which clinical demonstration in man of the lymphatic system was obtained by intralymphatic injection of contrast material. LEENHARDT and COLIN (1957), while studying the lymphatic circulation in the human, injected radioactive colloidal gold and an aequous solution of radioactive iodine into a lymphatic of the leg: they stated that some radioactivity was found in the first relay of nodes but none in nodes beyond. However they only used tracer doses and did not describe any therapeutic applications.

In 1958 JANTET gave an account of his early results of the clinical use of radioactive colloidal gold (^{198}Au) injected directly into lymphatic vessels as a method of producing internal irradiation of the lymph nodes in the human with various lymph node diseases. Working independently CHIAPPA et al. (1962) and JANTET (1962) described their encouraging results with intralymphatic radiotherapy: CHIAPPA et al. advocating using "Lipiodol F" tagged with ^{131}I in patients with primary malignant lymph node diseases and JANTET advocating using colloidal ^{198}Au in patients with malignant melanoma without clinical lymph node metastases for the treatment of micro-metastases in the nodes.

Since that time the technique of intralymphatic therapy has been further developed and is now in current use in many fields for the treatment of both primary and secondary malignant lymph node diseases. Most workers use radioactive agents but some trials have also been made with cytotoxic drugs.

Intralymphatic Radiotherapy

Choice of Material for Intralymphatic Radiotherapy

There is as yet no general agreement on the best substance to use for intralymphatic therapy. Consideration must be given to the choice of the radioactive isotope and also to the transport medium in which it is administered. The aim being to obtain irradiation of the lymph nodes and sometimes of the lymphatic vessels also but as little as possible of the surrounding tissues, the primary ionisation source must be a strong beta-emitter as these emissions have limited tissue penetration.

In order to study the distribution of the radioactive substance in the body after it has been injected into a lymphatic vessel, the presence of some gamma rays for external scanning is desirable or else the isotope must be combined with some radio-opaque medium for radiological examination.

An isotope with a short radioactive half-life is clearly better than one with a longer half-life as it minimises the effect of biological decay of the injected substance from the nodes and also reduces the time that protective precautions must be taken because of the danger of radioactivity in the patient.

The physical characteristics of the injected substance must be such that it can be given by injection but neither diffuse too rapidly out of the lymphatic vessels into the surrounding tissues nor pass too rapidly through the lymph nodes where it is essential that it should be concentrated (i. e. the biological half-life of the injected substance in the lymph nodes must be as long as possible).

Further requirements are that it should be non-toxic and safe to use, bearing in mind that some leakage into the general circulation is inevitable.

In selecting an isotope to use for intralymphatic administration, a review of the filtering function of lymph nodes and also of the available isotopes (JANTET, 1958) gave some guidance.

Filtering Function of Lymph Nodes

The lymph nodes are efficient filters of particulate matter. GILLCHRIST (1940) found that normal nodes of the rabbit or the dog would not pass a suspension of insoluble particles as small as one micron in diameter even with an injection pressure of 120 cm of water.

Experimental evidence on the filtration of lymph nodes reviewed by YOFFEY and
COURTICE (1956) led them to the conclusion that innanimate particles were held up
in nodes to a considerable extent.

Summarising this evidence, JANTET (1958 and 1962), who had been working on
lymphangiography with water soluble contrast media, concluded that a particulate
isotope must be used. Whereas CHIAPPA et al. (1962), who had been working with
oily contrast media, approached the problem by using Lipiodol F directly labelled
with ^{131}I — this material was known from its use as a contrast medium in lymphangiography to give good localisation in the lymphatic vessels and nodes; in this way
a therapeutic intralymphatic injection could be made which had the added advantage
of allowing at the same time a radiological means of following the effect of the
injection on the treated nodes.

Choice of Radioactive Isotope

1. Radioactive Gold (^{198}Au)

^{198}Au has a short half-life of 2.7 days. It emits beta-particles of only relatively
low energy (mean energey 0.35 MeV) and also some low intensity gamma rays.

Most of the previous reports concerning the use of beta-emitting isotopes to
produce irradiation of nodes deal with radioactive colloidal gold administered by the
subcutaneous, interstitial or intracavitary routes. It has been shown to produce
marked irradiation effects in the lymph nodes leading to fibrosis both in the experimental animal and in man (SHERMAN et al., 1950 and 1953; PUGET et al., 1955;
SHERMAN et al., 1951; ROMIEU et al., 1956; ALLEN et al., 1958; OKUHARA et al.,
1958). These reports also showed that the biological decay of gold from the nodes
was very slow; HAHN et al. (1956) state that the effective half-life of gold in the
lymph nodes can be taken as equal to its physical half-life and point out that it is
safe to use as it is non-toxic.

2. Radioactive Phosphorus (^{32}P)

Radioactive phosphorus is a pure beta-emitter with a mean energy of 0.7 MeV
(thus stronger than ^{198}Au). It has no gamma emission which makes it easier to handle
but more difficult to detect externally. Its physical half-life is however relatively
long (14.5 days). Considering the use of intralymphatic radiotherapy in the treatment
of the regional nodes in patients with malignant melanoma, radioactive phosphorus
is particularly appealing in view of its reported selective uptake by malignant
melanoma cells (MARCUS and ROTBLAT, 1950; BAUER and STEFFEN, 1955).

Radioactive colloidal chromic phosphate has been used in much the same way as
colloidal gold but the published reports have been fewer (ROOT et al., 1954; KUNTZ-
MANN et al., 1956).

3. Radioactiver Silver (^{111}Ag)

^{111}Ag is a beta- and gamma-emitter which has been used experimentally both
alone and also as a coating for radioactive gold particles (HAHN et al., 1952). It has
no advantages over ^{198}Au and its toxicity in the human is a disadvantage.

4. Radioactive Iodine (^{131}I)

^{131}I is a weaker beta-emitter than ^{198}Au (mean energy 0.19 MeV) and has a longer half-life (8.1 days); it is also a gamma-emitter so that external scanning of its distribution in the body is possible. ^{131}I has of course been used for some years mostly in the treatment of thyroid diseases.

5. Radioactive Yttrium (^{90}Y)

In many ways ^{90}Y represents the ideal isotope to use for intralymphatic radiotherapy. It has a short half-life of 2.7 days. It is a strong beta-emitter of high energy particles (mean energy 0.93 MeV). It does not emit any gamma rays however, making external scanning more difficult.

Radioactive Preparations Used for Intralymphatic Therapy

Although much work, both experimental and clinical, is still required before the ideal preparation is found, various preparations have been used and will be discussed below.

Animal Studies

The experimental work of WALKER (1950) using ^{90}Y has been discussed above.

Reviewing the available isotopes, JANTET (1958) suggested that ^{198}Au, ^{131}I and ^{32}P would be suitable for intralymphatic therapy. After a series of animal experiments (JANTET, 1962 and 1966 a) he came to the following conclusions. Human serum albumen tagged with radioactive iodine (^{131}I. HSA), although of large molecular size, did not localise to any significant degree in the lymph nodes following intralymphatic administration; its distribution over the body was the same as after an intravenous injection. He also experimented with colloidal ^{198}Au containing gold particles measuring 5—20 millimicrons (with a mean of 6 millimicrons) which on contact with the tissue proteins forms aggregates ranging in size from 1 to 5 microns (ANDREWS et al., 1953; YALLOW, 1956; BEIERWALTES et al., 1957): he found that the ^{198}Au localised well in the lymph nodes although there was some overflow into the general circulation. The best localisation of the ^{198}Au in the nodes was obtained by reducing the speed and the volume of the injection as much as possible; these findings were similar to those of WALKER (1950) using ^{90}Y. He also tested radioactive colloidal chromic phosphate (^{32}P) containing aggregates measuring up to 300 millimicrons; this suspension is said to form much larger aggregates than colloidal gold on contact with tissue proteins (BEIERWALTES et al., 1957). In his animal experiments he found that none could be made to pass beyond the first group of nodes. On the basis of these animal experiments, JANTET (1962) thus concluded that colloidal ^{198}Au was a suitable isotope for intralymphatic radiotherapy; although it produced relatively low energy beta-emissions it had the advantages of a short half-life, was readily available and was known to be safe clinically following its use by interstitial, intracavitary and intravenous administration. His animal experiments showed that following intralymphatic injection high concentrations of ^{198}Au could be made to localise selectively in the lymph nodes where it would remain for many days, biological decay from the nodes being very slow; radiation doses in the nodes ranging from 5,600 to 67,000 rads were obtained.

FISCHER (1962) also experimented with colloidal [198]Au and suggested that a more balanced distribution of the radioactive gold among the nodes "could be obtained by alternate intralymphatic injection of the colloid and a flushing solution, such as saline".

Following the introduction of [131]I Lipiodol by CHIAPPA et al. (1962) and of [131]I. Ethiodol by SEITZMAN et al. (1963), LIEBNER et al. (1965) made an animal experimental study of intralymphatic [131]I. Ethiodol. They found good distribution among the regional nodes; they showed that the spillover into the general circulation and thence into the lungs and to the thyroid could be controlled by reducing the volume of the injections and by monitoring the para-aortic nodes during leg injections so that the injection was stopped when the para-aortic nodes had filled; they also suggested blocking the thyroid by pre-operative administration of Lugol's iodine. Following intralymphatic injections of doses of 18—19 mCi of [131]I. Ethiodol they found that 29,000—49,000 rads had been absorbed by the regional nodes with subsequent necrosis and calcification; they also confirmed the findings of LENZI and BASSANI (1963) that the lymphatic vessels could tolerate extremely high doses of radiation and they showed that re-injection of these vessels could be done easily at a later date.

EDWARDS and KINMONTH (1966) conducted a series of animal experiments in which VX2 tumour was implanted into a leg of rabbits and the consequent regional node metastases treated by intralymphatic [131]I. Lipiodol. A control series of rabbits was prepared in the same way except that the intralymphatic injections were made with non-radioactive Lipiodol. These experiments demonstrated "the efficacy of [131]I. Lipiodol in destroying microscopic size metastases in lymph nodes".

KOEHLER et al. (1968) found that in the dog the lungs could be protected from overflow of the radiotherapeutic agent by simultaneously cannulating the thoracic duct following which volumes 3 to 5 times larger than normal could be injected. They showed also that a diagnostic lymphogram using Ethiodol did not significantly decrease the uptake of activity by the nodes in a subsequently performed radiotherapeutic lymphogram using [131]I. Ethiodol. They further demonstrated that there was no advantage to be gained by administering the isotope as a slow continuous infusion of a large volume of low specific activity rather than as a more rapid injection of a small volume of high specific activity, as in both cases the uptake by the nodes was not significantly different.

Clinical Applications

Probably the most generally used preparation is Lipiodol tagged with ^{131}I as will be discussed below.

Colloidal [198]Au has been used by JANTET since 1958 for the treatment of patients with malignant melanoma without clinical lymph node metastases (JANTET, 1958, 1962 and 1967); following the intralymphatic injection, tracing of the isotope is carried out by external scanning and good distribution among the regional nodes has been demonstrated.

CHIAPPA et al. (1962) introduced [131]I. Lipiodol F. in which the Lipiodol F is directly labelled with ^{131}I and have used it extensively in patients with primary and metastatic diseases of the retroperitoneal lymph nodes (CHIAPPA et al., 1966; BONADONNA et al., 1967).

American workers have mostly used ^{131}I. *Ethiodol* in which the Ethiodol is directly labelled with ^{131}I (SEITZMAN et al., 1964; ARIEL et al., 1964; LIEBNER, 1965).

More recently ^{131}I. *Lipiodol U.F.* became available [1] in which the ^{131}I is first incorporated into triolein which is then diluted with unlabelled Lipiodol Ultra Fluide [2]. This preparation has been used mostly by European workers (VECCHIETTI et al., 1963; EDWARDS and KINMONTH, 1966; VAERENBERGH and SIMONS, 1967, and WEISZLEDER et al., 1967).

ARIEL et al. (1964) recommended using ^{90}Y-*tagged Micromicrospheres* [3]. These spheres are made of ceramic or plastic and are completely inert chemically and physiologically; those used for intralymphatic administration measure 1 to 4 microns in diameter. These micromicrospheres act simply as carriers for isotopes which can be permanently bound to them: the isotopes used are ^{90}Y for therapeutic purposes and scandium — 46 for scanning. ARIEL et al. (1967) described their use in the treatment of malignant melanoma — the injection of the ^{90}Y micromicrospheres being combined with an injection of Ethiodol in order to obtain a lymphogram at the same time.

Radioactive phosphorus vehicled by Lipiodol Ultra Fluide, ^{32}P. *Lipiodol U.F.*, has been advocated by VECCHIETTI and ONNIS (1967): trioctyl phosphate is synthesised using ^{32}P and this compound is then dissolved in Lipiodol U.F. This preparation thus produces a radiotherapeutic and a radiological lymphogram; they describe its use in gynaecological surgery.

Conclusions

The aim of intralymphatic radiotherapy is to administer a high dose of radiation to a selected part of the lymphatic system; ideally there should be no effects on surrounding tissues and no spillover into the general circulation. Furthermore the injected substance should be traceable either by external scanning methods or by radiological examination: because of the added complication of protection from gamma-emitters, the latter alternative is preferable. The physical characteristics of the isotope and the nature of the vehicle are thus both important.

The originally used colloidal ^{198}Au has now been superseded by other preparations. ^{198}Au is not a strong beta-emitter and furthermore this preparation spills over into the general circulation (and thence to the liver) and can only be traced by external scanning. Some of these deficiencies were partly met by using a colloidal suspension containing gold particles of larger size (mean of 30 millimicrons) which reduced the spillover considerably (JANTET, 1966 a) and experimentally (HEINZEL and ROSLER, 1966) by carrying the colloidal ^{198}Au in Lipiodol U.F. Nevertheless suitable preparations of stronger beta-emitters are now available. Colloidal ^{198}Au is still useful however to obtain perilymphatic irradiation by intralymphatic injection (see below).

^{131}I. Lipiodol F, ^{131}I. Lipiodol U.F. and ^{131}I. Ethiodol are extensively used as they give excellent radiological lymphograms at the same time but ^{131}I is a weak beta-emitter with a relatively long half-life. Spillover into the general circulation and thence to the thyroid and the lungs has caused occasional pulmonary complications

---

[1] From the Radiochemical Centre, Amersham, Bucks, England.
[2] Supplied by Laboratoires André Guerbet, 82 rue du Landy, 75 — St. Ouen, France.
[3] Supplied by Nuclear Products Department, 3M — Company, St. Paul, Minn., USA.

(see previous chapter) but this can be almost completely controlled. Like ^{198}Au it is a gamma-emitter and suitable precautions must therefore be taken.

There can be no doubt that ^{32}P and ^{90}Y which are both pure strong energy beta-emitters are in many ways better isotopes for intralymphatic radiotherapy. Both however must be combined with a radio-opaque vehicle. This has been done very succesfully with ^{32}P. Lipiodol U.F. but the relatively long half-life of ^{32}P is far from ideal. ^{90}Y is the best available isotope from the physical point of view (strong beta-emissions, no gamma-emissions and short half-life) and if the early satisfactory reports of its use are confirmed, the ^{90}Y micromicrospheres carried in Lipiodol will probably prove to be the best available preparation for intralymphatic radiotherapy. It is hoped that further work in this field will continue, such as the search for a ^{90}Y compound which can be dissolved in, and thus combined with, Lipiodol or other suitable radio-opaque vehicle.

Technique of Intralymphatic Radiotherapy

The technique of exposure and cannulation of the appropriate lymphatic vessel is the same as for radiological lymphography ensuring that a leak-proof injection is obtained. When using gamma-emitters, suitable protective measures must be taken during the handling of the material and during the injection—such as shielding the injector pump by a 2 cm thick lead case (EDWARDS and KINMONTH, 1966) or by delivering the pump from the supplier already loaded and suitably shielded (VEISZ-LEDER et al., 1967).

The lymphatic vessel to be injected depends upon the group of nodes to be treated. Some groups, such as the inguino-pelvic, the retroperitoneal, the axillary and the cervical nodes are more accesible than others, the limiting factor being the difficulty in isolating a suitable afferent lymphatic trunk.

The volume injected depends on the volume of the nodes to be treated and on the specific activity of the material used. Normal axillary nodes require about 2 ml each side, while the inguino-iliac and para-aortic nodes require about 5 ml for each side. When the nodes are enlarged by disease, larger volumes may be necessary. Measures to prevent spillover into the general circulation have been discussed above.

When ^{131}I is used, the thyroid can be protected by giving Lugol's iodine, 15 drops 3 times a day for 3 days before the injection and for 2—3 weeks after.

When dealing with metastatic lymph node diseases it is important that the injection should be made, if it is at all possible, into a lymphatic trunk draining the site of the primary lesion as it is along this pathway that any metastases must travel; in this way the injected material travels along the same pathway and reaches the same regional nodes as any metastases from the primary (JANTET, 1962). Furthermore the mode of spread of the primary lesion must be taken into consideration when planning the technique of the injection. Thus in the treatment of malignant melanoma (JANTET, 1966 b) the injection is made into lymphatic trunks just proximal to, and draining the site of, the excised primary lesion; while in the treatment of testicular tumours (CHIAPPA and USLENGHI, 1966) an injection is also made into the lymphatic vessels of the testicular cord. In malignant melanoma, metastases occur along the course of the lymphatic trunks: to try and prevent this the perilymphatic tissues are irradiated by the same technique with a second injection (JANTET, 1966 b) after placing a tourniquet round the root of the limb and giving the injection rapidly to favour diffusion out of the lymphatic vessels. Edwards and Kinmonth (1968) have adopted this technique but monitor the injection by scanning and radiography to prevent spillover into the general circulation.

Vecchietti and Onnis (1967) aim at localising the injected material to the pelvic nodes, in the treatment of pelvic gynaecological cancer, by first ligating the efferent lymphatic trunks along the common iliac arteries at the time they excise the structure containing the primary growth and subsequently making an injection of radioactive material into a lymphatic in each foot.

Dose

In arriving at a figure for a satisfactory dose to inject, most workers have had to proceed by a method of trial and observation. Inevitably in the early patients cautious doses which were too low were given: the lack of any ill-effects has encouraged the administration of larger doses.

Jantet (1962 and 1964) calculated the theoretical doses required to produce different levels of radiation in the nodes from the beta-particle dosimetry formula given by Hine and Brownell (1956). This requires knowledge of the weight of the nodes which was arrived at from the weight of the patient (Yoffey and Courtice, 1956). Thus, aiming to obtain 30,000 to 75,000 rads in the nodes, doses varying between 20 mCi and 80 mCi of colloidal ^{198}Au were injected.

Chiappa et al. (1962) using ^{131}I. Lipiodol F started with a total dose of about 10 mCi, but are now giving 20—25 mCi in 10 ml on each side for inguino-ilio-aortic node irradiation (Ratti and Chiappa, 1966).

Seitzman et al. (1964), using ^{131}I. Ethiodol, limited their total injection to 30 mCi to avoid isolation precautions of the patient and administered this dose in a maximum of 12 ml to fill the retroperitoneal nodes.

Ariel et al. (1964) injected 20 to 50 mCi of colloidal ^{198}Au or 20 to 30 mCi of ^{131}I. Ethiodol for irradiation of the retroperitoneal nodes. Edwards and Kinmonth (1966), Edwards (1967) also using the beta-particle dosimetry formula, gradually increased the dose of ^{131}I. Lipiodol U.F. injected until satisfactory histological changes were found in the nodes; their dosage is 45 mCi in 4 ml for the lower limb and 30 mCi in 2 ml for the upper limb.

Vaerenbergh and Simons (1966), using ^{131}I. Lipiodol U.F., started with low doses of 5 mCi in 10 ml for each foot, calculated to give 7,000 to 8,000 rads to the lymph nodes; in view of the excellent tolerance, the dose was later increased to 10—15 mCi in 10 ml into each foot with no ill-effect.

Vecchietti and Onnis (1967) at first used ^{131}I. Lipiodol F in doses of 7 to 10 mCi in 5 to 6 ml into each foot: this produced an average of 8,253 rads at "the point of focus". With 1 mCi of ^{32}P. Lipiodol U.F. in 4 to 5 ml into each foot an average of 34,688 rads was obtained at the same point.

There is seen to be some variation in the dose administered but it must be remembered that tumours such as a malignant melanoma (Jantet; Edwards and Kinmonth), not being very radiosensitive, require much larger doses than the more radiosensitive primary lymph node diseases treated by the other workers mentioned above.

Effects on the Lymph Nodes

The final test of whether intralymphatic radiotherapy achieves its object will be in an analysis of the long term results when compared with proper control series: this is under way but few long term studies are yet available.

Indirect evidence of whether the method is likely to be effective can be obtained by showing whether the injected material has been concentrated in the nodes, by observing the clinical effects on the nodes and any histological changes and by calculating the doses received by the nodes.

The evidence reported by all workers in this field shows quite clearly, either by external scanning or by radiography, that the injected material collects and remains in the lymph nodes with very little biological decay so that the effective half-life of the isotope in the nodes is virtually identical with its physical half-life (JANTET, 1962; LUIGI et al., 1962).

Autoradiography of excised nodes also confirms that the activity is localised in the nodes (JANTET, 1962; LIEBNER, 1965; VECCHIETTI and ONNIS, 1967).

Following an intralymphatic injection of an isotope, the nodes become tender and swollen and after several weeks become fibrosed (JANTET, 1962). In limb infusions given under conditions favouring perilymphatic diffusion, the skin and subcutaneous tissues overlying the injected lymphatic trunk show typical post-irradiation effects with epilation and thickening (JANTET, 1966 b). In some patients mild oedema of the injected limb has developed from obstruction of the nodes by fibrosis. Nodes which have been involved by disease can be observed radiologically to become smaller when the material administered is radio-opaque (CHIAPPA et al., 1962; VECCHIETTI and ONNIS, 1967). These findings confirm that a radiotherapeutic effect is obtained in the lymphatic vessels and regional nodes following intralymphatic isotope administration.

The histological changes produced in the nodes have been described by SEITZMANN et al. (1964), LIEBNER (1965), JANTET (1962 and 1966 b), WINKEL et al. (1966) and VECCHIETTI and ONNIS (1967). Cancerocidal effects with necrosis of tumours have been observed but all these authors agree that in nodes involved by metastases no appreciable effect is obtained on the metastases if they are larger than micro-emboli because of the short penetration of the beta rays since the injected material only localises in the normal parts of nodes. On the other hand, nodes involved by primary lymph node diseases took up the material well and were very effectively irradiated.

The doses calculated (from the volumes or weights of the nodes) to have been received by the nodes vary with the dose administered but are all considered to be cancerocidal doses. BURAGGI et al. (1962) found 700 rads per mCi administered using [131]I. Lipiodol F., JANTET (1962) obtained 30,000 to 50,000 rads using colloidal [198]Au and SEITZMANN et al. (1964) 37,000 rads using [131]I. Ethodiol; LIEBNER (1965) studying 118 nodes from 12 gynaecological patients using [131]I. Ethiodol in doses of up to 20 mCi found 600 to 38,000 rads in the different groups of nodes with mean doses of 10,000 to 14,000 rads for the different groups; RATTI and CHIAPPA (1966) found up to 20,000 rads in their patients' nodes using [131]I. Lipiodol F, while VECCHIETTI and ONNIS (1967) calculated that 1 mCi of [32]P. Lipiodol F. gave doses varying between the various groups of nodes from 7,755 to 57,407 rads. EDWARDS (1967) calculated that after 45 mCi of [131]I. Lipiodol U.F. as much as 100,000 rads was obtained in individual regional nodes, while WINKEL et al. (1967) found radiation doses in the

lymph nodes ranging from 5,000 to 18,000 rads in 12 patients given 20 mCi of
^{131}I. Lipiodol by the intralymphatic route. LAHNECHE and VÉROT (1967) studied the
distribution in the body of ^{131}I. Lipiodol and ^{32}P. Lipiodol after an intralymphatic
injection in 30 patients and found that 66% was fixed in the visualised inguino-ilio-
aortic nodes, 33% in the lungs, 0% in the thyroid, less than 5% of the administered
dose was excreted in the urine during the first 15 days and that the maximum total
blood level (7th to 10th days) was 0.16% of the administered dose per litre of
plasma; from these figures they calculated that the dose at the centre of normal nodes
containing isotope equal to a concentration of 1 microcurie per Gram of node was
120 rads for ^{131}I, 720 rads for ^{32}P in nodes with a radius of 1 cm or over and 504 rads
for ^{32}P in nodes with a radius of 2.5 mm. Thus, if 66% of the administered dose
localises in 100 Gm of lymph nodes, the mean radiation dose at the centre of the
lymph nodes for each 1 mCi administered was 790 rads for ^{131}I and 4750 rads for ^{32}P,
showing the greater effectiveness of ^{32}P compared with ^{131}I; they found greatly
reduced levels of radiation in nodes containing metastases, ^{32}P however producing
better levels than ^{131}I, but with micro-emboli, tumour doses equal to 50% of the dose
at the centre of the node were found; they suggest using ^{32}P or ^{90}Y.

Complications

The introduction of large quantities of a radioactive substance into the lymphatic
system some of which spills over into the general circulation might well have been
expected to produce unwanted general effects. But in fact, complications have been
very few. CHIAPPA et al. (1962) did not observe any signs of bone marrow damage
with ^{131}I. Lipiodol F. On the other hand, JANTET (1966 b) using ^{198}Au and EDWARDS
and KINMONTH (1966) and EDWARDS (1967) using ^{131}I. Lipiodol U.F., each report one
case of radionecrotic ulcer at the site of injection due to leakage and some effects on
the haemopoietic system. JANTET found a temporary depression of all elements of the
bone marrow in two patients from which a complete recovery was made; he points
out however that the liver function tests remained normal in all cases. EDWARDS and
KINMONTH noticed an absolute lymphopenia in several patients with mild total depression of the leucocyte count at a later stage but state that the morbidity rate of this technique is low and that long term clinical studies have failed to show any deleterious effects
due to radiation of the lungs. Subsequent lymphoedema appears to be rare but JANTET
found that the fibrosis produced in the lymph nodes could make the subsequent clinical
assessment of these nodes difficult. No harmful effects on the thyroid have been reported.
SEITZMANN et al. (1964) report no adverse side-effects generally or on the haemopoetic
system in 15 patients treated with ^{131}I. Ethiodol but they were using lower doses. In a
series of 10 patients treated with various isotopes, ARIEL et al. (1964) commented on one
patient who suffered a temporary weakness and numbness of the hands and feet but
it is doubtful if this was due to the treatment; in no instance did they find any
changes in the blood picture or any untoward reaction. They consider that the procedure is safe when proper precautions are taken. RATTI and CHIAPPA (1966) do not
report any complications in 486 patients treated by intralymphatic radiotherapy using
^{131}I. Lipiodol F, nor do VECCHIETTI and ONNIS (1967) in 170 patients using ^{32}P. Lipiodol U.F.

Results

Intralymphatic therapy is still in its infancy and there are therefore few series to evaluate its long term value.

ARIEL et al. (1964) in a short evaluation of intralymphatic therapy treated four patients with ⁹⁰Y micromicrospheres: three patients with lymphosarcoma obtained relief of symptoms and reduction in the size of the nodes but in one patient with a malignant lymphoma no appreciable effect was noted. No long term follow up was given. LIEBNER (1965) employed intralymphatic radiotherapy with ¹³¹I Ethiodol as an adjunct to established surgical and radiotherapeutic techniques in a total of 51 patients; 38 patients with pelvic cancers (cervix, vulva, testicle, anus, etc.), 8 patients with lymphomas (Hodgkin's disease, lymphosarcoma, reticulum cell sarcoma), 3 patients with retroperitoneal tumours (fibrosarcoma, liposarcoma, pancreatic carcinoma) and 2 patients with lymph node metastases. He concluded that prophylactic irradiation of the regional lymphatic system before detectable metastases occured would probably be the best use.

RATTI and CHIAPPA (1966) reported on a large series of 486 patients treated with intralymphatic ¹³¹I. Lipiodol F in combination with other forms of treatment. The first group (275 patients) suffered from primary lymph diseases (Hodgkin's disease in 139 patients, reticulum cell sarcoma in 61 patients, lymphosarcoma in 41 patients, etc.). The results were difficult to assess as other methods of treatment were also given but the authors were impressed by the general improvement obtained in the patients and the reduction in volume of the treated nodes which could be observed radiographically. The second group (211 patients) consisted of patients with cancers of the pelvic viscera and lower half of the body (carcinoma of the cervix in 77 patients, carcinoma of the body of the uterus in 22 patients, carcinoma of the bladder in 44 patients, testicular tumours in 25 patients, malignant melanoma in 9 patients, etc.). Again the results were difficult to assess as the intralymphatic therapy was used as an adjunct to surgical therapy or other forms of radiotherapy. However they report that of 35 patients with a stage I carcinoma of the cervix treated in this way, 30 (85%) were alive and free from disease after three years; similarly, of 18 patients with a stage II carcinoma of the cervix 15 (83%) were alive and free from disease after three years. They compare these results with the results of standard treatment for patients with stage I and II carcinomas of the cervix in whom, according to the authors, "the frequency of metastases is never lower than 25%". They concluded that intralymphatic radiotherapy used alone would be particularly indicated in Hodgkin's disease affecting the lower half of the trunk.

CHIAPPA and USLENGHI (1966) treated 36 patients with testicular tumours with intralymphatic ¹³¹I. Lipiodol F administered via a testicular cord lymphatic together with an injection via a foot lymphatic followed by an orchidectomy on the affected side if this had not already beeen carried out and Cobalt therapy to the para-aortic and testicular nodes: the part played by the intralymphatic therapy was therefore difficult to assess. The authors propose that tumours of the testicles should be treated by testicular intralymphatic radiotherapy followed by bilateral foot intralymphatic radiotherapy and later by orchidectomy. In patients who are first seen after orchidectomy they advocate bilateral foot intralymphatic radiotherapy and external Cobalt therapy to the testicular nodes. For patients with clinical or lymphographic lymph node metastases they advise external Cobalt therapy.

18*

Jantet (1966 b) followed-up 18 patients with a primary malignant melanoma of an extremity with clinically uninvolved nodes and no distant metastases. These patients were treated solely by wide excision of the primary tumour and intra-lymphatic colloidal [198]Au given into a lymphatic vessel draining the site of the primary lesion. Fifteen patients (83%) were alive and free from recurrence after a period ranging from 2 months to 7 years: three patients died of the disease during that time, but only in one patient was disease found in the regional nodes. The latest follow-up review ranging from 1 year to 10 years, reveals that, in a total of 21 patients, the disease has recurred in 6 patients of whom 4 have died giving a 10 year recurrence-free rate of 71% and a survival rate of 81%; in only 2 of the patients who suffered a recurrence was disease found in the regional nodes. Thirteen of the 21 patients have been followed-up for 5 years or more; of these, 4 have developed a recurrence (but in none was it in the regional nodes) of whom 2 have died of the disease, giving a 5 year recurrence-free rate of 69.2% and a 5 year survival rate of 84.6%. Although these numbers are still small they compare very favourably with Gumport and Mayer's (1959) analysis of 126 patients with malignant melanoma treated by standard methods in which they found that in those with clinically un-involved nodes the 5 year recurrence-free rate was 51%. These figures suggest that intralymphatic radiotherapy improves the prognosis in these patients (see Table). However it is important that patients with malignant melanoma be followed-up for many years as recurrences can occur late: in this series only 2 recurred within 2 years and the other 4 after an interval ranging from 3½ to 7½ years.

Table. *Patients with malignant melanoma treated by wide excision and intralymphatic radio-therapy* (see text)

Regional nodes	Author	Results			
		length of follow-up	survival rate	recurrence-free rate	Controls (no intralymphatic radiotherapy)
Clinically normal: *no* block dissection of nodes	Jantet (see text)	5+ years	84.6%	69.2%	Gumport and Mayers (1959) 5 year recurrence-free rate: 51%
		1—10 years	81%	71%	
	Edwards and Kinmonth (1968)	1½—4 years	93.5%		Edwards and Kinmonth (1968) 5 year survival rate: 55%
Clinically involved: block dissec-tion of nodes performed	Edwards and Kinmonth (1968)	1½—4 years	52.6%		Edwards and Kinmonth (1968) 5 year survival rate: 10%

JANTET (1966 b) also describes the management of a patient with a lymphangio-sarcoma occurring in a lymphoedematous arm following a mastectomy; the only method of treatment was intralymphatic colloidal ^{198}Au into one of the lymphatic vessels of the affected arm. The patient died 18 months later with recurrences not of the lymphangiosarcoma but of the original breast carcinoma. The author has since treated, with other isotopes, patients with other malignant processes of an extremity which metastasize by the lymphatic system but the follow-up period is still too short to comment on the results.

EDWARDS and KINMONTH (1968) also treated patients with malignant melanoma by intralymphatic radiotherapy using ^{131}I. Lipiodol U.F., combined with a wide excision of the primary lesion as the only method of treatment if the regional nodes were clinically uninvolved (31 patients). Treatment of patients with regional lymph node metastases (19 patients) was similar except that they underwent, in addition, a block dissection of the regional nodes about four weeks after the intralymphatic therapy. They compared the survival rates after $1^1/_2$ to 4 years in the two groups with the survival rates of patients treated by surgery only, performed by various surgeons in the same hospital, arranged in the same two groups (42 and 10 patients). They found a survival rate of 93.5% in the first group with clinically uninvolved nodes and 52.6% in the second group with involved nodes: the comparable survival rates in the control groups treated by surgery alone were 55% and 10% (see Table). The follow-up period is relatively short but these results also are very encouraging.

Lamarque (1966) discussed his series of 41 patients treated with intralymphatic ^{131}I. Lipiodol: 28 patients had malignant lymphadenopathies (of which 23 were Hodgkin's disease) and 13 patients had treatment to the regional nodes draining a primary carcinoma elsewhere. He does not give any follow-up statistics but comments on the very good general and local response in patients with Hodgkin's disease. In those who only partially responded or who failed to respond, the treatment had to be completed by Cobalt therapy.

VAERENBERGH and SIMONS (1967) illustrated their clinical impression of the beneficial value of adjuvant intralymphatic radiotherapy with ^{131}I. Lipiodol by discussing the progress in a few patients with primary or secondary malignant lymph node diseases but gave no complete results.

VECCHIETTI and ONNIS (1967) gave full results of a series of 170 patients treated with adjuvant intralymphatic radiotherapy by their technique (see above). These patients were followed-up for up to 4 years: 42 were treated with ^{131}I. Lipiodol U.F. and 128 with ^{32}P. Lipiodol U.F. All the patients except one suffered from a primary pelvic gynaecological carcinoma, the exception being a carcinoma of the breast (carcinoma of cervix or body of uterus, vagina and vulva). In all cases the intralymphatic treatment was associated with surgery, other forms of radiotherapy or chemotherapy. The survival rate for up to 4 years was 89.4%. Owing to the short follow-up no definite conclusions could be drawn, but the authors advocate intralymphatic radiotherapy in gynaecological cancer as complementary to standard treatment.

A very good short term demonstration of the value of intralymphatic radiotherapy is described by BONADONNA et al. (1967). In 15 patients with a stage IV malignant lymphoma and in 1 patient with chronic lymphatic leukaemia all involving the retroperitoneal nodes, one chain was injected with ^{131}I. Lipiodol F and the other with plain Lipiodol F; intravenous chemotherapy was then started 24 hours later. On the side treated with [131]I. Lipiodol F, the shrinkage of the involved nodes was more marked and prolonged than on the control side; on the latter side 9 relapses occured in 2 to 5 months and only one on the other, [131]I. treated, side.

All these results offer strong presumptive evidence of the beneficial value in suitable cases of intralymphatic therapy but long-term results and controlled series are eagerly awaited.

Indications and Discussion

The technique of intralymphatic radiotherapy involves injecting substances into lymphatic vessels; the injected substance is then carried to the nodes of which the injected vessel represents an afferent trunk. It may thus by-pass completely adjoining nodes if they are not in the pathway of lymph coming from the injected vessel. Thus the indication, par excellence, for intralymphatic radiotherapy is in the treatment of metastatic nodes. If the primary lesion is so situated in the body that its lymphatic pathway is multi-directional, the method will be unreliable. Furthermore many primary malignant lesions are deeply situated so that access to the draining lymphatic pathway is difficult and the method becomes impractical in such cases. Poor radio-sensitivity of the primary tumour and its potential lymph node metastases is not necessarily a contraindication to this method of treatment, since, as has been shown above, very large levels of radiation can be obtained in the nodes. Again, it has been shown that the injected substance localises only in the normal parts of metastatic nodes, and not in the metastasis itself. Therefore with the beta-emitters used, large lymph node metastases will not be irradiated; this however does not apply to microscopic lymph node metastases. In short the ideal indication for intralymphatic radiotherapy is for the prophylactic irradiation of regional nodes in which metastases are no greater than microscopic size when the primary lesion is so situated that its draining lymphatic pathway is uni-directional and therefore easily accessible. In practice this means the prophylactic irradiation of the regional nodes in patients with either a malignant melanoma or an epithelioma of the upper or lower limb or in patients with testicular tumours, so that the injected substance follows the same possible lymphatic pathway as any metastases from the primary lesion. The published series suggest that this method may be sufficient as the sole method of treatment of the regional nodes in these patients. It must be pointed out however that this applies when the primary lesion is situated at a distance from the regional nodes when the alternative would be a block dissection of the regional nodes in discontinuity from the excision of the primary lesion. When the primary and the regional nodes are sufficiently close together that an excision of both in continuity can be carried out, it is felt that this is the better method of treatment.

When the regional nodes contain larger metastases (either palpable clinically or seen by lymphangiography) or when the primary lesion is deeply situated, as in pelvic gynaecological cancers, the technique appears to be a useful adjunct to other forms of treatment such as lymphadenectomy, external irradiation or chemotherapy: in the former case, preoperative intralymphatic radiotherapy will take care of any un-removed lymph nodes, or, because they can be seen radiologically, allows a search to be made for them at operation.

Lymph nodes affected by primary diseases such as Hodgkin's disease, lymphomas, lymphosarcomas, reticulosarcomas, etc., absorb and retain the injected material well, even when they are grossly involved unlike metastatic nodes. However these are systemic diseases, the development and spread of which is not necessarily dictated by the flow of lymph from one node to the next, so that intralymphatic administration of radioactive substances into a remote lymphatic vessel is very likely to by-pass many of the affected nodes. For this reason it is felt that in these cases this technique should be used only as an adjunct to other forms of treatment such as external irradiation or chemotherapy. These diseases are usually highly radiosensitive and the published series in which this technique was used in this way showed it to be a very useful and beneficial adjunct. The most common sites of injection in these patients are the foot and arm lymphatic vessels to reach the inguino-ilio-retroperitoneal and the axillary groups of nodes respectively but new techniques are being developed using head, neck and mediastinal routes.

The use of this form of treatment in lymphangiosarcoma has been reported above: this condition, being a malignant disease of the lymphatic vessels, seems ideally suited for treatment in this way and further attempts are indicated.

Further progress will be made with this technique as new substances for injection are developed, the field having been opened by the use of micromicrospheres the size of which can be varied and may allow accurate localisation in selected groups of nodes. Undoubtedly further applications of this method will be made particularly in the field of tissue transplantation but this is still in the experimental stage.

In conclusion, intralymphatic radiotherapy allows very high levels of irradiation to be administered selectively to the lymph vessels and nodes without any effects on surrounding tissues. This offers obvious advantages over other forms of treatment but the limitations of the method must be respected.

Intralymphatic Chemotherapy

Attempts to use the intralymphatic pathway as a means of delivering chemotherapeutic agents to the lymph nodes were reported by WALLACE et al. (1961) and MERIALDI and LAZOTTI (1961). The results were disappointing because the agents in aequous solutions diffused too rapidly and none of the drugs were soluble in oily vehicles (GOULD and SHAFFER, 1962; JACKSON et al., 1962)—no worthwhile results were reported (ARIEL et al., 1964). This approach was largely superseded by intralymphatic administration of radioisotopes.

HARTGILL (1966) combined intralymphatic chemotherapy with lymphadenectomy in the treatment of patients with carcinoma of the cervix of the uterus. He reported some histological effects on the nodes, and, following a series of animal experiments, applied the method clinically either by single pre-operative injections or by an indwelling catheter technique to obtain a perfusion. The most encouraging results were obtained with methyl hydrazine which is of particle size. No final assessment of this method has yet been given, but it is felt that radioisotopes in suitable vehicles are a better alternative.

Other Forms of Intralymphatic Therapy

Nodes affected by chronic inflammatory disease (e. g. tuberculosis) or infestations might lend themselves to treatment by the appropriate drug administered by the intralymphatic route, high local concentrations of the drug might be obtained.

References

ARIEL, I. M., W. FLYNN, and G. T. PACK: Second International Symposium on Regional Therapy of Tumours. Rome 1967.
—, M. I. RESNICK, and D. GALEY: Surgery 55, 355 (1964).
ALLEN, W. M., A. I. SHERMAN, and H. M. CAMEL: Radiology 70, 523 (1958).
ANDREWS, G. A., S. W. ROOT, H. D. KERMAN, and R. R. BIGELOW: Ann. Surg. 137, 375 (1953).
BAUER, F. K., and C. G. STEFFEN: J. Amer. med. Ass. 158, 563 (1955).
BEIERWALTES, W. H., P. C. JOHNSON, and A. J. SOLARI: Clinical use of radioisotopes. London: W. B. Saunders Co. 1957.
BONADONNA, G., S. CHIAPPA, S. DI PIETRO, P. MARANO, R. MOLINARI, and C. USLENGHI: N. Rev. franç. Hémat. 7, 381 (1967).
BURAGGI, G. L., P. D'AMICO, and G. FAVA: Tumori 48, 149 (1962).
CHIAPPA, S., G. GALLI, S. BARBAINI, and G. RAVASI: Tumori 48, 147 (1962).
—, and C. USLENGHI: In: Progress in Lymphology. Stuttgart: Georg Thieme 1967.
— —, G. BONADONNA, P. MARANO, and G. RAVASI: Surg. Gynec. Obstet. 123, 10 (1966).
EDWARDS, J. M.: Second International Symposium on Regional Therapy of Tumours, Rome 1967.
—, and J. B. KINMONTH: In: Progress in Lymphology. Stuttgart: Georg Thieme 1967.
— — Brit. med. J. 1, 18 (1968).
FISCHER, H. W.: Radiology 79, 297 (1962).
GILCHRIST, R. K.: Ann. Surg. 111, 630 (1940).
GOULD, R. J., and B. SHAFFER: Surg. Gynec. Obst. 114, 683 (1962).
GUMPORT, S. L., and H. W. MEYER: Ann. Surg. 150, 989 (1959).
HAHN, P. F., G. ROUSER, H. BRUMMITT, J. MOOREHEAD, and E. L. CAROTHERS: J. Lab. clin. Med. 39, 624 (1952).
—, E. L. CAROTHERS, G. W. HILLLIARD, L. BERNARD, and M. JACKSON: In: Therapeutic use of artificial radioisotopes. New York: J. Wiley and Sons, Inc. 1956.
HARRIS, W. H.: Proc. Soc. exp. Biol. Med. 29, 1049 (1932).
HARTGILL, J. (1966): In: Progress in Lymphology. Stuttgart: Georg Thieme 1967.
HINE, G. J., and G. L. BROWNELL: Radiation dosimetry. New York: Academic Press 1956.
JACKSON, L. G., S. WALLACE, and A. WEISS: Cancer 15, 955 (1962).
JANTET, G. H.: 9th Scientific Meeting. Surgical Research Society. London 1958.
— Brit. J. Radiol. 35, 692 (1962).
— (1966 a). In: New trends in basic lymphology: Symposium 1966. Exp. Suppl. 14. Basel und Stuttgart: Birkhäuser 1967.
— (1966 b). In: Progress in Lymphology. Stuttgart: Georg Thieme 1967.
— Second International Symposium on Regional Therapy of Tumours, Rome. Min. Med. 58, 4516 (1967).
—, J. M. EDWARDS, M. H. GOUGH, and J. B. KINMONTH: Brit. med. J. 2, 904 (1964).
KINMONTH, J. B.: Ann. Roy. Coll. Surg. 15, 300 (1954).
KOEHLER, P. R., E. J. POTCHEN, W. R. COLE, and R. STUDER: Lymphology 1, 33 (1968).
KUNTZMANN, J., A. CHEVALLIER, C. BURG, and D. RODIER: Mém. Acad. Chir. 82, 156 (1956).
LAHNECHE, B., and R. VÉROT: Second International Symposium on Regional Therapy of Tumours, Rome 1967.
LAMARQUE, J. L. (1966): In: Progress in Lymphology. Stuttgart: Georg Thieme 1967.
LEENHARDT, P., and R. COLIN: Presse méd. 68, 1534 (1957).
LIEBNER, E. J.: Amer. J. Roentgenol. 93, 110 (1965).
—, R. E. HAAS, and E. P. LEROY: Cancer 18, 827 (1965).
MARCUS, R., and J. ROTBLAT: Brit. J. Radiol. 23, 541 (1950).
MENVILLE, L. J., and J. N. ANÉ: J. Amer. med. Ass. 98, 1796 (1932).
MERIALDI, A., and G. LAZOTTI: Quad. Clin. ostet. ginec. 16, 840 (1961).
OKUHARA, M., R. MONMA, K. ONODA, T. TAKEDA, and T. HONDA: Amer. J. Roentgenol. 79, 988 (1958).
PUGET, R., A. BRU, and H. PLANAL: Bull. Cancer 42, 192 (1955).
RATTI, A., and S. CHIAPPA (1966): In: Progress in Lymphology. Stuttgart: Georg Thieme 1967.

ROMIEU, C., P. LEENHARDT, and R. COLIN: Montpellier méd. **50**, 128 (1956).

ROOT, S. W., M. P. TYOR, G. A. ANDREWS, and R. M. KNISELEY: Radiology **63**, 251 (1954).

SEITZMAN, D. M., R. WRIGHT, F. A. HALABY, and J. H. FREEMAN: Amer. J. Roentgenol. **89**, 140 (1963).

—, F. A. HALABY, P. FLANAGAN, R. WRIGHT, and J. H. FREEMANN: Surg. Gynec. and Obstet. **118**, 52 (1964).

SHERMAN, A. I., J. F. NOLAN, and W. M. ALLEN: Amer. J. Roentgenol. **64**, 75 (1950).

—, M. BONEBRAKE, and W. M. ALLEN: Amer. J. Roentgenol. **66**, 624 (1951).

—, M. TER-POGOSSIAN, and E. C. TOCUS: Cancer **6**, 1238 (1953).

VAERENBERGH, P. M., and M. SIMONS: Second International Symposium on Regional Therapy of Tumours, Rome 1967.

VECCHIETTI, G., A. ONNIS, and A. ROMAGNOLO: Attual. Ostet. Gin. **9**, 625 (1963); **9**, 659 (1963).

— — Attual. Ostet. Gin. **9**, 583 (1963).

— La radioisotopoterapia endolinfatica in oncologia ginecologica. Padova: Cedam 1967.

WEISSLEDER, H., P. PFANNENSTIEL, K. H. STRICKSTROCK, and G. HOFFMANN: Fortschr. Röntgenstr. **107**, 758 (1967).

WALKER, L. A.: J. Lab. clin. Med. **36**, 440 (1950).

WALLACE, S., L. JACKSON, B. SCHAFFER, J. GOULD, R. R. GREENING, A. WEISS, and S. KRAMER: Radiology **76**, 179 (1961).

WINKEL, K., H. SCHEURLEN, M. GEORGI, E. JAHNS, and U. HERZFELD: Second International Symposium on Regional Therapy of Tumours, Rome 1967.

YALOW, A. A.: In: Therapeutic use of artificial radioisotopes. New York: J. Wiley Sons, Inc. 1965.

YOFFEY, J. M., and F. C. COURTICE: Lymphatics, lymph and lymphoid tissue. 2nd Ed. London: Edward Arnold Ltd. 1956.

Appendix

The authors recommend the sources below as additional references:

ABBES, M., E. MARTIN, A. PELLEGRINO, V. PASCHETTA et P. P. PRAT: La lymphographie en cancérologie. Paris: Expansion Scientifique Française 1964.

ARVAY, N., et J. D. PICARD: Lymphographie; étude radiologique et clinique des voies lymphatiques normales et pathologiques. Paris: Masson & Cie. 1963.

DODD, G. D., and S. WALLACE: The hemopoietic lymphatic system. In: Atlas of tumor radiology. Chicago: Year Book Medical Publishing Company 1969.

FISCH, U: Lymphography of the cervical lymphatic system. Philadelphia-London-Toronto: W. B. Saunders Company 1968.

LAMEER, C.: Retroperitoneale Lymfografie. Asten: Schrik's Drukkerij 1965.

New trends in basic lymphology: Symposium 1966. Exp. Suppl. 14. Ed. by J. M. COLLETTE, G. JANTET, and E. SCHOFFENIELS. Basel and Stuttgart: Birkhäuser 1967.

Progress in Lymphology. Vol. I. Proceedings of the International Symposium on Lymphology in Zurich 1966. A. RÜTTIMANN (Ed.). Stuttgart: G. Thieme 1967.

Progress in Lymphology. Vol. II. Proceedings of the International Symposium on Lymphology Miami Beach 1968.

REIFFENSTUHL, G.: Das Lymphknotenproblem beim Carcinoma colli uteri und die Lymphirradiatio pelvis. Direkte Bestrahlung des Beckenlymphsystems mit Isotopen. München-Berlin-Wien: Urban und Schwarzenberg 1967.

DE ROO, T.: Lymphografie. Assen: Van Gorcum & Comp. 1964.

RÜTTIMANN, A., u. M. S. DEL BUONO: Lymphographie. In: Ergebnisse der medizinischen Strahlenforschung. Neue Folge: Diagnostik, Therapie, Nuklearmedizin, Biologie. Hrsg. H. R. SCHINZ, R. GLAUNER und A. RÜTTIMANN, Band I. Stuttgart: G. Thieme 1964.

— Erkrankungen des retroperitonealen Lymphsystems. Lehrbuch der Röntgendiagnostik. Vol. 5. Stuttgart: G. Thieme 1965.

SIEBER, F.: Die Lymphographie in der klinischen Praxis. Leipzig: G. Thieme 1966.

VIAMONTE, M., and A. RÜTTIMANN: Atlas of Lymphography. Springfield: Ch. Thomas (in preparation).

WELIN, S., and S. JOHANSSON: Lymphography. In: Handbuch der medizinischen Radiologie. Bd. VIII. Berlin-Heidelberg-New York: Springer 1968.

Subject Index

Type-setting, printing and binding:
Konrad Triltsch, Graphischer Betrieb, 87 Würzburg, Germany

Monographs already Published

In Production

In Preparation